DOING THE RIGHT THING

DOING THE RIGHT THING

*Taking Care of
Your Elderly Parents
Even If They Didn't
Take Care of You*

Roberta Satow, Ph.D.

JEREMY P. TARCHER / PENGUIN
A MEMBER OF PENGUIN GROUP (USA) INC.
NEW YORK

JEREMY P. TARCHER/PENGUIN
Published by the Penguin Group
Penguin Group (USA) Inc., 375 Hudson Street, New York, New York 10014, USA • Penguin Group
(Canada), 90 Eglinton Avenue East, Suite 700, Toronto, Ontario M4P 2Y3, Canada (a division of Pearson
Penguin Canada Inc.) • Penguin Books Ltd, 80 Strand, London WC2R 0RL, England • Penguin Ireland,
25 St Stephen's Green, Dublin 2, Ireland (a division of Penguin Books Ltd) • Penguin Group (Australia),
250 Camberwell Road, Camberwell, Victoria 3124, Australia (a division of Pearson Australia Group Pty
Ltd) • Penguin Books India Pvt Ltd, 11 Community Centre, Panchsheel Park, New Delhi–110 017,
India • Penguin Group (NZ), Cnr Airborne and Rosedale Roads, Albany, Auckland 1310,
New Zealand (a division of Pearson New Zealand Ltd) • Penguin Books (South Africa) (Pty) Ltd,
24 Sturdee Avenue, Rosebank, Johannesburg 2196, South Africa

Penguin Books Ltd, Registered Offices: 80 Strand, London WC2R 0RL, England

First trade paperback edition 2006

Most Tarcher/Penguin books are available at special quantity discounts for bulk purchase for sales
promotions, premiums, fund-raising, and educational needs. Special books or book excerpts also can be
created to fit specific needs. For details, write Penguin Group (USA) Inc. Special Markets, 375 Hudson
Street, New York, NY 10014.

The Library of Congress catalogued the hardcover edition as follows:

Satow, Roberta.
    Doing the right thing : taking care of your elderly parents
even if they didn't take care of you / Roberta Satow.
        p.   cm.
    Includes bibliographical references and index.
    ISBN 1-58542-392-0
    1. Aging parents—United States.   2. Aging parents—Care—United States.   3. Adult children
of aging parents—United States.   4. Intergenerational relations—United States.   5. Caregivers—
United States.   I. Title.
    HQ1063.6.S28   2005   2004058870
    306.874'084'6—dc22

ISBN 1-58542-462-5 (paperback edition)

Printed in the United States of America
10 9 8 7 6 5 4 3 2 1

Book design by Lovedog Studio

For Richard, Matthew and Jason

CONTENTS

ACKNOWLEDGMENTS

My agent, Gail Hochman, believed in this book from the moment she read the first draft of my proposal. I will always be grateful to her. Mitch Horowitz has been a wonderful editor, offering his support and good judgment throughout.

Geri DeLuca, Jennifer McCormick and, more recently, Nancy Hoch read chapters and revisions of chapters endlessly. They believed in me and they made me believe in my writing. They always heard my voice and encouraged me to strengthen it and let it ring out.

My sister, Florence Isaacs, and friends Jo Dobkin and Randy Lehrer read several chapters and offered helpful comments. My husband, Richard Wool, and sons, Matthew and Jason, suffered through my obsessing about the book for over three years.

I could not have done my interviews with caregivers without the help of Anne Potter, director of Senior Citizen Services, and Nancy Lindoerfer, Senior Services counselor for the town of New Milford, Connecticut; and Bonnie Walson, executive director of Heritage Day Health Centers in Columbus, Ohio. They offered their offices for interviewing caregivers and did everything they could to make my research possible.

Most of all I would like to thank the caregivers who opened their hearts to me and shared their loving feelings as well as their pain. Thank you all.

PREFACE

THIS BOOK IS PERSONAL. It is about middle-aged care-giving as a stressful stage of life that many of us—myself included—are confronting, but for which we are often un-prepared. In it, I talk about my feelings about my mother and father as well as other people's feelings about their parents. I discuss the struggle to be conscious and not fall back into old patterns—what psychoanalysts call "the repetition compulsion." You may ask yourself: How can she help me when she has these feelings herself? How can she help me when she is just like me—struggling against the compulsion to repeat old patterns?

I have asked myself these questions—and others. Should I write like an authority who is above having these conflicts and struggles so that the reader can feel confidence in me? Or should I disclose personal material that my patients and readers may see and that may affect their feelings about me? I have struggled with all these questions—yours and mine—

while I was writing this book. I came to the conclusion that disclosing my own struggles was worth the risk because I am trying to communicate that the struggle described here is an ongoing one.

There is no one day after which we no longer have to contend with the compulsion to repeat old patterns that keep us stuck and unhappy. A major theme of the book is that old patterns and conflicts that remain either unresolved or incompletely resolved reemerge throughout our lives—especially during stressful times such as caregiving. If we do not resolve them, the best we can do is reach a point where we are more conscious of the telltale signs that presage their reemergence. We can get to a point at which a red flag goes up when we are about to plunge into the depths of despair like a helpless child; when we are about to do something self-destructive; or when we are about to say something hurtful. We can get to a point at which we can realize the meaning of what we just said or did and not let our lives or our selves get out of control. Or we can do even better than that. We can resolve the underlying conflicts that cause us to repeat painful experiences.

I could not write this book as if I did not also have these struggles, share these feelings and struggle to resolve underlying conflicts. Therapists and patients are not qualitatively different types of people, but simply people at different stages in the quest for consciousness and resolution. I tell my patients that putting their feelings into words makes their feelings more conscious and makes them less likely to act them out in ways they will regret. In this book I have tried to put my feelings, and those of the caregivers I interviewed, into words for those people who have not been entirely able to do so themselves.

Some of the fifty caregivers I interviewed for this book had done or were doing a substantial amount of work to become more conscious about what they were experiencing in the process of caregiving. They were able to resolve some old issues with their parents and experienced caregiving as an important stage in their own emotional development. Others were unable to move beyond entrenched patterns. I want to thank all of them for sharing their conflicts, love, wishes, fears, anger, guilt and hope with me. I found their stories compelling, and knowing each and every one of them has enriched my life and the experience I have been able to bring to this book. Their names and identifying traits have been altered to protect their privacy.

INTRODUCTION

IT'S 7 P.M. AND I HAVE just walked into the house after a weekend away in the country. As I put all my packages down, I notice that my son Jason has left a message for me: "Grandma's in the hospital again." I feel alternately mad at her for ruining my evening (I'm so hungry), bad for her that she's alone and probably feeling out of control, frightened that she is dying, and furious that she's probably *not* dying— just nauseated again. I think to myself that soon 911 will be saying: "Oh, it's Sarah again." I have to go or I won't be able to stand myself, but I hate to drive alone at night and my husband, Richard, has just driven three hours from Connecticut in traffic and I don't want to ask him to drive me. I call my sister in hopes that she will come with me instead. When I call she says her husband thinks he has a blood clot in his leg again. He has to go to the hospital and probably will have to cancel his business trip. I can hear the anxiety in her voice. To my great relief, Richard offers to drive me to see my mother.

An hour later I find my mother in the emergency room at Maimonides Hospital in Brooklyn. It's familiar to me. The room is full of Hasidic Jews and Hispanics with nurses and aides milling around. I look through all the curtains set up around the nurses' station until I find her. She is opposite the cubicle where I found my father at 11 p.m. on the rainy night before he died. "Hi, Mom," I greet her, and she smiles at me. Part of me is angry at her because I came all this way and didn't eat dinner and she's smiling at me. "I thought I had a heart attack," she says, "but I didn't. I had pains in my right arm and with a heart attack it's your left arm." While I am relieved that she didn't have a heart attack, I am also furious that I came all this way and she *didn't* even have a heart attack! What kind of daughter am I?

Uncle Morris, my mother's brother-in-law, is standing next to my mother's bed in the cubicle. He lives in the same apartment building as my mother and called 911; he came with her in the ambulance. "Hi, Uncle Morris. Thanks for bringing Mom here," I greet him. "Have you had dinner?" No, he tells me, but waves as if to say: I'm all right, don't worry. But if I'm not going to have dinner, I'll be even angrier if he stays here too and there would have been no reason for me to come. So I thank him and Richard walks him to the bus down the block. After Morris and Richard leave, my mother says casually: "You know, I think Morris has my keys," and starts shuffling through her purse. Sure enough she doesn't have her keys. I realize that my mother, who is not likely to be discharged until after Morris is asleep, won't be able to get into her apartment. I start running to the bus stop to try to reach Morris, but he is gone by the time I get there and I am left gasping for breath.

I find Richard back in the waiting room and tell him the sad story. "Don't worry," he reassures me, "you can call him in a little while and ask him to leave the keys for you." But there's no place for Morris to leave them because there's no doorman in their building. We will have to get the keys from Morris and return to the hospital. After half an hour I call Morris on my cell phone, but he isn't home. I keep redialing until I notice the sign: "No cell phones." Maybe it causes someone's pacemaker to skip or something. I start wondering if I've unwittingly killed someone here with my phone. I go looking for a pay phone and call. Finally, Morris is home and I tell him I've been calling a long time. He says he stopped to get a bite to eat, but I can come now and get the keys.

Richard and I drive to Morris and my mother's building. Richard waits in the car. I sprint up the three flights of stairs because I'm too nervous to wait for the elevator. I ring the bell and . . . no answer. I keep ringing the bell, but there's no answer. How could he not be home? I just called him five minutes ago. Oh, my God, I think to myself, he must have died after I called. He's in there lying on the floor. He's not used to eating so late. Maybe he got so hungry that he had a heart attack. He died of hunger.

He probably didn't die of hunger. Maybe he went out again. So I run down the stairs and find someone at the door. "Did you see Mr. Weiss?" "Yes," he says, "he came in a little while ago." So he's in there, he didn't go out. I sprint up the stairs again and ring the bell and knock on the door concurrently. Still there's no answer. He's a little deaf. Maybe he didn't hear the bell. But probably he's dead. I continue knocking and ringing frantically and start worrying that the neighbors will think that I'm a lunatic.

I'm torn between which is more upsetting to me—my uncle lying dead on the floor or having to take my mother home to sleep at our house. Just then I hear his European-accented voice. "Roberta, I'm here, I'm here." He opens the door, pulling up his pants, and says apologetically, "I was in the bathroom." Guilt attack! I'm so crazy and selfish, I dragged this eighty-five-year-old man out of the bathroom because I'm so afraid I'll have to take my mother back to my apartment.

Morris gives me the keys and I return to Richard in the car. I find myself thinking that he should have been worrying that I was raped and/or murdered because I was gone so long. But he isn't. It reminds me of when I was in primary school. I delivered prescriptions for Perlman's drugstore on Sundays. I sat in the chair next to the phone. When calls for deliveries came in, I walked to various parts of the neighborhood making deliveries. I wished my mother worried about me—but she did not. She never directed me not to go into someone's house or not to go to certain parts of the neighborhood. She didn't worry about me—and neither did Richard.

With my silent disappointment, Richard and I head back to the hospital. I've got the keys. I just need to get my mother out of the emergency room.

AFTER READING this anecdote, you may see me as a selfish and unsympathetic person. Perhaps you feel critical of me for feeling imposed upon and angry at having to take care of my elderly mother. You may feel I'm a bad daughter. Several friends read this story and said: "If I didn't know you, I wouldn't feel sympathetic toward you." The expectation that we should love our parents and not feel angry and resentful toward them when they are old makes coping with our ambivalent feelings toward them more difficult. It's painful to feel anger and guilt toward our elderly parents, but what makes it worse is the injunction to be silent. Victoria Secunda calls this injunction the "Bad Mommy Taboo."[1]

Social arrangements, like there being no public provision for the care of the elderly, induce a range of feelings, and "feeling rules" are one way that society exerts control over our feelings. Feeling rules define what we *should* feel in a particular circumstance; they serve a social function by shaping our subjective experience as it is evoked in different spheres—like taking care of elderly parents. Our culture protects the image of the Good Mother—especially when she is old. In many parts of the country and among certain cultural groups, the admission that you don't love your mother or don't like her is met with a cold stare or a gasp of horror. We are supposed to *want* to take care of our parents when they get old—it's not enough that *we do it*. We are supposed to do it because we *love* them. We can't help it if we break these feeling rules because we can't control what we *feel*, we can only control what we *do*. Yet, we feel guilty if our feelings don't fit the rules.[2]

Feeling guilty adds to the stress of middle-aged caregiving—a stage of life that many of us are confronting, but for which most of us are unprepared. My mother and Uncle Morris are part of the fastest growing segment of the population, people eighty-five years of age and older. While the total population increased by 13.2 percent from 1990 to 2000, the population over eighty-five increased 38 percent.

Half of those who are eighty-five or older need help carrying out at least one activity of daily living such as eating, bathing, going to the bathroom, dressing or getting in and out of bed. More than one-third of them depend on an adult child for this assistance.[3]

Medical advances have transformed many acute illnesses into chronic ones. Between 1990 and 2000 there was a 35 percent increase in centenarians (people one hundred years old or older). The increase in life expectancy means that elders will require care over a longer period of time and the decline in fertility means that adult children will have fewer siblings to depend upon when elderly parents need care. In addition, there is a trend toward deinstitutionalization of all but the most medically needy—the percentage of people eighty-five years or older living in nursing homes declined from 24.5 percent in 1990 to 18.2 percent in 2000. More elderly people requiring help are remaining in the community.

With so many of our parents living so long, middle-aged caregiving can last into *our* old age: Seventy-year-olds are caring for their ninety-year-old parents. In addition to all of the practical difficulties that middle-aged caregivers face, often the most painful part of caregiving is the reemergence of feelings from our childhood that seem to erupt inappropriately and make us feel out of control. The past intrudes on our experience of today. Many social workers and counselors who work with caregivers tell them not to think about the past—just deal with today. In this book I argue that we *must* think about the past to deal with the conflicts we feel and in order to do the psychological work necessary when confronted with this awesome burden.

For example, Richard and I could have had a sandwich before rushing to the hospital. But no matter how hungry I was, how could I eat when my mother might have had a heart attack? I would be breaking the "feeling rules." The adult part of me knows that things go very slowly in the emergency room and there was no need to rush—she would certainly still be there when we arrived. If we had dinner before going, I would have felt calmer and less angry. I responded in a way that *made* me feel deprived and angry— exactly how I felt as a child.

MEMORIES OF MY CHILDHOOD THAT INTRUDE

My mother never kissed me; she never put her arms around me and hugged me or told me she loved me. I often say to my sons when I hug or kiss them: "Do you know I love you?" I often ponder that. It's curious. Why isn't it enough for me to say: "I love you"? I think it's because it's so impor- tant to me that they *feel* it—because I never did. I never re- member my mother holding my hand, although she must have when we crossed the street. When the other kids all ran after "Pop," the ice cream man, pushing his cart down our block in Brooklyn on warm summer evenings in the 1950s, my mother wouldn't give me the money to buy ice cream. She made a point of telling me it wasn't because she couldn't afford it (which was often true), but rather she would say: "You don't need it!" I could have tolerated not having ice cream like the other kids if the news came with a hug and the reality that money was tight for us. But instead, I felt that I was bad for wanting it—*wanting* was bad. I felt guilty for wanting and angry at her for making me feel guilty.

My childhood was spent in fear of her, hiding from her, avoiding her critical gaze. When I was still wetting my bed at ten and eleven, I never went to her in my distress. I knew she'd yell at me and announce disgustedly in front of my older sister and brother that I had wet the bed. I remember getting up in the middle of the night, after one of my repetitious dreams of sitting on the toilet and urinating. I stripped the bed, changed the sheets and mattress pad and hid them under the bed until she went to work the next day. All this I did behind her back—in terror. Each time I was sent to the store to shop for food because my mother was working, I knew I was in danger. It seemed inevitable that the A&P would have the right brand in the wrong size and the right size in the wrong brand. I would be faced with a Solomonic dilemma. I knew that when she came home from work, tired and frazzled, she would yell at me either way.

Much of my childhood was a series of similar dilemmas— trying to figure out how to avoid my mother's slaps across my face or her screaming reproaches. I didn't dust right or vacuum right or cook right or shop right. I never felt anything I did was right, so I was always trying to cover up and hide so she wouldn't find out. Sometimes I still wake up in the middle of the night, as I used to then, fearing that there is something I've done wrong, but I'm not sure what it is. There's always something. Part of me is still involved in trying (and failing) to *earn* her love.

I started planning my getaway when I was in the seventh grade. I got a job delivering sandwiches and coffee to the hordes of Jewish women who had their hair done every Saturday. No Jewish women had gray hair in Brooklyn in the 1950s; they were blonds, brunettes with blond streaks, and redheads. They spent all day Saturday reading magazines under big metal dryers with dye and rollers in their hair. I brought them coffee and bagels when they came in; I brought their lunch; and I brought them cigarettes. I saved my money in a bank account that I opened when banks offered free gifts, such as cheap cameras, if you opened an account with $25. I had accounts all over Brooklyn and I would visit the banks on my bike. I used the camera to take pictures of automobile accidents, children who got run over and other "news" that I would call in to the *Daily News*. I would get a check for my "reporting." I saved every penny and dreamed about going to college and getting away from my mother.

But after a lifetime of being angry at my mother for not taking care of me, I find myself in a position for which I am not prepared—having to take care of *her*. Despite the popular misconception that formal institutions have replaced the family as the main source of care for the elderly, in reality families provide 80 to 90 percent of the care of the elderly living in the community.[4] My view is that caring for an elderly family member is a new stage of life.[5] Of course people have always taken care of elderly or infirm parents. However, now there is a very large generation (the baby boomers) who are facing the same task simultaneously. Additionally, it is usually done for an extensive period of time because of the increase in life expectancy. Nearly half of all caregivers assist between one and four years; 20 percent provide care for five years or more.

The period spent caring for an elderly parent is not just a stage of life—it is a developmental stage because it is an opportunity for continuing the process of separation and further consolidating our sense of self.[6] During the years of our parents' decline we have yet another opportunity to integrate our parents' experience of themselves and us with our sense of self in relation to them. We have another opportunity to connect with our parents in a deeper or, sometimes, even new way.

For many caregivers it is that opportunity that motivates them. In some cases the caregiver is able to experience growth through working out unresolved feelings from childhood with the accompanying feelings of remorse, sadness and loss. In other cases the caregiver is stuck repeating the same dynamics that were so painful in childhood. I am going through this developmental stage now. I am *once again* dealing with: feelings about my brother getting special dispensations because he is a boy; my wish to have my mother appreciate me; and feeling angry at my mother for being so needy and wanting me to take care of her.

But not every middle-aged person with elderly parents becomes a caregiver. Some siblings end up the primary caregivers while others do not. Certainly, factors such as geographic proximity and employment are important. Social class and ethnic group play an important part in whether elderly parents are invited to live with their children or caregiving takes the form of paid homecare, assisted living or nursing home care. However, my purpose is to understand how family dynamics from childhood, often related to gender expectations, affect who becomes the primary caregiver in a family and how that caregiver feels about their position in the family and their relationship with the elderly parent(s).

In my case, I am the youngest of three siblings. My sister is eight years older and my brother is four years older than I am.

I was not my mother's favorite. On the contrary, I have always known that I was not a planned pregnancy. In addition, it seems that my parents wished for a Robert, but got me instead—hence I am Roberta. Clearly, my role as primary caregiver for my mother is not a result of having been her special child. My brother was the clear favorite in the family. My father attended his Saturday baseball games while my sister and I were left to clean the house under my mother's critical eye.

Since my brother was never expected to do the domestic chores that my sister and I were forced to do, he has no sense that he should be an equal participant in caring for my mother other than financially. Several years ago, I brought up the unequal distribution of caregiving responsibility between us, my brother responded: "Well, you're her daughters!" My sister seems to concur with him. She does not seem to have the same expectations of a brother as a sister.

Since women are more likely to do the hands-on nurturing of caregiving, as a dependent parent's need for assistance progresses from a need for practical help to a need for more personal care, daughters are more likely to move into a primary role.

My sister, on the other hand, has had her hands full because her husband has been seriously ill and for several years she was the primary caregiver to our elderly uncle, who was particularly kind to her at crucial and difficult moments in her life. I did not feel a similar obligation to him because he was not equally kind to me. My sister also feels that she was compelled to be "the good daughter" for many years when I was not similarly compelled. Thus, she feels it is my turn to take over. Ironically, then, I am left with the primary responsibility for my mother.

Whatever the pragmatic difficulties of caregiving, it's the interpersonal and intrapsychic factors that take the highest toll. Bonnie Walson, executive director of Heritage Day Health Centers in Columbus, Ohio, told me: "When people are involved in the acute level of caregiving, it is a huge amount of *emotional* as well as practical work. They feel like they no longer have their own lives."

I have seen many of my patients, friends and interviewees relive childhood experiences when they care for their elderly parents. My usually mild-mannered friend Carl, a specialist in pain management, was telling me about his difficulty in getting his parents to accept the help he is trying to provide for them. Finally, he burst out with: "Goddamn it, when I was a senior in college I drove my father to Alcoholics Anonymous every day for thirty days and at the end of it *he called me up drunk.*"

You may feel that my story and the stories of many of the caregivers I present are extreme examples. But the majority of people I have interviewed are living through extremely difficult situations with their parents and struggling to care for their parents while managing their own emotions and maintaining their own families and/or jobs. In Anna Quindlen's novel *One True Thing,* the daughter, Ellen, who returns home to care for her dying mother, says:

> Everyone makes up their little stories and then they wonder why their own lives aren't like that. It makes life so much simpler if we can get rid of all the loose ends. Ellen is such an angel, loved her mother so much she couldn't bear to see her suffer. Or, Ellen is such a witch that she walked over her mother in spikes to get what she wanted.

I can't be responsible for other people's stories. I have enough trouble making sense of my own.[7]

I have learned from years as a psychotherapist that there are always loose ends. Even people who seem very successful and well put together on the outside often have lived through and/or are living through very extreme experiences. One theme of this book is that caregiving *is* often an extreme situation that lasts a long time and dredges up our conflicts from a lifetime—with our parents, siblings, children and selves. It is a major challenge. But it offers us the opportunity to make sense of our *real* stories.

THE UNSEEN CAREGIVER

The National Family Caregivers Association (NFCA) estimates there are 25 million family caregivers in the United States.[8] More than one-half of all family caregivers are children and 77 percent of us are female.[9] As Gail Sheehy points out in *The Silent Passage,* more and more women are being put on "the daughter track," possibly for a decade or more, just as we emerge from "the mommy track."[10] Just as most women and men assume a woman will be the primary parent, we also assume that a daughter will be the primary caregiver for a parent—unless there are no daughters.

Fathers and mothers choose different solutions to the conflict between parenting and paid work. Similarly, daughters and sons also choose different solutions to the conflict between waged work and informal caregiving. Daughters are likelier to curtail labor force participation, while sons are more likely to reduce caregiving responsibilities. Daughters are more likely than sons to relinquish paid employment, reduce work hours and take time off without pay. Hence, daughters are more likely than sons to experience caregiving as stressful.[11]

Often, emotional stress is expressed physically because the caregiver is too guilty to tolerate her own anger. The NFCA members survey found that since their caregiving activities began: 27 percent reported more headaches; 24 percent reported more stomach disorders; 41 percent reported more back pain; 51 percent reported more sleeplessness; and 61 percent reported depression.[12]

The majority of American women between the ages of forty and sixty-four are employed. Current estimates are that between one-quarter and one-third of the workforce *also* takes care of an elderly parent. We have to deal with the demands of our jobs, children, spouses, friends *and our elderly parents*. At the same time as the need for caregiving is increasing, the difficulties in providing that care are multiplying. Increased numbers of women in the labor force, high levels of divorce and more geographical mobility make it more difficult for adult children to care for their elderly parents.[13]

I am one of those caregivers. I am fifty-eight. My father is dead. My mother is ninety-one. She's had a few small strokes so her short-term memory is not very consistent. Sometimes she is perfectly lucid and other times she can't remember how to use the telephone or what month or year it is. Despite her limitations, my feelings toward my mother are not entirely sympathetic because of my childhood relationship with her.

THE GOOD NEWS AND THE BAD NEWS

The caregiving experience offers both bad and good news. The bad news is that caregiving is a stressful stage of life for which most middle-aged people are unprepared. Just when you finally feel you've reached a plateau in your life—that is, your children are grown or you have attained success in your career or financial security and you have more freedom to enjoy life—you have to turn your attention to caring for your parents. When you feel you've finally separated from your parents and developed "adult" relationships with siblings, you have to reengage with them in ways that make you regress to your old and usually painful ways of relating to them. A sixty-year-old grandfather reexperiences his yearning for his ninety-year-old father's approval. A fifty-year-old woman gets enraged at her mother with Alzheimer's disease who asks her each day: "Why haven't you called me?"

But the good news is that caregiving can be a life-affirming experience. If you had a warm and loving relationship with your parents, it is an opportunity to show your appreciation of them and add a new level of reciprocity and intimacy to your relationship. On the other hand, if your relationship with your parents has been difficult, caregiving is a developmental stage that offers us another opportunity to work out some of the unresolved issues that are still lurking in us from childhood. During the years of caregiving, you can separate out your past and present and put your parents' way of relating to you in the context of their parents' way of relating to them. You can forgive yourself for being angry toward your parents for what they didn't give you by giving them what you didn't get. If your expectation of yourself as a caregiver combines empathy and reality, you can experience the pleasure of meeting your own expectations of yourself. And if you have enjoyed a warm relationship with your parents you may be in the enviable position of deepening and strengthening these bonds in the last years of your parents' lives.

In the course of interviewing caregivers, I have found people who have developed constructive ways of dealing with their complicated feelings about caring for their elderly parents. I have also found people who, in contrast, are stuck repeating patterns from the past that continue to make them feel bad about themselves. What distinguishes those who have experienced caregiving as a growth experience from those who are stuck? One crucial factor that distinguished those caregivers who were able to take advantage of the opportunity to once again grapple with unresolved issues from those who got caught in a downward spiral was their ability to set limits. We need to decide what we can reasonably do and then set limits on what we agree to do.

Of course, people need to set different limits at different points—there is no set recipe. It depends on the realities of your life, your comfort level and the degree to which you feel firmly separate. Setting limits in a healthy way involves balancing generosity and self-preservation and learning to accept what you have to offer as good enough. It sounds easy. But it isn't. As we shall see in the chapters in Part I, setting limits is one of the most difficult aspects of caregiving, but it is also one of the most important.

SETTING LIMITS AND FEELING SEPARATE

The ability to set limits is rooted in the process of psychological separation which is at the heart of what is most difficult about caregiving. Setting limits is a behavioral reflection of feeling separate and clear about your boundaries. The process of separation reverberates throughout our lives; it is not a one-shot experience. It begins at birth with the physical separation from the mother's body and continues throughout our lives until final separation—death.[14] If we have a good-enough mother who cares for us as infants, but allows us to experience a tolerable amount of frustration, we realize that she is separate from us in a deeper way—we begin a process of psychological separation.[15] If she is clear about her own boundaries and allows us to go off and explore the world and return to her as a safe haven, we continue to develop a sense of ourselves as separate at the same time that we feel love and attachment.

Adolescence offers still another opportunity to work out this balance between attachment and separation. It is the period during which we attempt to adjust to puberty and integrate our sexuality into our sense of ourselves as well as renegotiate our relationship with our parents. During the end of the second year of life ("the terrible twos"), the child tries to make a distinction between self and non-self by saying "No." During adolescence the process of separation and developing a sense of identity takes the form of experimenting with behaviors that are "me" and "not-me"; rebelling against authority; testing the limits of authority and the self.[16]

If we become parents ourselves, we are challenged by yet another level of balancing attachment and separateness. We have to allow our children to become more and more autonomous while at the same time offering them love and support. Sarah, a publishing executive, recounted a story about how difficult it was for her to allow her daughter to be separate. A friend made a date with her eleven-year-old daughter and canceled it at the last minute. Sarah found it difficult to tolerate her daughter's disappointment. She wanted to make her feel better by calling the girl's mother and telling her to tell her daughter she can't break appointments at the last minute. She wanted to control her daughter's reality to protect her. Her husband made the point that their daughter needs to learn to deal with disappointment and learn that she can bear it. A simple hug or "I'm sorry things didn't work out" or the combination of both would express caring, but allow her daughter to feel separate and have her own feelings.

Paradoxically, the more difficult our childhood relationships with our parents, the less likely that we were able to develop a sense of being firmly separate from them. Since each stage of separation echoes previous ones, childhood separation issues remain with us as adults. For example, Rebecca is a successful public relations executive but her feelings about herself are tied to her childhood experience of her mother's response to her. Rebecca's mother was depressed when she was a young child because Rebecca's father was hospitalized with manic-depressive disorder. Her mother was unable to respond to Rebecca's excitement about the world around her—she was withdrawn and distracted. Rebecca assumed her mother's lack of response was because *she* was not interesting enough to warrant her mother's attention. She was too young to understand that her mother's lack of interest in her was a symptom of her depression.

When Rebecca began treatment with me she told me a dream that expressed her experience of her mother. In the dream Rebecca was trying to get into a pawnshop that was locked. Inside were beautiful antiques and jewelry that she could see through the window, but the shop was closed and she couldn't gain access to any of the riches inside. Rebecca internalized an image of herself as not good enough to engage her mother and an image of her mother as full of goodies that she was withholding because Rebecca was undeserving. She had spent her life trying to be smart enough, funny enough, interesting enough to engage her mother and all of the mother substitutes in her life.

Separation involves seeing your mother as *not you* and her responses to you, if they were less than adequate, as a result of *her experiences, not of you.* Separation means acknowledging how limited *her* choices were. In Rebecca's case, she has come to appreciate how difficult it was for her mother to cope with the demands of a young child and a manic-depressive husband. From my psychoanalytic work, I know that there are several steps in the process of psychic separation and a great deal of resistance to taking them. Caregiving is a stage of life that involves balancing attachment and separateness; it is an opportunity to prepare for the final separation from our parents. As I will discuss in the chapters in Part II, it is generally more difficult for daughters to separate from their mothers than it is for sons to separate from mothers, daughters from fathers and sons from fathers. Since most children who are caregivers for elderly parents are daughters, I am using the term "daughters" instead of "children" or "daughters and sons."

Separating from your mother involves separating from an image of yourself as "bad daughter." If we are lucky and we had a "good-enough mother" who was able to help us separate, we feel good about taking care of our selves as well as those we love—we are able to feel that we are good-enough daughters. The worse our childhood relationship with our mother, the more important it is for us to preserve an image of her as a "good mother."[17] Otherwise *we are alone and we have no mother.* In the most extreme cases, the mother is consciously idealized—the child cannot allow any ambivalence for fear that the hate will completely overwhelm the love. In less extreme cases the good mother–bad daughter split may be less conscious. The daughter may be able to talk about the mother's faults, but keeps trying to get the impossible—to get mother to love her.

In order to protect "the good mother," we take on the burden of "the bad daughter." It gives us a fantasy of control—after all, if the problem is *me* then there's some hope for things getting better. I can try harder, do more and say the "right" thing. But if the problem is my mother's inability to mother, then there is no chance of getting what I need. This sets up the dynamic of repetition—trying to please mother (or mother substitutes), failing and feeling angry and hopeless and unlovable.

As long as you hold on to the image of yourself as "bad daughter," you cannot separate from your mother. I sometimes sit with patients whose mothers neglected or even abused them and I wonder: Why do you resist giving up such a painful image of yourself? And then I remember that giving it up feels like *being a child and having no mother*. Accepting that we cannot get what we want from our mother means giving up hope and facing a black hole. I try to remind my patients that they might be able to get some of it someplace else if they were not locked in this internal battle that depletes all their energy.

In order to separate from your mother you have to recognize that childhood feelings remain intact from when you were totally dependent on her. Although we are now adults with careers and perhaps husbands and children, we simultaneously live on another level of which we are not conscious unless we have been in psychotherapy. Our early relationships get internalized inside us and they are evoked in situations that are reminiscent of childhood experiences. When I saw a revival of Sam Shepard's play *True West,* I was struck with how much he was able to capture the power of regression. In the play, a son, who is a writer and has a wife and children, returns to his mother's home to finalize a business deal and finds his brother there. In the process of their interaction, the writer regresses and is soon overwhelmed by his feelings of sibling rivalry and desire for approval from his brother, who appears to be an aimless wanderer.

Many caregivers report similar regressions when they visit their elderly parents or have them move into their home. Karen, a sixty-two-year-old high school principal, feels humiliated when her eighty-year-old mother says: "You got a haircut, right?" and doesn't follow it with: "It looks good." She feels like a rebuked child. All her childhood insecurity and need for her mother's approval comes up in a rush.

As Victoria Secunda points out in *When You and Your Mother Can't Be Friends,* time may have moved on, but not childhood feelings and fears, trapped in a grown daughter's memory.[18]

You have to recognize the feelings and accept them as legitimate—we are not responsible for what was done to us as children. We are as entitled to feel angry as we are to feel loving. Of course, this is easier said than done. There is a clear cultural mandate to put a good face on your childhood and not expose your grief and rage. Religious leaders often reinforce this cultural mandate rather than helping congregants work through and resolve difficult feelings about their parents so that they will be more able to provide caregiving.

One of my patients explains that the Roman Catholic schools she attended taught that feelings and actions are the same—angry feelings are as sinful as angry acts. It is very hard for her to accept the legitimacy of her feelings and distinguish between *feeling* angry and *doing* something harmful to another person. I point out that we do not have control over what we feel, only what we do. But, it is difficult to give ourselves permission to feel whatever we feel (without a therapist's or group's support).

You have to recognize your resistance to separating. My own experience and those of my patients and friends indicate that the process of separating from your mother is never-ending—it is a continuum of separation. Our relationships with our mothers turn up in our relationships with our spouses, friends and children—it's a matter of degree.

When a daughter cannot separate from her mother, and when she *will not* or is *unable to* examine why, her unresolved feelings turn up in all her other relationships—

what she could not get from her mother surfaces as an un-realistic need and expectation. She becomes all want, little give; all disappointment, little optimism; all appetite, little confidence. And so she may, in the saddest sense, indeed become more like her mother every day.[19]

Some people's relationships are a replica of their relation-ship with their mother, and they have no consciousness of the repetition. For others, it is a never-ending process of see-ing repetitions and trying to catch them before they have gone too far. For example, my unresolved feelings about my mother emerged the night of the hospital episode with my mother and my uncle Morris.

When I returned to Richard waiting for me in the car after my lengthy adventure trying to get my mother's keys from my uncle Morris, I was disappointed that Richard wasn't worried about me. I could have asked him to come with me instead of sitting in the car. I was perfectly capable of climb-ing the stairs to the third floor and ringing the bell. Instead, I fell back into an old pool of disappointment and was yearning unconsciously for a more involved and concerned mother. I had displaced my feelings about my mother to my husband by feeling upset that he wasn't more worried about my safety. This was a vivid reminder of the impor-tance of working through separation problems in the care-giving process.

You may experience significant others as if they were your mother and at other times treat those same people as you were treated as a child. This can feel good when you have had a secure early childhood, but if you have very ambiva-lent feelings toward your mother, recognizing that you are acting like her can be very painful—even loathsome. Ironically, the more you refuse to see your mother in yourself, the more you become like her. This book is an exploration of what we need to know in order to make a difficult caregiving process a positive developmental stage in our lives.

I BEGAN this book when I was fifty-four and my mother was eighty-six. In the intervening five years, I have become increasingly comfortable with my feelings about her. As she slips deeper into senile dementia, there is a blissful calm about her. She smiles when I arrive but sometimes thinks I'm her sister and other times her niece. Occasionally there are glimpses of her former angry self, but they are rare.

During these five years my understanding of my relationship with my mother has deepened through the process of coping with the intense feelings provoked by the progression of her dementia. I have become able to comfort my mother as well as myself because I have been more able to remember that it is *normal* and *okay* to feel ambivalent at times about my role. This book is not a "how-to" guide in the ordinary sense because each caregiver has to find her own level of comfort in the role. However, I hope it will offer you some of the support and insight necessary to find that niche for yourself.

Part I

THE
INTERNAL
STRUGGLE

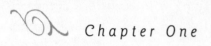 *Chapter One*

SETTING LIMITS

When you confront an ocean of need, bring a cup.

—*The Reverend Michael Moran,*
First Congregational Church, New Milford, Connecticut

WHEN PEOPLE CONFRONT an ocean of need they feel anxiety. Some run for their lives; others jump in and drown. Both reactions are rooted in the inability to stay separate and set limits in a healthy way that balances generosity with self-preservation. I have seen this dynamic in myself in my therapy practice and with my mother. Often, when patients feel so needy that they are desperate for me to take their neediness away, I feel overwhelmed by anxiety. I feel helpless and afraid of drowning; the feeling makes me want to withdraw. Sometimes I do, temporarily. In order to offer patients *something*, I have to be able to accept that I cannot take away their ocean of need, but I can bring a cup and offer *some* relief. I cannot do that until I am able to feel securely separate from them—clear that I am not going to drown in their neediness.

Similarly, when my mother had a series of small strokes and was increasingly unable to take care of herself, I felt overwhelmed by her neediness. She was going to a dozen different doctors who were not communicating with one another; she was losing weight and constantly complaining of nausea; she had stains on her clothes; she couldn't remember her keys or that she had just found them; she couldn't remember if she had sent her rent check or not; she couldn't remember if she had taken her medication or not; and she couldn't remember my husband's name or my birthday. She called me all the time—to ask me the same questions over and over. My sister said it was my mother's anxiety; she often felt angry toward her. My sister is the eldest child and *her* anxiety about drowning in our mother's neediness made her feel so overwhelmed that she needed to withdraw from our mother. She could hardly bear to visit her. In addition, my brother rarely visited and never indicated when he was going to. I felt guilty and frightened. What could I do? I felt that my only alternatives were doing nothing at all or letting her take me over (that is, live in my house; change my relationship with my husband and my children; interfere with my work, my friends and my routines).

I had to face a new phase in my own development. For a long time I dealt with my mother by trying to keep my distance. During high school and college I imagined whom I would go to for help if I got pregnant—my mother was definitely out. When I was in college I had mononucleosis and I was in the university hospital. I did not tell my mother. As a young married woman, I never talked to her about anything personal that mattered to me. It was easier to report on facts of my children's lives, Jason has a cold or Matthew got an A on his English paper, or day-to-day activities and events in my life, I spoke to my cousin or I went to the dentist. My withdrawal from my mother was a result of my insecure attachment to her—and that remained inside of me, sometimes consciously and sometimes unconsciously.

The early insecure attachment creates a wish to be comforted and a wish to run away from danger. The problem is that the person from whom you want comfort and the person who is dangerous is the same person—that creates an often lifelong conflict. The mother you yearn for is the mother you withdraw from; the mother you are afraid of is the mother you cling to. Children with school phobias offer a good example of this paradox—the inability to leave home is often a response to a perceived threat from the parents. Thus withdrawal and clinging are two different anxiety responses resulting from an insecure early attachment to the mother.[1]

Often, the withdrawal and clinging are split off and transferred to people other than your mother.[2] In my case, I avoided my mother, but clung to friends, lovers and my analyst. I didn't experience separation anxiety from my mother, but from my analyst and my husband.

Ever since I returned to New York from college in California at age twenty-one, I took a minimalist approach to seeing my mother. I saw her and spoke to her as little as possible. My sister enjoyed shopping with her, but I never did. I never felt good about myself in my mother's presence because I was always struggling with yearning for her to be what she could never be and being angry with her for being unable to be that. I guess what I wanted her to be was a mother with whom I could feel like a good daughter. But that was not possible.

About two years ago I realized that my mother could not take care of herself. She forgot to make entries in her checkbook, although she had been a crackerjack bookkeeper when I was a girl. She could add a long list of numbers in her head and never lose track of the total. Now she couldn't figure out where to enter the amount of the check. Her clothes were dirty and she was steadily losing weight. I had been denying it. But I couldn't deny it any longer. I had to find some way of helping my mother cope with living while maintaining my own life—bringing a cup to relieve some of her feeling of helplessness, but not drowning in her neediness.

Setting limits is difficult for most people—it's a common problem in many areas of our life, not just caregiving. It's hard to say "no" or "enough" without feeling guilty. It's difficult to tell a friend she can't borrow money or tell your son he can't have another toy he can't live without. I had a terrible time toilet training my elder son. One of my friends used to console me by saying: "Don't worry, by the time he gets married he'll be toilet trained." The more you project your own neediness onto someone else and then identify with the person to whom you are saying no, the harder it is to do it without feeling bad about yourself. I would start off feeling like a separate adult and saying: "Okay, now you're going to use the toilet." As soon as Matthew started yelling that he didn't want to use the toilet, I would start identifying with him. How can I force him to do what he doesn't want to do? I'll be acting like my mother. I'll wait until he *wants* to use the potty. Except he never got to that point. He was three years old and they wouldn't let him into nursery school in diapers so I went to a child psychologist for help. She said: "Your son does not have a problem. You do; you are not like your mother. You can tell him he is going to wear underpants and throw out his diapers and he will be fine." I followed her advice and he never had an accident again. She made it clear to me that the problem was all mine. I was so afraid of being like my mother that I couldn't set limits and stick to them. I couldn't distinguish between being sadistic and helping my son master a developmental task that would make him feel better about himself.

If we feel needy and deprived because we have an insecure internal attachment to our early mother then it is hard to say no or enough to somebody else. People who have difficulty saying no often get angry at people who ask them for anything. After all, asking them for something sets off their conflict. Thus, setting limits with needy elderly parents can be extremely difficult if we are needy ourselves—which we usually are if we had needy parents. We vacillate back and forth between identifying with their neediness and feeling we have to save them; and feeling angry at them for needing so much from us and wanting to run away so that we do not drown. Adults with a secure attachment do not feel needy—or are able to work their way out of that feeling fairly quickly. They have needs, of course, but they are not "needy." The feeling of being needy is a feeling of desperation for someone else to save you and to provide sustenance. In addition, it easily gets projected onto other people so it's hard to stay clearly separate. Caregivers who have an internal sense of secure attachment have secure boundaries and have less difficulty saying no or enough in a way that does not necessitate hitting the other person over the head with it or running away from a person who is needy. They can say: "I wish I was able to do that for you, but unfortunately I'm not."

SIBLING RIVALRY

Rose is not afraid of drowning. At forty-nine, Rose wants to be a good daughter and is angry with her mother for making her feel that she's horrible and inadequate. She wants her mother to appreciate all that she sacrifices for her.

> I'm just constantly running . . . I can't do anything right—
> no matter how much I do for her . . . She thinks I have
> nothing to do all day . . .

Rose's eighty-two-year-old mother came to live with her, her husband and two teenage children more than three years ago. Her mom had broken her hip and was discharged from the hospital after two days. Rose's brother had been living with their mom before the accident, but felt unable to care for her in her house. Medicare would have paid for her to go to a rehabilitation center to recuperate, but Rose decided to bring her home instead. After she moved in, her mom began having congestive heart failure and needed oxygen twenty-four hours a day.

When I arrived at the house to interview Rose I was ushered into a very large sunken living room. I could hear the noise of the oxygen machine from the next room, where the nurse was caring for Rose's mother. One corner of the room was taken up with the largest TV screen I have ever seen outside a theater. In each of the other three corners of the room were chairs facing the screen, rather than one another. In the center was a huge space. I imagined people sitting in each of the chairs having to yell to each other across the large expanse of the room. Clearly this was not a room in which people spoke to one another.

Rose told me that she has always prided herself on *not* being like her mother. She feels her mother did not set any limits for her brothers and encouraged their acting out with alcohol and drugs.

> My brothers . . . got in trouble, they stole, and they drank. One of my brothers is messed up with drugs and alcohol every day. He just moved to Florida and came up to visit. It was a total disaster. He came and asked my mother for money and she was going to write him a check. I said, "Mom, that's a mistake. He'll cash the check and go to the bar and spend it." And that's exactly what he did.

Rose has tried not to repeat her mother's mistakes in bringing up her children.

> My brothers would come home falling-down drunk and she would just give them something to eat and put them to bed. Tell him to get out. It's called tough love.

However, in her attempt to be different than her mother, she set so many limits on her daughters that she has difficulty allowing them to separate.

> My daughter is a great kid. I told her she has to go to the local community college. She had her heart set on going to the University of California. I said no, she has to go to

community college for one year and then she can transfer. She's never been anywhere. No, she can't go away for the first year.

Despite all her protestations, Rose is living out her childhood script and passing it on to the next generation. Her need to be the opposite of her mother keeps her tied to her. And Rose keeps her daughters tied to her by overcontrolling them and not allowing them to develop their own inner limits and sense of judgment.

Using the language of Alcoholics Anonymous, Rose says her mother was an "enabler" for her father's alcoholism and irresponsibility.

> My father was an alcoholic and no matter what time he came home she got up and made his dinner and put him to sleep. He'd wake up the whole house when he came in because he was so loud when he was drunk. He spent all his money on drinking and then she worked sixteen hours a day to support us. I'm sorry, there's no way in hell that I would do that.

Rose feels bitter that her mother allowed her father's alcoholism to control the family. She resents her mother for not standing up to her father and protecting her children.

Rose has given up seeing friends, having vacations and going out with her husband because her mother doesn't like it. This increases her sense of deprivation and rage. She refuses to use the $600 a month allotted to them by the state for housing her mother, which further intensifies her feeling unappreciated and used.

There's certain things she needs and she doesn't buy them because she gives the money to everybody else [that is, to Rose's brothers]. The only thing we take out of that money is she pays for half of our electric because of the cost of the oxygen machine going twenty-four hours, the TV is on twenty-four hours, and the air conditioning is on because it takes so much energy for her to breathe that she's always hot. My electric bill is sky high.

Rose allows her mother's neediness to control her family's life. Unfortunately, Rose doesn't see the parallel with how her mother supported her father's alcoholism.

Once I tried going out for half an hour and leaving her alone. She's got Life Line. There's no reason she can't be alone for a while. Oh God! She called our neighbor and she wasn't home so she pressed the button on Life Line and the cops came. So we don't go out alone. We pack her up and take her with us.

Her mother's message was: "You cannot have a separate life from me. You have to take care of me." Her mother's tactic worked—Rose no longer goes out without her mother. Her mother never insisted her husband stop drinking or bring home his paycheck; she just organized the family around his abuse. She worked two jobs to compensate for the money he spent in bars. The family ate dinner without him; his drunken yelling awakened the children nightly. Similarly, Rose angrily accepts her mother's abuse and organizes her family's life around it.

Rose seems to think that she has protected her children

from the effects of having her mother living with them. But she can't protect her children from the effects of her feeling like an unloved child: "Sometimes I would take it out on them and I have to stop and think: 'Hey, they didn't do anything wrong.'" Rose has given up going shopping with her daughters because her mother doesn't like to be alone. She relents because she cannot tolerate her mother's displeasure. All these sacrifices increase Rose's sense of deprivation and rage at her mother.

Rose's mother did not have a separate identity herself. She sacrificed her life for her alcoholic husband and so she remains a still-dependent child at eighty-two. Never having had a mother who protected her, Rose insists on making unnecessary sacrifices for her mother/child. For example, she and her husband built her mother a huge room to live in without discussing it with her. When the room was unveiled to Grandma, she said no thanks and Rose felt unappreciated for her effort to please her mother. Despite that experience, Rose continued to try. She had her husband build a deck around the house so that her mother could sit outside, but her mother doesn't *want* to sit outside and that makes Rose feel that her mother doesn't appreciate anything she does for her.

Rose is stuck in an old pattern—trying to get her mother to appreciate her instead of taking care of her "no-good" father and brothers.

It's a guy thing. I go in and she is grumpy and nasty, but one of the boys goes in and she's all excited . . . She gets social security and a pension and it goes into her account and she writes checks to my brothers.

Rose keeps trying to get her mother to see how bad "the boys" (ages fifty-five, fifty-one and forty-eight) are. Rose is pained when they come to the house drunk and say "She's an asshole" behind her mother's back.

> The boys come here spacey and drunk and she writes them a check. Why doesn't she make my brother pay back the Visa card? He could pay $100 a month or something. She thinks I'm horrible.

When Rose complains about her brothers her mother tells her: "If you kept your damn mouth shut they wouldn't bother you." Rose feels slashed by her mother's sadism toward her, but blames her "no-good" brothers instead of her mother. Whenever she complains about her mother's sadism toward her, she immediately disavows it or blames it on her brothers.

> There's a senior center nearby and the people there have oxygen or other kinds of problems and she could spend some time there, but she wouldn't have anything to do with it. She didn't want to give me that little break. *It's not her fault that she's in this situation . . . It's not her fault that she's on oxygen. If only my brothers would help.*

Rose is caught in a tragic bind. The mother, who she desperately wanted to protect her as a child, neglected and abandoned her. Her mother always made it clear that Rose's needs were unimportant in comparison to the needs of her alcoholic father and out-of-control brothers. The insecure attachment to the person she was totally dependent upon is still central in Rose's life. She clings to the mother who still refuses to consider her needs; she feels like a little girl who cannot survive without her mother's love and protection. As Judith Viorst points out in *Necessary Losses:*

> It doesn't seem to matter what kind of mother a child has . . . or how perilous it may be to dwell in her presence . . . Separation from mother is sometimes worse than being with her when *she* is the bomb.[3]

Like so many children who had mothers who did not take good-enough care of them, she has not been able to develop as an autonomous person. Since her actions look so outwardly selfless and gallant, it's hard to see that it's not related to getting her mother the care she needs, but rather to Rose's own need to cling to her rejecting mother. Rose has no conscious understanding of her conflict. In fact, she told me that she has been having panic attacks for a few years, but she did not connect it to having her mother living in her house. She was seeing a psychotherapist to help her cope with the panic attacks, but the therapist's approach did not relate the panic attacks to Rose's early relationship with her mother. Hence, the panic attacks were getting better, but the therapy was not helping her understand why caring for her mother was so agonizing.

Professionals from an addiction/recovery background would discuss Rose's insecure attachment to her mother and consequent inability to separate in terms of codependency.[4] Rose needs to be needed. She watched her mother organize her life around the chaotic moods and needs of her father. In the language of recovery, Rose's mother was an "enabler."

Typically, codependent caregivers are, like Rose, the children of alcoholics, drug addicts, depressed or mentally ill parents.

Melody Beattie, author of *Codependent No More,* says that caregiving is a major characteristic of people who are co-dependent.[5] They feel compelled to solve other people's problems and anticipate their needs because they feel safest when they are giving. They willingly abandon their routine for somebody else because they don't expect anyone to want them for their intrinsic worth. They try to make themselves indispensable and often end up feeling unappreciated and used by others. While all caregivers have to make some sacrifices to care for their elderly parents, codependent caregivers sacrifice their happiness for others even when sacrifice *is not required.* For example, Rose complained about being exhausted, but believed she was suffering for the sake of her family. She insisted on getting up with her husband and making his breakfast at 4 a.m. despite the fact that he told her he was perfectly happy picking up coffee and a doughnut on his way to work.

My view is that what is called "codependency," in the recovery perspective, is a set of symptoms that reflect a separation problem. Rose has not been able to separate from her mother. She still yearns for approval and recognition from her and is embroiled in an old crusade to prove that she is more deserving of her mother's love than her "bad boy" brothers. Why can't her mother see how good she is and how bad the boys are? Rose is eaten up with anger and frustration because of the unfairness of it all. On a deeper level, Rose cannot give up the battle to get her mother to mother her; she cannot face the loss of the mother she unconsciously feels she cannot survive without. Rose wants her mother to fulfill a need that was never satisfied when she was a child and for which she still yearns—the need for what psychoanalysts call "mirroring." Mirroring is the mother's smile back when the baby smiles; the smile of pleasure that comes over a mother's face when a child says something cute or does something for the first time; the mother's words of recognition when the child feels hurt or is treated unfairly. Mirroring builds up our sense of self so that we can later perform that function for ourselves. Unfortunately, Rose did not get enough of it as a child and she is still trying to get it from her elderly mother, who is incapable of giving it. She's still looking for the smile of appreciation on her mother's face to confirm that she's good.

At the same time that she desperately wants her mother's appreciation, Rose is angry with her mother for not taking care of her. But she cannot admit that directly, so she focuses on her mother's failure to take care of her sons by setting limits for them. In an attempt to give her daughters what she and her brothers did not get, she over-mothers them— which is probably experienced by her daughters not as protective as much as anxious.

Listening to my interview with Rose over and over again, I thought about what I might say to her if I had the opportunity—and I thought about how she might respond. I would try to help Rose understand how much *she* wants from her mother. Rose did not seem to be in touch with wanting anything from her mother. Indeed, she refused to use any of her mother's money to prove she didn't want anything from her. Rose finds it hard to accept that we can be grown up mothers in reality and still have feelings from when we were little girls. It's that little girl who built a big room for her mother and waited for the smile of appreciation—which still hasn't come.

ACCEPTING HIS MOTHER'S LIMITS AND SETTING HIS OWN

Paul is a sixty-two-year-old retired lawyer. He has been married for thirty-seven years and has a thirty-year-old daughter and a twenty-eight-year-old son. I met Paul's mother, Clara, at the assisted living facility where she has lived for the past two years. She is an eighty-eight-year-old woman, shrunken by severe osteoporosis, who walks with a walker. I asked several seniors at the center if they thought their children might be willing to be interviewed and Clara told me that her two daughters, sixty-eight and seventy years old, live in Florida, but she volunteered her son's phone number because he lived nearby. Paul and I met at the facility and had our first interview there. He is a paunchy man with a thick head of dark brown hair and an air of gruffness about him. As he talked, I initially felt his speech was stilted and that he was not being very open about his feelings about his mother. To my surprise, a few days later, he called me and we had a long phone conversation during which Paul expressed much more of his ambivalence toward his mother. Still unsatisfied, Paul sent me a handwritten letter clarifying some things that had come up in our two conversations. In the letter, Paul talked about the issues that were most painful to him: the time he stopped speaking to his mother and the violent relationship between his parents. Clearly, it was very important to Paul that I understand the complexity of the emotional struggle he has gone through in trying to come to peace with his ambivalent relationship with his mother.

Paul told me that his father had been a professional boxer, a proud man, a macho guy who owned a bar. He was sort of the neighborhood strongman who protected everyone. When he first bought the bar there was this gang of thugs who used to hang out there. For months he had fistfights with these guys and was taking weapons away from people. He said that his mother was a domineering woman who did not complement his father's machismo—their personalities were in total conflict. "It was like living in an arena, not a house." Paul explained that his mother had a weight problem and went to a doctor in New Jersey who gave her pills. He said that when she ran out of pills, she would lie in bed for days.

> I realized only recently that the doctor was giving her amphetamines. She became paranoid and would spy on my father. She was in a paranoid state for a lot of years.

Paul explained that his sisters moved out as soon as they could, but he was six years younger than the younger sister and was left alone to deal with his mother's drug addiction and his parents' violent relationship.

> After my older sisters moved out, my father would be away for months at a time. When he came back they would be like lovers when they first saw each other, but I knew the shoe would drop and they would get into violent fights. I would step in between them. I don't believe in men hitting women, but I don't know how he could have

avoided hitting her because my mother would get in his face and say the most awful things to him, curse at him. He would try to leave so he wouldn't hit her and she would jump in his way and not let him leave. I don't condone his hitting her, but I understand it.

His mother threw things at his father or hit him in addition to constantly cursing at him. Paul says he often thought his mother was masochistic because her behavior provoked his father to hit her.

My father was not without fault either. When things were going well and times were good, he often made stupid, inciting remarks concerning his lack of fidelity. I sometimes got the impression that he was trying to create a situation that would justify his leaving the house. They were totally incompatible from the beginning.

Then Paul gets very sad and says with deep feelings of regret:

It had a profound impact on my personality. I became the arbitrator, the peacekeeper. When I first got married, I couldn't get out of that role. When my wife had problems with how my mother treated her I would try to keep the peace. I couldn't stand up for my wife. When we had a baby, we moved into an apartment near my mother. She would stop by every day and criticize my wife; she would tell her everything she was doing wrong. My wife was respectful, but she would ask me to intercede, but I couldn't do it. It took me many years to start setting boundaries for my mother.

Social workers at the assisted living center told me that Paul
is the most loving of all the caregivers who visit their parents. But he was quite matter-of-fact in describing all the
things he does for his mother—the mother who never took
care of his needs; the mother who provoked his father to hit
her; the mother who almost destroyed his marriage.

> I try to see my mother at least twice a week. She's a very
> needy person. She either can't or won't do things for her-
> self. At the beginning I tried to get her to take care of
> things that she could. But I have given up. I take her to
> doctors and dentists. I buy her things in the drugstore. I
> balance her checkbook and pay her bills. I used to take her
> to lunch a lot, but she seems more comfortable eating
> here.

Paul went on to describe how painful his relationship with
his mother has been his entire life. He said that his mother
believes that she is the center of the universe. She has trouble caring about other people. Paul feels that she tries hard
to act as if she cares, but she doesn't—and she has always
been this way. He told me a story about something that
occurred before his mother went to an assisted living facility and that exemplifies the degree of his mother's self-
centeredness.

> My mother called Friday night and my wife answered the
> phone and told my mother I was having chest pains and I
> was waiting for my doctor to call me back. My mother said
> to my wife: "Don't hang up, don't hang up, this is very im-
> portant, you have to cancel the cleaning woman."

Clara did not express any concern about Paul having a heart attack. It was a false alarm, but Paul was hurt. Soon after that, Clara got enraged because Paul told her she couldn't sleep at his house and then she attacked his wife and daughter for not taking good enough care of her. Finally, Paul exploded and told her she was getting what she gave.

> I accused her of never really being a mother or a grandmother. I proceeded to itemize all of her abusive and neglectful behavior all the way back to my early childhood and stormed out of her house, telling her I never wanted to see or speak to her again.

She responded, in disbelief, "My God, you hate me." Paul did not speak to his mother for a year. When his sisters told him she was sick, he called her. He and his sisters decided Clara needed to be in an assisted living facility. He wanted her to move to one in Florida, where his sisters live, so they could oversee her care.

> I felt I had borne the brunt of dealing with her for so many years and welcomed a shifting of the burden to my two older sisters. Mom claimed she hated Florida and always felt sick there and refused to go.

Paul says that, at first, he undertook her care with great ambivalence. Then he realized he had to set limits on what he did for his mother.

> I spent four or five nights in the emergency room with my mother. The doctors told me she just wanted attention.

Finally I told her that she should call me from the emergency room when she was finished and I'd pick her up. She stopped calling me. If she calls and I have time, I help her. I evaluate how serious it is and decide what I will do. If I'm busy I just tell her I can't do it.

Paul set limits in other ways as well.

I let her know that I couldn't spend a lot of time with her, given her never-ending negativity. I found her very unpleasant and told her so, chastising her for her constant moaning, groaning and complaining. Over time, she has tried very hard to change, at least in my presence. She is very quick to respond favorably when I point this out to her. She has become very careful with me now. I am her only lifeline. I continually let her know I will not tolerate her unpleasantness and have, more than once, left her quickly when she became intolerable.

Setting limits with Clara has allowed Paul to feel better about her because her behavior has improved.

This has allowed for a warmer and more comfortable relationship. As a result I have spent increasingly more time with her. We have learned to make our time together more pleasant and, even at times, fun. As a result, new warmth in our relationship has emerged.

Paul understands his mother cannot feel empathy for him. He said: "Her insignificant needs are more important to her than other people's important needs." But, since his mother has been ill, he has come to terms with who she is and how she became that way.

Author Wendy Lustbader points out that the more hurtful our parents were when we were children, the more crucial it is for us to try to ascertain the wounds inflicted during their own upbringing as a way of putting our relationship with them in context. Otherwise their weaknesses become black holes into which we pointlessly pour our resentment.[6] Pouring our resentment into that black hole does not help in our healing process, but rather exacerbates the feeling of being bad. Paul has been able to feel better about himself by understanding that his mother has terrible feelings of insecurity and can't tolerate being wrong. He explained that she needs to be right and the smartest. He told me that she's so competitive that she competes with little kids to show how smart she is. He has come to appreciate her childhood miseries and how they constricted her ability to mother him.

Paul explained that his grandmother was abusive, treated his mother as a servant and clearly favored his mother's brothers over her.

My grandmother was pregnant when she was eighteen years old and had an arranged marriage to a man she never loved. It was a terrible marriage. My grandmother told my mother that her father—my grandfather—whom she loved dearly, was not her biological father. When my mother was ten, her mother kicked her father out of the house and he died when she was fourteen. She was devastated by the loss of her father. She still visits his grave twice a year, and he died almost seventy-five years ago.

Paul's grandmother took up with a man who was ten years her junior and only eight years older than his mother. His grandmother and her lover played poker day and night. Paul explains that his mother married at seventeen to get out of her mother's house, but never separated from her.

> When I was young my mother was so attached to this mother who was so hateful to her that she went to visit her in Florida when I was fourteen or fifteen and left me in the care of my sisters for the entire winter. My sisters are five and a half and eight years older than I am. When she was home, I never saw her either. She slept all day. She never gave me breakfast before I went to school or lunch to take to school. Now I realize that she was going to this Dr. Feelgood doctor in New Jersey and he was giving her speed. When she would crash she'd stay in bed all day. She forced me to go to bed early because she wanted to go out and play cards. She was never there for me.

Paul says that neither of his parents was particularly warm or loving, but he feels that whatever warmth was available was directed toward him. For example, he remembers cuddling with his parents, but his sisters say they never got that. They say he was both parents' favorite. As little nurturing as Paul got, his sisters seem to have gotten even less and hence are not eager to help him care for his mother.

Clara has not changed.

> I took her to the eye doctor's office in the city. It was horrible because I couldn't park. I had to leave the blinkers on and take her into the office and ride around until she was

finished and then run in and get her. It was terrible. So I found one closer and I took her there. She called me over and whispered that the other ophthalmologist's chairs were more comfortable. She has to find something to complain about. I buy her clothes and she complains and makes me return them. She calls and complains about gifts she gets. She can't accept anything gracefully.

But Paul has been able to continue to care for her by setting limits: "If she moans and groans I leave."

Paul doesn't *forgive* his mother, but he understands her within the context of her own deprivation and neglect. That allows him to take care of her in a way that is responsive to her real needs, but protects him from being overwhelmed by her neediness and his anger.

THE IMPORTANCE OF RECIPROCITY

Isabella has been able to take care of herself and her children while being a caregiver to her parents. Isabella is a forty-five-year-old mother of two sons—ages fifteen and twenty-one. She was born in the Bronx and grew up in a working-class Italian neighborhood. When she got married she and her husband were eager to get out of New York City and moved to a rural area of Connecticut. She lives in a working-class subdivision that was created from farmland. There are no beautiful old trees or flower gardens around the house—just dried grass. It is a large characterless house with plenty of living space. When Isabella ushered me into the house, I was struck by how perfectly clean and orderly it was despite the fact that she works two jobs.

When she was divorced nine years ago, she needed to work to support her two young children. She also felt that she was soon going to have to take care of her mother, who had been diagnosed with cancer, so she bought a two-family house. Her parents had a separate apartment and watched her children while she was at work. Isabella explains that the arrangement with her parents was reciprocal and there were limits built in from the beginning: "I was there for them and they were there for me. It was an exchange for the most part."

Isabella's mother died three years ago after a series of bouts with cancer. During the six years that her mother shared her house, Isabella had a lot of difficulty dealing with her.

> My mother still did that Italian Catholic guilt trip that I remember so clearly from childhood. She'd make me feel bad if I wasn't there for her because she refused to take responsibility for her own needs.

It's clear that Isabella was very angry at her mother for trying to control her and it seems that her mother used to accuse *her* of being controlling and demanding when she set limits. It seems life with mother was a perpetual power struggle with each pot calling the kettle black: "*She* was the demanding one . . . the controlling one . . . She tried to get me to do things *her way*. She never gave up." The emphasis on "she" implied to me that Isabella used to have trouble sorting out who was who. Was she bad for wanting to have a self, separate from her mother? Did her mother want things from her that she could not supply? Isabella had a needy mother who looked to her daughter to satisfy her needs, but during the caregiving experience Isabella began to understand, in a way she had not previously, that there are some things no one else can supply for you. She was coming to grips with her own neediness and it made her clearer about her mother's.

Isabella wants me to know that her mother did not succeed in molding her in her own image and the thought of being like her mother is disturbing.

> I have a twenty-one-year-old who lives on his own. If he calls, he calls. If he doesn't call, I call him. I don't give him a guilt trip about why he didn't call me like she did.

It seems that Isabella was able to work out some of her separation issues with her mother during the time she cared for her before she died.

> One day she said to me: "You've changed." And she was right . . . I said to her: "You're right, I'm not that person who, when you were upset with me, I'd look for any which way to make you happy because I couldn't stand you being mad at me." It wasn't that I didn't care, but I allowed her to be upset and I'd say: "Oh well."

Isabella was able to tolerate her mother being upset with her because she came to understand that her mother's wishes and her own needs were not the same. Being separate means you have to tolerate your mother's anger when your needs conflict with hers: "I grew and became so much stronger because of the connection—actually the reconnection."

Isabella must have felt very dependent and helpless as a

child, and perhaps that carried through to her marriage. But when she left her husband and had to support her children, she seems to have found a strength she didn't know she had. She was able to take care of herself and her children, and she liked that. She also liked feeling more equal to her mother, who she had always experienced as powerful and domineering. She enjoyed having her own power and not feeling dependent: "I was the breadwinner and I was the one who ran the show and we were in it together, but I was the one they counted on."

She describes her caregiving experience as a growth experience that, at times, made her angry and frustrated. But she felt that it was the best way to take care of her children, her parents and herself.

One indication that she is right in her assessment is her younger son. Bobby, fifteen years old, came home while I was interviewing Isabella. He didn't come in the front door, but entered through his grandfather's apartment. He went to say hello to Grandpa before he came upstairs to greet his mother. As he came up the stairs, before realizing I was there, he called out a warm hello to his mother. Bobby is a polite and confident teenager—very comfortable with himself. He looked me straight in the eye and shook my hand when he greeted me and came out later to say goodbye.

Part of Isabella's strength seems to come from her faith. She believes her mother is in heaven and her image of heaven seems to be a place in which people are able to come to terms with things they didn't understand in life.

When she died I knew she got it. There was no more anger and disappointment. I felt she was up there and she got it.

I knew she got what all the issues were. I couldn't get her to understand it when she was alive, but when she died I knew she got it . . . I knew she was watching from above. I was at peace and she was at peace.

Since her mother's death, Isabella's father has lived alone in the apartment downstairs. After I interviewed her, she took me downstairs to meet him. At eighty-one, he is relatively healthy. But he depends on Isabella to pay his bills, drive him to doctor appointments and shop. Isabella and Bobby have dinner with him most nights and that night he was cooking *pasta fazul.* Yet Isabella seems to be able to have a full life herself—she told me she just met a wonderful man and that she's in love.

SETTING LIMITS is not an act of selfishness, but involves caring for yourself *and* your parents. Setting healthy limits means not sacrificing personally fulfilling activities and pursuits. Feeling angry frequently is a good indicator that there is a disparity between the limits that have been set and what you need. You may be feeling angry at your parent or fighting with your spouse about your parent—either way, that's a tip-off that a renegotiation is probably in order. Rose was not able to set any limits and was chronically angry with her mother as a result.

In contrast to Rose, Paul stopped being chronically angry with his mother when he began setting limits. When she complained or said something negative about his wife or children, he told her that was unacceptable and left. Setting limits entails recognizing and accepting what you can and cannot realistically do for your parents and communicating this information to them in an empathetic and clear manner.[7]

There is no rule to follow about setting limits—each of us is comfortable with different lines in the sand. The first task is to identify your comfort level and the comfort level of your family. You may have space in your house for your mother to live with you, but that does not mean you could stand having her there—or that your husband could. The issue is not simply what you could objectively do, but also what you can emotionally tolerate. You may be happy to have your father live downstairs or close by, but not actually *in* your house. Isabella was clear that she could help her parents *and* herself by buying a two-family house and having her parents live downstairs, but not in the same apartment. She needed to retain her privacy. They were able to offer childcare and she was able to offer them emotional support and help with finances. On the other hand, you may feel good about having a parent live in your house, but not about handling the finances. There is no one-size-fits-all answer.

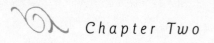 *Chapter Two*

GETTING ANGRY AND GETTING OVER IT

My father's old and helpless and I take care of him. It makes me furious that he never took care of me . . . It would be easier if I felt more loving toward him, but it all feels like obligation.

—*Joan, a fifty-year-old psychotherapist*

WHY IS FEELING ANGRY such a central part of the experience of caregivers? If you have had a predominantly positive relationship with your parents as adults, their increasing frailty or illness means you lose some of the joys and benefits of that relationship. You can no longer go shopping and out to lunch with your mother. She doesn't send a check for each of the kids on their birthdays because she can't remember the dates anymore. Your father can't pick up the kids at school or drive to your house to visit. Instead of looking to your parents for help, they need *your* help. These are real losses that may make you sad, but also angry. And you may feel guilty for being angry at those losses: Perhaps it makes you feel as if you are being selfish. You may get frightened when your mother can't remember what you told her last week. Just for a minute it feels like she's not paying attention to you and it makes you angry. Then you realize she's losing her short-term memory and it's frightening. You realize it's going to get worse and you start worrying about getting old yourself.

For example, my mother insists on walking around with hundreds of pennies in her purse. They are mixed with old cookies and bananas she takes from meals in case she gets hungry later. When I visit her I find myself getting angry because no matter how many times I clean out her purse, when I return it is heavy and smelly again. However, these twinges of anger and guilt are not the most difficult to handle. The most difficult feelings are usually related to *old* hurts and losses that get revived during the caregiving experience. This anger may feel irrational, out of control and out of place.

The cycle of anger and guilt is common among caregivers and is often related to our difficulty in setting limits. As psychologist Harriet Lerner, author of *The Dance of Anger,* points out, we often talk about the problem as if it were our parent who "makes" us angry or guilty, but no one can "make" us feel something.[1] Feeling that a parent "makes" us angry and guilty puts the responsibility on the parent to change, which is unlikely, and keeps the caregiver feeling like a helpless child. My friend Susan is caught in this bind. Susan is an attractive fifty-year-old college professor and writer who is married with two children. She writes me:

My holiday has mostly been very nice. My kids are home, which has been fun. However, my mother did manage to be hospitalized for gas. The doctor's diagnosis was: "You're full of shit!" When she called me she said: "Get me out of this hellhole. I'm dying here." Then when I arrive, "What took you so long?" That's how the day was. Two ambulances and I didn't get home until 9 p.m. She'd like me to carry her on my back.

Susan's mother feels angry that Susan will not let her live with her. Her mother does not simply want to be taken care of—she insists on being taken care of *by Susan*. Like many elderly Italian-Americans, Susan's mother expected to live with her daughter when she got elderly and infirm. Susan's mother experiences going to an assisted living facility, or even living in her own home with health-care aides, as shameful rejection.

However, having her mother live in her house would require Susan changing her life. She would not be able to wake up in the morning and work on the book she's writing; she would not be able to have dinner alone with her husband; she would not be able to have time away from her mother unless she left her house.

In my conversations with Susan it has become clear that if she moves her mother into her house she will feel continuously angry at her because her mother will not be satisfied with the level of attention and will continue to complain that Susan is not doing enough. Susan will also feel bad about herself for feeling angry and intruded upon. Her mother wants something that is not possible for Susan, but what *is* possible? Susan can talk to her mother's doctor about taking antidepressants; she can suggest counseling; she can pay an aide to pay special attention to her. But she cannot *make* her mother happy. But how can life be made tolerable for both mother and daughter?

If Susan can realize that giving up her life to try to alleviate her mother's neediness is both impossible and corrosive to her, she may be able to feel less angry toward her mother for wanting it. Susan's mother has a great deal to be unhappy about: getting old and frail; the loss of her husband; her daughter Laura's premature death of cancer; and the deaths of old friends. Unfortunately, no matter how much Susan wants to, she cannot take the losses away.

We do not, as many writers have claimed, become our parents' parents; no matter how old we are, we remain our parents' children. We may do things for them when they are elderly and infirm that we do for children (soothe them, even bathe and diaper them), but we remain their children in their minds and our own. Therefore, experiences in the present when we are adults and our parents are elderly and frail resonate with experiences from the past when we were helpless children and they were the adults we counted upon.

If we had a loving relationship to our parents and they were "good-enough" parents, it may make us angry to see them unable to take care of *themselves,* let alone *us.* We may want them to feel comfortable and happy and feel angry toward them if we can't make them comfortable and happy. That is painful. But, if we were neglected or abused as children, we may respond to our elderly parents in ways that make us feel guilty and loathsome.

For example, recently I visited my mother at the assisted living facility where she lives. She was very upset when I arrived because they had served chicken chow mein for dinner and she felt she only got a little bit of chicken and she doesn't like Chinese food. My mother told me the story in a tone of voice that was a mixture of outrage and hurt. The woman next to her, Faye, told me that you're supposed to mix up the little pieces of chicken with the noodles—it's not supposed to be a whole chicken breast. I understood completely. But my mother has always taken offense at not getting what she wants—she feels it is a personal affront. I felt angry at my mother for all the times she took offense at things that were not personal. And I felt angry at her because I often do the same thing and hate myself for it afterward. I am only able to console myself because my children will point it out to me and I see it and I apologize. Then, at least, I feel I must have given them something she didn't give me because they are able to tell me I'm being paranoid. After all that, I was able to hug my mother and tell her we'd get some chocolate ice cream for dessert and she felt much better.

When you get overly angry at an elderly parent, you need to identify the trigger that makes the anger flow and try to figure out if it is a response to something in the present or a reexperiencing of something in the past. Perhaps something in the present is upsetting, but the extremity of your reaction can be a key to realizing that something from the past is being evoked. Sometimes it is not possible to separate out past and present without getting some professional help. If your reaction is a repetition from the past, it's important to identify it before you can get over it. Some of my patients want to skip this step—they want to protect themselves from getting in touch with earlier hurts or they want to protect the parent by not getting in touch with painful childhood experiences. But, in my experience, this step cannot be skipped. It's only by knowing what hurt us and experiencing it that we can console ourselves and move on. One patient, Carla, often says: "I'm just an angry person that's all." She means that it's part of her inborn character to be angry rather than a response to experiences that hurt her. I disagree with Freud's view that aggression is an instinct. I believe anger is always a response to hurt or neglect. I tell Carla that no one is born an "angry person." She is angry because she has been hurt. Only by understanding *how* she was hurt and what it is that makes her angry can she "work through" the anger and move on.[2]

As Paul showed us in Chapter 1, understanding how our parents' experiences shaped them can be an important part of working through our anger at our parents. Whatever their history, *it does not excuse them* if they abused us or neglected us, but it helps us make sense of our own experience. Sometimes the caregiving period gives us access to our parents as people so that we are not driven to react blindly against them and repeat their hurts in our own lives—hating ourselves for what we hate in them.

Turning the furor of our reactions into a quest for understanding can be made easier if we understand our parents' histories—but it cannot replace getting in touch with the early experience. After we have experienced the hurt, understanding our parents' histories allows us to get past our fantasy that they were in control of their lives and their emotions (the angry part) or that the reason they hurt us was because we were "bad" (the guilty part).[3]

The more hurtful our parents were when we were children, the more crucial it is for us to try to understand how our parents got that way so that we can put our relationship with them in context. For example, my mother always made it clear that my father and my sister, brother and I were not her prime concern. Her first concern was getting the approval of her mother and older sister Gus. I felt angry that our feelings did not seem to matter to my mother, only what Aunt Gus or my grandmother wanted. My mother could not separate from her mother and my aunt Gus, and my grandmother could not separate from her mother either. I came to understand this when I was thirteen. My parents went to Miami Beach to celebrate their twenty-fifth wedding anniversary and I was sent to stay with my aunt Hannah, who had moved from the house next door to us, on Webster Avenue under the elevated train, to a brand-new prefabricated pastel-colored house on Long Island.

In contrast to my feelings about my aunt Gus, I loved Hannah dearly and was delighted at the prospect of spending a solid block of time with her to talk endlessly about all of the members of the family and the history of their relationships. Sure enough, Hannah and I spent the week sitting in her backyard looking at the newly planted trees and the backs of the other pastel-colored prefabs, gabbing endlessly. I was in heaven! Hannah was my mother's and Gus's older sister and the family oral historian. It was during that week that she told me a family secret that made me understand my mother in a way I never had before.

My grandmother was the eldest daughter of four siblings. I knew that. But I didn't know that my grandmother had a different father than the other three. She was born in Russia and her father was the man to whom my great-grandmother was matched—though she was deeply in love with another man. My grandmother's father drowned and her mother then married the man she loved. When Great-Grandmother had three more children with the man she loved, she clearly rejected my grandmother. Indeed, when she died she left all her money to the three children from the second marriage. If my grandmother had any doubts that her mother did not love her, her mother clarified it in her will.

So, it seems, my grandmother had a very ambivalent connection to her mother—she was overtly rejected by her. She spent her life trying to please her mother, but never could, and, in her turn, my mother grew up trying to please her mother. My grandmother asked my parents to lend her money to pay for my mother's youngest sister Mitzi's wedding. It was the money my parents had saved to put a down payment on a house; at my mother's insistence they loaned my grandmother the money. She never paid them back and they never bought a house. My mother never allowed my father to ask my grandmother to repay the loan. My mother couldn't separate from her mother. She yearned for her love and approval and my father, sister, brother and I suffered the consequences.

FINDING OUT WHAT THE ANGER IS ABOUT

Sally is a fifty-four-year-old social work administrator and mother of two grown sons. She and her husband live in a modest house they built when they got married soon after graduating from Ohio State University. Sally is the oldest of three children. Her mother is seventy-seven and has lived alone since her husband died in 1989. Sally describes her

mother as a very intelligent woman who was a history teacher. Sally says that her mother deferred to her husband in all
decisions because he was very controlling, and if she did not
defer, he would not speak to her for days at a time. Sally says
that he used that technique on her as well: "That's probably
why I became the good girl; because I had it figured out that
if you were the good girl, you didn't get cut out."

When Sally's father died, her mother quickly decided to sell
their house and move to Columbus, Ohio, where her three
children were living. Sally says that her mother was financially comfortable and bought a condominium that had many
residents her age and was close to her children and grandchildren. Nevertheless, her mother was depressed.

> There was a lot of "This isn't working out," "This isn't
> what I had in mind," "They don't appreciate me." She'd
> say to me: "You call every day, but you don't visit me—
> calls aren't good enough."

Sally began to experience her mother as demanding and controlling.

> She had some real health problems—she took antiseizure
> medication because she was having epileptic seizures; she
> had heart difficulties and she had stomach problems. But
> another way of exhibiting control is to not attend to those
> things, or to attend to them only partially. Then she would
> need intervention from us.

When Sally's mother had a valve replacement, she rejected
the idea of recuperating in a long-term-care facility. She in-

sisted that any rehab would be done in her own home. Sally, her brother and sister went along with their mother's request, feeling that it was reasonable. They knew she'd be more comfortable in her own home and believed they could arrange or provide all the care that she needed, but soon they realized that although her physical care needs were manageable, their mother's psychological needs would not be satisfied by this arrangement.

An aide came in the morning to help her mother get out of bed, get her medications in order and fix her some breakfast. Sally's brother came in the middle of the day for a visit; Sally visited in the afternoon; and her sister came before bed. There was company in attendance for most of her waking hours, but Sally's mom insisted that it wasn't enough. Her perception was that she was alone a great deal of the time.

> We started to feel angry and resentful, but how can you get angry at someone so vulnerable and frail? My sister and I thought we could fix it. We wanted to make her understand how much we were helping her, how much we wanted to help her, and that we were doing the best we could, and that we were really stressing ourselves. And after that period of time there was a long period of recovery, because she didn't believe physical therapy was necessary. So, instead of a three-month recuperation, there was a three-year recuperation, and not a return to the strength that someone of her age could have gotten.

Sally's mother's pattern of refusing to do what would help her get the care she needed and thus requiring *more* care continued when she moved permanently to Florida. She arranged, almost immediately, to have cataract surgery there, which meant she would be released from the hospital unable to see and without anyone to help her at home and no friends in the immediate area. Sally and her siblings then felt obligated to fly to Florida and stay with their mother in shifts.

Most recently Sally's mother was diagnosed with stomach cancer. After the surgery she was temporarily unable to speak or respond when spoken to. Sally had what seemed to her at the time an irrational reaction.

That inability to respond represented to me that what I give her will never be enough, and it infuriated me. I have always, because of my relationship with my dad, avoided anger, never been honest about anger, because when you were honest about anger, it triggered his anger, and he withdrew, so you never wanted to do that. He'd shut me out, and I didn't want that to happen. So, I'm a person who can be so angry that I can't even speak, but I don't often express that in a good, healthy way.

Sally's caregiving experience brought up old feelings that she had repressed about her early experience with her mother.

Before she had the surgery she said something very hurtful, and my thought was, It doesn't matter what I do for you, it will never be enough.

I asked her about the attention she received as a girl.

Just of not being nurtured, not being held, not being talked to the way I talk to my children. She never partici- pated in my life as a parent. I just don't think of my mother as parenting. My mother had a friend who adored me, who would brush the hair out of my eyes. I remember her friend who had two boys holding me and loving me, and I remember sort of comparing that tactile, clear demonstration of mothering to my mother because they were friends.

I asked if she remembered her mother hugging her. She said: "No. I think she couldn't."

Sally never understood why her mother couldn't show af- fection to her. She didn't think about it. She went off to col- lege at eighteen, met her husband and never lived in her parents' house again. She distanced herself and focused on her own family. But the experience of caregiving has been bringing up the feelings she has tried not to think about all these years. She never felt mothered and she felt it was be- cause she wasn't able to make her mother happy. Sally as- sumed it was something about her that was the cause of it. She just accepted it unquestioningly all these years. But dur- ing a recent visit, her mother told her a story that was a psy- chological turning point for Sally. It explained to Sally why her mother could not love her.

Sally's grandfather was a civil engineer and her grand- mother was a businesswoman at a time when being a busi- nesswoman was a very unusual thing. They had two children, Sally's mother and her uncle John. When John was eighteen months old and Sally's mother was six years old, they were sent to an orphanage.

The children remained in the orphanage for two years and Sally's mother told her they never knew why. Although John and Sally's mother had what seemed to be a loving relationship, they weren't really close until the end of her uncle's life when they finally discussed it. It seems that each of them had been afraid to let out their feelings about being sent away, yet everything else must have seemed trivial in comparison. It must have been like trying to have a conversation with an elephant in the living room. When they did discuss it, neither of them could explain it to the other one. The mystery remains unsolved.

Nevertheless, Sally finally came to understand her mother's coldness; her mother had never been able to get over her own childhood trauma. Therefore, her mother truly wasn't there for her when she was growing up, and it wasn't because Sally herself wasn't good enough. This realization has allowed Sally to forgive in large part her mother's neediness and unresponsiveness. She says:

> How do you have a legitimate relationship, a trusting relationship with other people if you were simply sent somewhere with your baby brother? There's good reason why she would have trouble fostering a caring relationship. There's good reason why she would want to be cared for and directed.

In situations when her mother is unreasonable, Sally is able to say to herself: "Well, but it must be very hard for her. She wants to be taken care of, but she keeps setting up situations in which she feels sent away or abandoned." Being able to forgive her mother has made it less frightening to be angry with her. Sally is also more able to be direct with her mother: "We cannot take care of you if you live in Florida and we live in Columbus. We have families and jobs. If you move to Columbus, we will be able to take care of you much better." I think it might be helpful if Sally were also able to share some of her insight with her mother. She could explain to her that she cannot take care of her entirely in the way her mother wishes, but if her mother is physically close to her children she can get much more from them than if she is Florida. She can point out to her mother that moving to Florida was like sending herself to an orphanage.

Sally is using caregiving as a growth experience. She is finally understanding why she has been afraid of being angry her whole life. When her mother was unresponsive to her she turned to her father for the love and affection she could not get from her mother. But her father made it clear that she would only get his love and attention if she behaved like a "good girl" according to his rules. She understood that meant she could not show any anger.

I've gotten to the point where I can say that I don't like the fact that you don't nurture me, that you didn't nurture me. I don't like the fact that you don't nurture other people. I don't like her very well. She's not the kind of person I would pick out. I've discovered a huge thing. I don't like my mother. I don't like her at all.

Ironically, the caregiving experience, although painful, has allowed Sally to work through her longstanding problems with anger. She has been able to get in touch with her anger toward her mother and work it through in a way that makes it tolerable—she does not have to deny it and she does not have to run away from her mother.

GETTING STUCK: HANGING ON TO ANGER FROM THE PAST

I first met Beverly in the living room of a former student of mine who is a geriatric social worker in the Bronx. Beverly is bright, psychologically minded and quite articulate. I immediately liked her and assumed she was a social worker who was going to be an informant talking about caregivers with whom she worked. I was delighted to find out that she was also a caregiver herself because I was sure that she would be articulate about her situation. She began by telling me that although she is a college graduate, she works part-time, at minimum wage, as an aide for elderly people. An only child, Beverly is fifty-five years old and single and lives with her eighty-seven-year-old mother.

> Ten years ago I lived in my own apartment and had a successful business. But my aunt and uncle who I loved dearly both had dementia and he died. I felt I had to take care of my aunt. She had no children and I loved her very, very much. She was very nonjudgmental in contrast to my parents.

Beverly experienced taking care of her aunt as an opportunity to finally have the "good mother" she always wanted (in contrast to her own mother). She rented a house for herself and her aunt and gave up her own apartment in another city.

Once Beverly relinquished her independent life because of her aunt's illness, however, she was drawn back to her own mother as well.

Before my uncle died I had pulled away from the family. But after his death, it was like, boom, I was back in the bosom of my family. All the work I had done in therapy just went down the drain. I screwed up my business. It was a jewelry business and I was doing well and then I just lost control of it.

Beverly stopped putting time and energy into her business. She stopped going on buying trips, stopped opening the store every day and stopped paying her bills. She was drawn further and further into her childhood wish to feel like a good daughter. After her father died, her mother, who is arthritic, diabetic and nearly blind, couldn't live alone.

So I decided that my aunt, the homecare person and I would move into my mother's house. So the next thing is I'm completely enmeshed in this situation. I knew when I took on my aunt that I was opening the door for my mother.

Perhaps Beverly imagined that her aunt (her "good" mother) would offset her own mother (her "bad" mother). But, instead, old resentments toward her mother suddenly surfaced with renewed force. Caregiving reactivated her childhood feelings of dependency and undermined her sense of competence and adulthood.

The first few years I lived with my mother we had some really fierce arguments. I wanted to smack her. I knew I had an enormous amount of anger there.

Beverly feels that she cannot separate from her mother until her mother dies. Her mother has to do the separating; Beverly feels she can't.

I do have the feeling that my relationship with my mother is very toxic, but I don't see myself pulling out of it. I don't see my life resuming until my mother is not here anymore. I realized last week how that pool of anger toward her is all still there and I can't pull myself out of it until she dies.

Beverly feels powerless in relation to her mother because she still feels endangered if she leaves her. Beverly's childhood feelings remain intact from when she was entirely dependent on her mother. Failing at her business and living in her mother's house intensifies her feeling that she is entirely dependent on her mother, as she was when she was a child.

She still has a lot of power over me. For example, last week my dog died. I was so upset that I didn't want to come home right after work. I wanted to wait until the vet came and took the dog away. My mother could not tolerate my feelings and my refusal to come right home. She didn't want to have to deal with the vet herself. She said, "If you do that it will be the biggest mistake of your life." And that was powerful. It took me way back. My mother used to say that all the time when I did something she didn't like. When my mother would say that I always felt it *was* going to be the biggest mistake of my life. She always had a power over me and she still does.

Her mother's power is based on Beverly's wish to be comforted by her and have her approval. So Beverly resists separating because she still has hopes that she will finally get what she has always wanted from her critical mother.

I never grew up and never cut the apron strings. Am I still trying to get my mother's approval? Probably, even though I know I'll never get it.

Beverly understands that her mother never got her needs met by her parents or her husband and looked to Beverly to fulfill her wishes. Intellectually she understands that her mother's responses to her were a result of *her own experiences.*

My mother's parents were very kissy and huggy and always walked arm and arm and my mother felt very left out. When she married my father, she very quickly learned that he was in his own world and he wasn't going to give her what she wanted. So when I was born all her hopes were on me.

Beverly understands her mother's neediness, but she still feels that she has to satisfy it and drown or be a bad daughter. As a young woman, she felt she had to run away to preserve her sense of self, and then yearned for a fantasized connection with her mother. When she came back, she hated her mother for being so critical and needy and making her feel like a bad daughter all over again. She goes back and forth between longing for her mother and having to run away out of fear of being gobbled up by her.

Before she moved out of her apartment and rented a house to share with her aunt, Beverly was in therapy. What did that therapist say to her when she told her what she was going to do? Of course, I don't know. Maybe the therapist warned her that giving up her apartment was not a good prognostic indication. She could have made sure her aunt was well taken care of and visited her frequently without giving up her apartment (and her own life). The therapist might have said that and Beverly did it anyway. She ended therapy when she moved in with her aunt and later her mother.

Beverly feels that the pool of anger toward her mother is all still there and she can't pull herself out of it until her mother dies. She feels that she cannot set herself free—only her mother has the power to set her free, by dying. Beverly explains by saying she feels she "should" take care of her until she dies. If she does not take care of her she will be a "bad daughter." However, Beverly *is* taking care of her mother and still feels like a bad daughter because she is constantly angry and guilty.

Beverly feels that no one ever asked her what she *wanted*—she was just told what she should do. She feels like she has no choice. However, the reality is that Beverly does have a choice. The choice is between continuing to feel like an angry helpless child living with her mother and hating her vs. moving out of her mother's house, hiring an aide for her and getting a job that is appropriate to her education and skills. It seems like a no-brainer. Why does Beverly opt for the self-destructive choice? There must be something that Beverly gets out of choosing to continue the sadomasochistic dynamic with her mother. Perhaps Beverly feels that this is the only way to have *any* relationship with her mother. If she gives up feeling angry and helpless in the face of her powerful and sadistic mother, what will she have? She will feel alone.

Beverly thinks that when her mother dies she will be free of her. But that's not true; she is tied to a relationship to her mother that will outlive her mother. She can move away, her mother can die but the internal relationship to her will live on. Beverly's mother will be alive and well inside Beverly when her mother is long dead, unless she is able to understand her need to hold on to being the angry, victimized, misunderstood daughter of a needy, dependent, yet powerful "mother." The image of herself vis-à-vis her mother will outlive her mother. For example, why is Beverly so underemployed? She is a highly intelligent college graduate with years of business experience, but she works as a minimum-wage health aide. She needs to remain the tortured, undervalued daughter in order to hold on to that inner relationship with her mother.

How would this understanding of her situation help Beverly? If she were aware of her own part in perpetuating this old masochistic relationship with her mother, Beverly might be more able to make choices about her life. If she saw that she *could* move out and get a job and have her own life, but that she is *choosing* not to do that, it would be harder to continue feeling like her mother's victim.

Beverly's caregiving experience caused a major regression and repetition of her early experiences with her mother. She is stuck feeling enraged at her mother and unable to work through her anger in a way that would allow her to separate from her mother and have her own life. What might happen if Beverly *did* leave? What would happen to her mother? She has money and could afford to hire aides to live in the house and care for her. She does not have the same expectations of aides that she had about Beverly. Just as Beverly's angry feelings are evoked by her mother, her mother's needy and angry feelings are evoked by Beverly. They are locked into an interaction with each other that they keep repeating. If Beverly moved out she might find she *wanted* to visit her mother and make sure she was cared for; it might feel like a choice rather than a duty she cannot escape. It is possible to use the caregiving experience in a more life-affirming way—to use it as an opportunity to work out problems that have been left unresolved or simply to resolve them more completely.

GETTING OVER THE ANGER BY SETTING LIMITS

Paula is a fifty-four-year-old round-faced woman with graying hair that's curled unevenly. She looks like a woman who cannot be bothered worrying about how she looks—her values lie elsewhere. She is a fund-raiser for a large nonprofit organization.

Although Paula has five children and works full-time, she is the caregiver for both her mother and father—they were divorced right after Paula graduated from high school so she has to deal with them entirely separately. Paula's mother is eighty-four and her father is eighty-seven. Her father is an alcoholic and twelve years ago he had surgery and got pneumonia and was incapable of living on his own. He lived with Paula and her family for six months and then they got him an apartment in an assisted living facility.

Paula's mother had a recurrence of breast cancer six years ago. She lives in independent housing, but her dementia is increasing and Paula says that the next time her mother is hospitalized, she is going to put her in a nursing home afterward. When she goes to the doctor, she cannot remember why she's there. She's safe right now, but only because Paula keeps her medication and gives it to her every day. Paula's mother goes to the senior center three days a week. But Paula is increasingly concerned about her safety the rest of the time.

Paula says she had "an abnormal childhood."

My father was always an alcoholic and it was an elephant in the room—no one ever talked about it. My dad was home every night because my mother worked as a waitress at night. But he was not emotionally there.

Paula says she always felt like she had to be the mother. She did the shopping and cooking because her mother wasn't there and she was the eldest girl. When her parents' marriage fell apart, Paula felt that she had to be even more grown-up.

My father was never a falling-down drunk, but when my mother left him he started to drink more heavily. She was a waitress and she had an affair. I knew it. It was very painful. My junior year in high school, I saw my mom and a man go into my aunt's apartment. I knew what was going on.

Paula's mother kept saying: "Someday you'll understand."
Paula says:

> To be candid, I never did. I don't agree with the way she
> handled the whole situation. She's not real brave. She's al-
> ways had to rely on a man. She's never had the strength to
> be on her own. She left my sister and me with my dad and
> moved in with my aunt and eventually married the man
> she had the affair with. It was very difficult.

Paula says that her mother's two sisters were very supportive
of her affair. She felt shocked by her aunts' reaction. One of
them called Paula and yelled at her for not being supportive
enough of her mother after her mother left the family. Paula
shakes her head in disbelief as she tells me about it. She doesn't
completely understand why her life is so stable considering
what she's been through. Clearly, Paula's "plain Jane" presentation of self is in contrast to her mother's overt sexuality. As
a young woman, she says she was petrified that when she
got married she would want to have affairs like her mother.
She can chuckle about it now, but it's clearly taken years
for Paula to work through her feelings about her mother's
infidelities. Paula says:

> She's eighty-four years old and she's still a flirt. She's flirt-
> ing with the sixty-eight-year-old van driver who takes her
> to the senior center. She wanted to invite him over and I
> said: "Sure, let's have Earl and his wife over." She looked
> like I punctured her balloon. She was so disappointed. It's
> comical. It's also interesting. As we age we become more
> of who we are. She's a youthful and attractive eighty-four-

year-old. She has to have her hair done every week. You might go out on the weekend, you never know. My kids say: "Grandma's getting more action than we are."

Paula doesn't feel her siblings fared as well psychologically as she has. Paula says her brother was her mother's favorite child. During World War II when her father was overseas, her brother lived with his mother and aunts. He was the only child and a boy at that. When his father returned, his aunts left and his mother turned her attention to her husband. Then she got pregnant with Paula. Paula feels her brother's privileged position came to an abrupt end and he never got over it. He and her father fought constantly, so as soon as he graduated from high school, her brother joined the army and went away. He doesn't talk to either of his parents or Paula. She said he occasionally talks to their younger sister. Like his mother, he started having an affair and left his wife, a close friend of Paula's, and two children to marry his lover. Paula did not support his affair the way her aunts supported her mother's and as a result her brother doesn't talk to her.

Paula says her younger sister is in worse shape. Her mother used to openly refer to her sister as "the accident." Paula says that even as a kid she knew that was not right. Her sister got married at sixteen—no doubt to get out of the house, but she got divorced two years ago. She suffers from severe depression and has tried to kill herself twice.

Paula feels angry and resentful that she is the caregiver for both her parents. She says simply: "I feel responsible. I always have." Paula feels her sister is incapable of helping, but she feels angry toward her brother.

Knowing that I have a brother who is wealthy and could make their lives easier—they both live on social security and live in subsidized housing. They're on Medicaid assistance. I don't feel as resentful toward my sister. I am stuck.

Then Paula makes an unconscious slip. She says: "I do have other children." Obviously, she feels she has to parent her parents as well as her children.

Paula has had to struggle with her anger at her father as well as at her brother and mother. Her father's drinking makes her angry. She says:

Two years ago we went to pick up my dad to go to church on Christmas Eve. We had this tradition that everyone comes to our house for Christmas. We got to his house and he had been drinking to the point that it was obvious. I said: "We're not going to do this." He was furious that he was left alone on Christmas Eve. That was really tough.

Paula felt that she had to protect herself and her own family.

I felt guilty, I'm a Catholic, and it's terrible to leave someone alone for Christmas and Christmas Eve. But I realized that God wouldn't want me to be angry and resentful on Christmas. It's a balance. I knew I was doing the right thing for me.

Paula explains more about her father. She says her father can just "go off" on anything. He's even more difficult to be with than her mom. Paula says:

He's always complaining. He has an entitlement mentality. He never says: "Gee, it's nice to do this." Instead he says: "Why didn't you ever do this before?" It was making me nuts.

After her father moved in with her family, about thirteen years ago, Paula went into therapy because it was such a demanding experience. She was depressed. She describes her father as very authoritarian—the kind of father that hit you with a belt. She says it's hard to separate the effects of the alcohol and his personality. "We were supposed to be quiet little girls and say: 'Yes, sir' and 'Yes, ma'am.'"

Paula says therapy helped her realize the depression was about anger.

I was always that kid who wouldn't say "shit" if I had a mouthful of it. Therapy helped me accept my angry feelings and realize that I had choices and options.

The burden of caring for both her parents and trying to deal with the anger it evokes is intensified by Paula's concern about her older daughter's health. Her daughter had melanoma in three locations. Paula says, tearfully:

Here's this beautiful girl with a beautiful baby and she has cancer. I didn't tell my mom because I knew she would forget right after I told her. I would be very angry at her for casually saying: "How are the kids?" I knew my father would call her and keep asking her: "How *are* you today?" He would hound her. So I didn't tell him. My daughter goes for checkups every six months and she's okay. But dealing with

the day-to-day trivial things for my parents feels more an-
noying when I'm thinking about my daughter.

For example, Paula's mother ends up in the emergency room
all the time. She calls 911 and they send an ambulance and
Paula ends up having to go there and spend hours and hours
waiting until they determine that nothing is wrong.

One time, after spending eight hours in the emergency
room because she decided she was bleeding internally, it
turned out she had taken Pepto-Bismol and that caused
the black stool.

Paula came to realize that she was either going to have to
stay away from her parents, which was what her brother did,
or set some boundaries.

I used to feel that every Sunday I had to have one or both
of my parents over. Then I said: "Why am I doing this?" I
finally decided to do it every three weeks or so. I was becoming the victim. There's a fine line in my mind between
feeling angry and resentful at situations and becoming the
victim. I felt that the only way not to feel like a victim and
hate them was to carve out that niche for myself and say:
"I will set the terms."

Paula asked herself: "Do I want to walk away like my
brother?" She decided she wouldn't be able to live with herself if she did. So she has learned when to take her mother's
complaints seriously and when to let things go. There are
days when Paula can't get to her mother's house and she

misses her medication. Paula has learned to accept that it won't kill her mother. She is able to keep her priorities very clear.

TO VARYING DEGREES, Beverly, Sally and Paula were able to work through their anger at their mothers (and for Paula, her father as well). While Sally and Paula were able to get in touch with their feelings, accept them and then move on, Beverly remained stuck.

Both Beverly and Sally felt they were bad children. Beverly was very aware of the feeling her whole life, but Sally didn't realize she felt it until she started to care for her mother and got in touch with it. Ironically, the child who has a "bad" mother usually turns her into a "good" mother. That necessitates feeling that you're a "bad" child. That does not feel good, but this defensive process that defines as "good" the person you are dependent on serves an important psychological function for a child who needs that mother. If the child can turn to the father or grandmother or older sibling, she may be able to tolerate more ambivalence toward her mother, but if there is no one else to turn to, the child may prefer to feel that *she* is bad, not Mommy. I have seen this in many of my patients. The alternative is to feel your mommy is bad and you are helpless, alone and orphaned. Sometimes the feeling alternates—"I hate Mommy" and "I'm bad." However, the process that might have served them well as a child becomes an impediment to feeling good about themselves as adults.

Beverly's situation was, and is, more dire than Sally's. Although she was fond of her aunt and uncle they did not play a large role in her day-to-day life. She was dependent on her mother as a child and still is as an adult. At fifty-five, Beverly is still hating her mother and hating herself.

On the other hand, Sally was able to turn to her father for love when her mother was unresponsive to her as a child. That allowed her to feel more ambivalent about her mother, and she did not have to defend against her negative feelings toward her mother by feeling like a bad daughter; she just had to be a "good girl" to keep Daddy's love. Caring for her mother allowed Sally to understand her relationship to her mother and father much better. It freed her so that she could stop being a good girl and become a mature woman.

Similarly, caring for both her parents allowed Paula to stop being a good girl as well. She realized that she would have to set limits with both her parents in order to protect herself from feeling like a victim and to protect them from her need to run away.

Chapter Three

FEELING GUILTY AND FORGIVING YOURSELF

I'm forty-one and have been the caregiver to my mother for the past thirty-one years. I have some nursing help during the day so I can keep my job, but I'm at my limit. I had to refuse better jobs because they're too far away for me to dash home if there's a problem. I'm on medication for nerves and depression and my own health is suffering. I've pretty much decided that it's time to call it quits and place my mom in a nursing facility. But she wants to die at home and I cannot honor her request. I am sure she will use every guilt tactic in the world. How can I deal with the guilt that comes with saying: "I give up and I have to disappoint my mom."[1]

AS CAREGIVERS, we often feel guilty for not rescuing our parents from the pain and discomfort of old age. But we cannot rescue them; we can only offer our love and support and hope they accept it. Yet, many of us *do* offer that to our elderly parents and *still* feel guilty. What is this guilt about?

In my experience and in my discussions with other caregivers I have found a variety of complex experiences that we refer to as "guilt." Some forms of guilt have to do with not meeting other people's expectations, while other forms have to do with not meeting our own.

There is the guilt we feel when we don't do things that we think we should. These "shoulds" are injunctions that we have not completely internalized as our own. When you say, "I should visit my mother every day," it really means you imagine someone else thinks you "should." Perhaps you imagine your relatives think you should visit your mother every day.

When you think, "I should make dinner for my family instead of visiting my mother after work," you are not saying you think that's right or that's what you wish to do. Rather, you are expressing the feeling that other people, perhaps your husband, thinks that's the right thing to do. Conflicting "shoulds" can be quite anxiety provoking, making you feel torn in many directions.

Then there is separation guilt—the guilt that communicates: "I am a separate person, I have different values or different needs than you do. We are not one." Separation guilt may emerge as a result of physically separating from your parent, moving to a different city, for example. But separation can be symbolic as well as physical. Making different choices about how to live your life can give rise to separation guilt as well. Each move toward self-development can feel like betrayal of your mother because you are living your own separate life.

And there is guilt as a result of having an envious mother. One of my patients feels guilty for having anything more than her mother. Her mother did not enjoy her daughter's achievements; she was contemptuous of them because she was envious. Having sensed her mother's envy beneath the contempt, my patient feels guilty for going to graduate school when her mother left school after high school to care for her sick father. My patient finally admitted she was even guilty for not having arthritis and cancer as her mother did.

On the other hand, there is moral guilt—a response to a violation of our own moral code. If you've spent your life believing elderly people should be kept in the community and decide to put your father in a nursing home, the guilt you experience is "moral guilt." Moral guilt is painful because it shakes your sense of self and involves a reconsideration of beliefs you took for granted.

There is also the guilt that one experiences as a result of ambivalent feelings toward a parent. If you are angry toward your mother when you have to decide whether to put her in a nursing home, there is always the question of whether you are doing what your mother needs or if you are trying to hurt her.

And then there is the guilt of feeling you are the special one who can offer comfort and solace, but other exigencies of your life (like living far away) make you unavailable to do so. Sometimes it is true that you are the only one who can offer comfort and solace, perhaps you're an only child and your parent is widowed. That is a painful conflict when you have other obligations that are equally compelling—young children or a sick husband. However, in some cases feeling that you are the only one who can offer comfort is *a wish to be special* rather than reality. In that case, as painful as the guilt is, it is the price for feeling special. Feeling less guilty involves the realization that you are not the only person who can provide some comfort for your mother, allowing you to mobilize other people to do so.

Although I have tried to delineate various types of guilt, we usually experience more than one type at the same time and the common thread among them is that they all make us feel bad about ourselves. When psychoanalysts talk about guilt they are usually referring to "neurotic guilt"—a feeling about a wish or fantasy rather than an action that caused damage to another person. According to Freud, the neurotic sense of guilt arises as a result of conflict between the superego, an internalized set of expectations, and infantile sexual or aggressive wishes. While the types of "guilt" I have discussed go beyond what Freud was talking about, they all involve turning aggression inward.

My friend Susan suffers from "shoulds" and from separation guilt. Susan's mother was born in Italy and feels that daughters are obligated to have their parents live with them when they get old. She feels angry that Susan will not let her live with her and Susan feels guilty. Susan feels she "should" invite her mother and if she were a good daughter she would. But Susan was not born in Italy. She is an American-born writer with a Ph.D., and she does not believe that daughters are obligated to have their parents live with them; she just feels like she "should." In addition, Susan suffers from separation guilt. When she says, "No, you can't live with me," to her mother, she is also saying, "I am a separate person, Mom, I have different values from yours. I don't want to live my life the way you did."

What might help Susan allay her guilt and forgive herself? She has to think about whether she agrees with those shoulds. Who is it that thinks she should do this or that? What does she believe is right? If what she believes is right does not coincide with the shoulds, then she has to decide if she wants to mold her life around what others think she should do. Susan knows that if her mother moves into her house she will feel perpetually angry toward her because her mother will not be satisfied with the level of Susan's attentiveness to her. Susan will also feel bad about herself for feeling angry toward her mother for intruding in her life and violating her privacy. Her mother wants something that Susan does not want to give. Susan has set a limit.

If Susan cannot give her mother all that she wants, what *can* she do for her? She can fulfill her own moral standard by finding a warm, safe environment for her mother where she will have social contacts and be taken care of. She can talk to her mother's doctor about prescribing antidepressants. But she cannot *rescue* her mother. She will only drown trying.

THE BURDEN OF TRYING TO SAVE YOUR MOTHER

Sharon is a forty-three-year-old social worker for the New York Department of the Aging. When I met Sharon at the entrance to the senior center, she seemed rather cold. I was surprised because a mutual friend told me that she would be happy to talk to me. However, as soon as I closed the door of the interview room I realized why she had been cool when shaking my hand. She was trying to control a flood of emotion—she started to cry as soon as she sat down to talk about her mother.

Sharon explained that her mother had died about six months ago. Her guilt was evident immediately.

> I couldn't be there every day. She was far away in another state. She and my father moved to Pennsylvania in 1993 to be closer to my sister.

Sharon feels that she "should" have been there every day, even though her mother lived in another state and her sister lived nearby.

Sharon is the youngest of four children. Her eldest sister died four years ago of breast cancer at fifty-two. Her brother is nine years older and another sister is four years older. Her surviving sister, Joan, lives in Pennsylvania and her parents moved there to be near her and her two boys. Sharon's father died suddenly two years ago and her mother began sliding downhill. She had heart problems for many years and became more and more isolated after her husband died.

> It became more difficult for Joan to spend time with Mom. When Dad was alive they used to go to the boys' games and things like that. But Mom wasn't interested in those things herself and it was hard for Joan to take time out from work, commuting and her kids to spend time with Mom separately.

Sharon's mother was too high functioning to be in assisted living and the only senior center was far enough away that she'd have to drive there, but she couldn't do it and Joan could not take her mother there and pick her up. Sharon is conflicted about her sister Joan. On the one hand, she is protective of Joan—she made it clear to me that the limited attention Joan could offer her mother was perfectly understandable: "She called her every morning." On the other hand, Sharon seems to feel that Joan invited her parents to move close to her (which was farther from Sharon than their original family home) for selfish reasons and did not intend to take responsibility for their care.

> My sister made a commitment to my parents when they moved near her, but she didn't think about what it would be like when one of them was gone. When my father was there it was fine. He played with her kids and went to their ball games.

One morning Joan called her mother and there was no answer. When she rushed to her house, she found that her mother couldn't get out of bed. She couldn't move; she had a severe kidney infection and it caused terrible back pain. Soon after her mother was hospitalized she became depressed and Sharon, who feels particularly responsible for making decisions about her mother's care, decided to ask her mother's doctor to prescribe antidepressants. Her mother came home from the hospital and stayed with Joan for a few days and then went back to her condominium. Sharon went down to stay with her and talked to her about assisted living.

Sharon soon found a beautiful assisted living facility with different levels of care for her mother and she was doing pretty well. Sharon drove from New York to Pennsylvania to visit her every few weeks and stayed several days each time.

Then her mother had two falls; she was having some issues with balance and it wasn't clear why. Sharon got her mother a walker and thought that was really positive, but then her mother started showing signs of Alzheimer's disease.

> I had done all this research on Aricept [the memory-enhancing drug for Alzheimer's patients]. Here in New York people think it's a wonderful drug, but in Pennsylvania they don't think that. My sister's personal physician did not feel very good about it. I called all the specialists I know and they all thought it was good and so I pushed for trying it. I thought it would help to get her back on her feet so she could adjust to assisted living.

Sharon was sobbing when she explained that her mother got up in the middle of the night, climbed over the bed's protective bar, only to fall and smash her pelvis. The physician said it was so severe she'd never walk again. Sharon's mother became increasingly confused and lost more and more weight. At this point in the interview, Sharon was crying so hard that she could hardly speak. Sharon is clinically depressed as a result of her guilt. She feels that she should have known that Aricept could cause dizziness. She imagines people must think she's a terrible social worker because she made that decision.

> I feel very guilty that I didn't just take off and stay with her for six weeks until she was in good enough shape to move into her apartment and also that I was the one who pushed for her taking Aricept. My sister looked to me to make these decisions because I'm the professional in the field. If

I had lived there or I had taken her home to live with me it wouldn't have happened. I *could* have done that.

At this point in the interview I was struck by Sharon's feeling that she could have saved her mother. I pointed out to her that she seems to blame herself for something she could not have possibly known. After all, she had spent a lot of time and energy finding her mother an appropriate place to recuperate and researching the pros and cons of Aricept.

After the fall, I was so miserable. I couldn't sleep. I was going to bring her up here. But then my sister would have a hard time coming up here and my brother could see her more easily in Pennsylvania and my mother's one and only brother lives in Baltimore. It would be much easier for him to get to Pennsylvania than New York. I decided it would be selfish to bring her here. I visited her as much as I could.

I remarked to Sharon that she seemed to feel *she* had to take care of her mother, but do it in a way that would be convenient for everyone else. She seemed to be making excuses for everyone else and didn't consider her own needs at all. Then she explained:

My mother had a long history of heart problems. Throughout my childhood I lived in tremendous fear that my mother would die. My mother worked in a factory and she was often taken out of the factory by ambulance. She worked three shifts and there were lots of times she wasn't home for dinner and my Dad and I would fend for ourselves.

Although Sharon is a social worker and does counseling, she seemed to be completely oblivious to how that childhood experience of being terrified her mother would die had affected her. She did not realize the connection between that childhood experience and how responsible she felt for caring for her mother. The little girl in her was desperate to keep her mother alive.

I never anticipated that my mother's illness and death would do this to me. As a child I was a caregiver. I knew even when I was a kid that I wanted to be a social worker and help old people. She'd come home from the hospital and I'd cook and take care of her. Every time my mother got sick as an adult and went to the hospital, my father would call me. It's really the only time my father would call me.

Sharon feels like a failure because her mother died. She failed at her raison d'être—saving her mother.

My sister has none of these feelings. I think she wasn't the caregiver that she could have been, but she doesn't feel guilty. My brother has never been involved in my parents' lives. He doesn't feel guilty. My sister did not see sacrificing to care for my mother as an obligation. I would never have asked my teenage boys if Grandma could move in like Joan did. They said no. I would have told them she's moving in.

Sharon knows that she felt responsible for her mother in a way her sister and brother did not. But she does not understand that it is a result of having spent her childhood feeling responsible for keeping her mother alive. That is a huge responsibility for a child; it is both a terrible burden and a special position of power. Sharon's sense of self was built around being a powerful caregiver—perhaps that had something to do with her choice of profession.

Sharon feels that as an expert in her field she should have been able to save her mother. However, I view the situation differently. Sharon's sense of being able to take care of other people was based on her feeling of potency from caring for her mother. Being unable to save her mother strikes at the heart of Sharon's sense of self. She has not only lost her mother, but her image of herself. Sadly, Sharon told me that for the last six months she's been wondering about whether she wants to leave the field of gerontology: "I'm a professional. This is what I do. I should have done the best job for my mother."

She also suffers from separation guilt. She did not bring her mother to live with her, nor did she leave her job and move in with her. She had a separate life and continued to live it. That makes Sharon feel guilty. If she were a "good daughter" she feels she would have given up her life to care for her mother. Finally, she is guilty because she feels she did not live up to her own moral values.

I have been so against institutions all of my life. It's such a value to me. I never should have let her leave home. I should have gotten live-in help for her.

ANGER AND GUILT

Sara is a forty-six-year-old university administrator. She and her husband live in a nineteenth-century building in one of Manhattan's most beautiful neighborhoods. Ringing the bell, I admired the beautiful wood door in the entry area. I loved the mahogany in the halls and the beautiful moldings. When she greeted me at the door, Sara seemed much more relaxed than when I had called her to set up our interview.

As I gushed about the beautiful apartment, Sara explained that her husband, Chuck, bought it five years ago—just before they met. Most of the furniture was his—the large burled mahogany coffee table and matching end tables, the dining room table and chairs. As we settled down to talk, I sank into the couch facing Chuck's extensive pottery collection while Sara sat in a chair facing me.

While Chuck was married before and has children, Sara never lived with anyone before Chuck. She has spent much of her adult life caring for her parents. After a long illness, her father died two years ago and her mother passed away a little more than a year later. In those last two years, Sara had to make life or death decisions for both parents. Interestingly, she feels little guilt about removing her father's respirator, but has not been able to resolve the guilt she feels about not putting in a feeding tube for her mother.

Sara's father worked until he was seventy-nine and needed bypass surgery. He never fully recuperated from that surgery. The nursing staff did not make him get out of bed and walk around. He didn't get any exercise while he was in the hospital. He got an infection while he was in the hospital as well.

He went downhill over a period of two years. He was hospitalized four times and went into rehabilitation each time, but ended up losing his foot. He never went back to work.

At the same time her father was in the hospital, Sara's mother was in the early stages of Alzheimer's disease.

He couldn't really go back to their apartment and have my mother care for him, but I didn't realize that. In fact, he may have gotten the infection that caused him to have his foot amputated because of poor homecare. She would leave the apartment for hours and we didn't know where she was.

Her father went back to the hospital and then to a rehabilitation hospital. Sara says:

I ended up going to visit my mother at the apartment and then to the rehab hospital to visit my father. But I didn't know where my mother was sometimes. She would wander onto the highway. I called every hour. I didn't know where she was. I was a wreck. She wouldn't accept any homecare. Her house smelled like feces and the refrigerator was full of rotten food.

Finally, Sara knew she had to get help for her mother. She contacted a homecare agency, interviewed various aides and chose one.

I took the day off to take her to my mother's house. They spent time together alone and I also watched them interact and I hired the woman. As soon as I got home there were two phone messages from the agency and two from my mother. She took this woman's things, threw them into the hallway and locked her out of the house.

Sara was intensely frustrated. She knew her mother needed help, but she would not accept it. She got a geriatrician to do a home visit and he suggested giving her a tranquilizer that would calm her down so that she would accept help. He said she had Alzheimer's and that people with cases less severe than hers were institutionalized. He said she couldn't be left alone. She either needed homecare or a nursing home.

I thought she'd be happier at home and my father would be coming home soon. She loved the doctor and I explained the pills to her and then I went home and called her and asked her about the pills and she said, "What pills?" She had taken all of them. I realized I needed to institutionalize her.

Sara had to make the decision to send her mother to a nursing home while her father was in the ICU on a respirator. Making the decision alone was very difficult. Sara was concerned about how to get her mother to go. The geriatrician said she should tell her she had an appointment with her regular doctor, whose office was across the street from the nursing home. He suggested that the doctor would then give her mother a sedative so that Sara could take her across the street to the nursing home.

One of the hardest memories was her dressing up to go to the doctor's office. When I was taking her to the nursing home I knew it was the last time she would be in her house. It was terrible. I got her to the doctor's office and he was really unprepared. He didn't have the medication that was going to make it easy to get her over there. I had to go to the pharmacy to get the drugs. She had to sit in the office and wait and the other patients were complaining that she smelled.

In the Alzheimer's unit in the nursing home, she was sometimes aware of what was going on around her—that was painful for Sara to witness. Then there were times her mother would slip into oblivion and needed the services that were available. She kept trying to find ways to get out.

When I was leaving her in the nursing home she was chasing after me: "Don't leave me here! Don't leave me here!" It would have been a hard thing to do if I really felt loving toward my mother, but it was even worse because I didn't.

Sara was wracked with guilt and anger. She knew her mother had to stay in the facility but felt guilty because she wanted to leave her there. She wanted someone else to care for her.

Sara had good reason to be angry with her father as well, but she was more able to express her feelings to him and be heard toward the end of his life. She explained that when her father moved from her childhood house to an apartment in the city, she went there and packed up the things that were most important to her and put them aside in a box. Her father, after forty-six years of living there, just threw everything away. When she went to get the box it was gone. Sara says:

I was deeply hurt. These were the things that were most important in my life. All my toe shoes were in the box. He didn't protect me. I was furious. For all the things I did for him, he didn't protect the little bit that I care about. But after he moved, I met him for lunch one day and he gave me a pair of toe shoes. All his therapy finally paid off. He was saying: "I know what's important to you. It *does* matter to me."

When Sara had to make a life and death decision about removing a ventilator from her father, it was harrowing but she never felt guilty about letting him die because she felt loving toward him. She had had the opportunity to tell him how she felt about him and he was able to respond in a way that made her feel heard.

They said he wouldn't last more than three minutes without a ventilator. I asked them to remove it. They pulled out the tube and he started gagging. It was horrible. I'm holding his hand. "Daddy I love you, Daddy I love you." It went on for *an hour.*

Eventually, after her father died, Sara's mother developed an infection and needed to be hospitalized. In the hospital, she forgot how to swallow and they asked to put in a feeding tube. Sara didn't know what to do. The doctor said: "Why don't you talk to some of your mother's old friends and see what they think?"

That was the best advice. They reminded me who my mother was and that she wouldn't have wanted this. I put her in hospice and the understanding was that there would be no feeding tube. She didn't eat for ten days and I felt that I was starving my mother to death.

Soon after her mother went to the hospice, Sara went to dinner with some colleagues and one woman said: "I would never put my mother in a nursing home." Sara felt guilty and horrible about her decision. But then there was another woman who helped Sara gain perspective.

I had a bad cold that day and she said: "You know how you're sick now and you're just pushing your food around on the plate, but you don't really want to eat? If I forced you to eat what's on your plate, that's what it's like putting a feeding tube in a person who's dying." It let me have a visceral idea of what it would mean to put the feeding tube in. The next day I got the phone call that she died. But the lingering feeling is: "Did I starve my mother to death?"

Sara feels guilty about her decision not to put in a feeding tube. Her anger makes her question her own motives. She asks herself, "Did I starve her to death because she starved me emotionally my whole life?" When you make life and death decisions for a parent, feeling angry increases the guilt if the choice is death. If you are feeling loving, as painful as it is to choose death, it is easier to feel that you are doing the right thing for your parent as well as yourself.

Sara explained that she wrote on her father's tombstone: "He got happy." Her father wasn't happy when he was young. But in the few years before he died, he found an assisted living facility and moved to the city. He went to the theater and made friends. These were things he never did before. Sara felt she had a part in her father being happier before he died because she was also able to work through some painful issues with him before he died. But she felt differently about her mother.

> With my mother [deep sigh], I haven't put anything on her gravestone yet because I can't think of anything positive to say. I went to her grave and asked her guidance for what I can say. But all I come up with is negative things. I have to lie, say nothing or say something very obtuse. There's no closure.

Her mother's Alzheimer's foreclosed the possibility of Sara working anything out with her mother before she died.

> When she first got Alzheimer's I went through a kind of mourning. I realized that I was never going to have the relationship with my mother that I always wanted. Once she had Alzheimer's I knew that was never going to happen. I wondered what I'd feel like when she died. To some degree it was a nonevent. There wasn't an "Oh, God she's dead."

Sara was left yearning for a relationship with her mother that she never had and never would have: "I see mothers and daughters on the subway chatting away and I know I will never have that."

Sara began to recall that her mother, who was a teacher, was always very depressed and that, as a child, she tried to take care of her mother.

I always felt I was the adult in the house. I'll take care of you, I'll entertain you; I'll make sure everything is okay. I remember sitting around the table—with my two aunts and feeling the tension. I felt that I had to make them get along. I had to make things right. I cooked dinner every night from the time I was eight or ten. I helped her grade. If something broke I fixed it. If we needed something, I'd run out and get it.

Sara understands that her mother's depression was rooted in a childhood experience. She explained that her mother was the apple of her grandfather's eye and then he lost his money in the Depression and was no longer functional. They had to move out of their house and relatives had to support them. Sara feels that experience of loss was a formative experience for her mother.

Sara went on to say that her mother was a business-woman, but gave it up when she got married. She became a teacher so that she and her husband, who was a teacher, could have summers off together. But Sara explains that while her father loved teaching, her mother hated it. Her mother seems to have experienced giving up her career as another thing that she loved being taken away from her. She came home each day tired and angry; her mother acted out her feelings of resentment on Sara.

She had me grading her papers when I was a kid. My older sister was a rebel and she and my mother were always in battles, so I felt I had to be extra good to compensate for all the trouble my sister caused. Mom never said anything good to me. No matter what I did it was never good enough.

Sara tried to please her mother, but she never succeeded. Rather, her mother envied Sara because she loved dancing. Her mother couldn't stand Sara doing something she loved when she felt so deprived herself.

> I was a dancer as a kid. I was in a semiprofessional group. I loved it. She had this thing about me dancing. They wouldn't pay for dance class. I had to work in the dance studio to pay for my classes. She promised if I got good grades I could dance and then she didn't follow through. In the area that was my self, my center, she didn't support me—she got in the way.

Sara cried as she described her mother's broken promise. Her feelings of resentment toward her mother posed a particular problem when Sara had to make the decision about the feeding tube. The doctor said: "Just tell her you love her." But Sara couldn't do that; she felt too angry with her mother. She was angry for always having to be good to compensate for her sister being bad and not getting any appreciation for it anyway. She felt hurt and angry with her mother for not allowing her to dance. But the experience that seemed to hurt the most was her mother's response when her sister had a psychotic breakdown.

Sara had been very close to her older sister, Tammy. After the birth of her third child, at age thirty-one, Tammy had a postpartum depression. She called Sara and said her husband was tapping the phone and trying to kill her. Then her brother-in-law called Sara and told her all the insane things Tammy was saying. Sara flew to Chicago the next day and hospitalized her sister. Sara describes it as something she did entirely alone—without the help of her brother-in-law or either of her parents. Tammy didn't want to be hospitalized; she jumped out of the car and tried to run away. Sara says:

> It was the hardest thing I've ever done. When I came back, my mother said I hospitalized my sister because I was jealous. It was sibling rivalry. Later my sister had a second break and my mother finally went out there to visit her. Imagine, it took two psychotic breaks for my mother to go out there and see her. She still wouldn't believe her darling daughter was psychotic. It's very difficult to make care choices for someone you're angry with.

When her mother was in the nursing home, Sara's cousins told her she was giving her more love and caring than her mother ever gave her. Indeed, Sara had a second wedding ceremony at the nursing home so that her mother could be at her wedding. But she is still left with the nagging question: "Did I put her in the nursing home because it was the best thing or because I was angry? Did I decide to not give her the feeding tube because I wanted to kill her?" Making that decision for a parent is painful and difficult no matter how much you love them, but if Sara had a well of love to draw on, she might feel more confident about the answer. She might feel sad and pained rather than guilty.

Sara told me that she's had a recurrent dream for many years—she dreams that she is buried alive and people are walking around above not knowing she's there. That is how Sara felt about her parents—each one was walking around without knowing she was there. Neither of her parents was able to see Sara's needs—her need to be a child and not take care of her parents, her need to be told the truth and her need to dance. Her mother was sadistic toward her and her father did not protect her. Sara's anger toward her mother never got resolved, leaving Sara with guilt about putting her in a nursing home and not putting in a feeding tube. Her anger toward her father, on the other hand, was resolved, so the decision to remove the ventilator was difficult, but did not leave her with guilt.

THE GUILT THAT GOES WITH BEING THE SPECIAL ONE WHO IS FAR AWAY

"My guilt is that my mother is dying alone . . ." Tom is a fifty-three-year-old editor who lives in New York. About six months ago, his eighty-one-year-old mother, who lives in Denver, had a stroke and went to the hospital and then to a nursing home. She lost her speech as a result of the stroke and then developed pneumonia in the nursing home and is now back in the hospital suffering from kidney failure. When I interviewed Tom, he and his family were making a decision about whether to put his mother on dialysis or let her die.

Tom has three younger sisters, and it is his middle sister who is the primary caregiver. She lives close to their parents and is currently unemployed. She was with her parents when her mother had a stroke. She visits her several times a day and picks up her father every day, takes him to the hospital and drives him back home.

Tom feels that his mother is dying "alone" because he feels that he is the only person who understands her and the only one who can comfort her. He says:

You can see she's trying to smile, she tries to formulate a question, but it comes out as a grunt. In the four days I was there, she got better. When I arrived, she rolled over and said clearly: "I love you." My mother and I never had much of a physical relationship, but when I visited her I told her stories, rubbed her neck and her arms. My sister put cream on her arms, but this was different.

Tom explained that his father has never offered any comfort to his mother. He was physically and emotionally abusive to his wife and his children. Tom's mother was pregnant with him when she married his father and Tom does not think they would have gotten married otherwise. He describes his father as a "falling-down drunk." Although he told me that his mother did not intervene to stop his father's drinking or allow anyone else to, Tom identifies with his mother as a victim of his father. Tom says his mother never expressed her needs and his father viewed her entirely as existing to fulfill his. When she started to show symptoms of Alzheimer's, Tom's father wouldn't believe she didn't know something or couldn't remember it.

While Tom views his father as ignoring his mother's needs, he views himself as the person who always understood her. It is ironic that she lost her ability to talk because, as Tom says:

Even when she could talk, she never expressed her emotions. I only saw my mother cry once or twice in my whole life.

Nevertheless, Tom always felt that he intuitively understood his mother.

Once my mom was in the hospital, knowing my mother the way I do, she was probably very frightened about what was happening to her. Part of her mind was active and alive. I could see it when I visited her.

Tom's father says he can't stand seeing his wife unable to speak or understand anything so he doesn't like to visit her. He goes every day, but Tom feels angry toward him because he stays very briefly and clearly doesn't *want* to be there. Tom says:

He's so self-involved he can't imagine that she has a need to see him. The last day I was there I tried to explain this to him. I told him: "When you're there, she's responsive." But he's so self-involved, he says: "Nobody understands how hard this is. My body can't take it." He *never* in his life thought about anyone having needs except him.

Tom feels guilty that he is not with his mother because he feels that he could comfort his mother in a way that his father refuses to do.

I said: "Why can't you just sit in the hospital room and watch television together?" He says: "You don't understand how hard this is for me."

His guilt is intensified by his knowing the eldest of his sisters doesn't visit his mother and he feels that the middle sister, who visits her mother several times a day, cannot offer her the kind of comfort that he can offer. He chuckles when he tells me that his sister's boyfriend is named Tom and when he goes to visit his mother she smiles and is very responsive to him. He fantasizes that she thinks it's her son Tom.

> I had to help the nurse turn my mother over. I found myself holding my mother, she looked up at me and I knew she was comfortable, she felt safe. It was such a familiar feeling to be with her like this. I felt it was a regression back to this early place where we were together. I felt that I understood my mother on a level that my father and sisters never did.

Feeling that he has a special bond with his mother makes Tom feel guilty because he feels that he is the only one capable of offering her any comfort.

> There's a part of me that wanted to be there when my mother died. I felt guilty coming back to New York. I can't afford to take off from work and stay with her. I don't know how long it will take. Is it just my *fantasy* that my mother is alive and well inside this shell? I can't imagine anything worse than to go through the process of dying totally alone.

Without him, he feels, his mother is totally alone.

IT WOULD BE wonderful if as adults we could appreciate our own compassion and attempt to do the right thing for our parents. But despite their heroic efforts to take care of their parents, Sharon, Sara and Tom are all plagued with often crippling guilt. Their deep, unresolved feelings about their mothers leave them unable to get over the guilt. Sara's guilt is the result of unresolved anger toward her mother, while Sharon and Tom's guilt is based on feeling they didn't do enough for the loved parent for whom they have felt responsible since childhood. Each of them struggles with different degrees of guilt, unable to forgive themselves. Sharon can't forgive herself for not saving her mother. She is stuck in the relentless self-punishment of "If only I . . ." Sharon won't be able to forgive herself until she is able to empathize with the little girl who felt that her mother's life was in her hands.

Sara, on the other hand, does not torture herself with the wish to undo the decisions she made. She accepts them. She feels she would make the same decisions again. But making those decisions while still angry has left her with anxiety about her sadistic wishes toward her mother. She's left asking herself: Did I act on them? Sara won't be able to forgive herself until she is able to separate her wishes and her actions toward her mother. She may have wished, at moments, to hurt her mother. But her actions toward her mother were not sadistic. She did what she could for her—more than many daughters. She made a decision about the feeding tube based on her mother's quality of life *as well as her own,* but the latter doesn't cancel out the former. Adult children often feel guilty for decisions that give consideration to their own life circumstances. But relationships involve weighing the needs of both people—we do that with our children and we have to do that with our parents.

Tom feels guilty for not comforting his mother in her dying hour in a way he feels only he had the power to do. Tom has always felt merged with his mother—as if they are one.

Tom will only be able to forgive himself when he accepts his mother's separateness. He was able to say goodbye to her. She knew he came to say goodbye. That's all we can do for another person—even our mother.

While we all deal with feelings of guilt about cruel things said or inconsiderate behavior, neurotic guilt is not based on actually hurting another person. Yet, neurotic guilt can be debilitating and, because aspects of it are often unconscious, it is very difficult to talk someone out of it. It's neurotic! Then what can we do to reduce crippling guilt? How can we make peace with ourselves? Taking care of our elderly parents exacerbates our neurotic guilt, but using this stage of life as an opportunity to reduce it enriches us and enhances the rest of our lives.

Often we vacillate between anger and guilt, so trying to work out angry feelings with a parent reduces guilt. Of course, the most ideal way of working out those angry feelings is *with* the parent before he or she dies. Sara was able to do that with her father. Unfortunately, that is often impossible either because the elderly parent is no longer lucid or because he or she is unable to take any responsibility for hurting you. Feeling angry toward a parent with Alzheimer's is particularly difficult because their inability to comprehend your anger increases the guilt. In that case you may need a therapist to help you work out the angry feelings.

Second, when we hear ourselves use a lot of "shoulds" that is a tip-off that we are trying to meet other people's expectations of what we should do. It might be helpful to ask yourself: What do I think is right? What do I need to do in order to make peace with myself? There is no one prescription for dealing with difficult life milestones with an elderly parent. You have to find your own level of tolerance and clarify your own values.

For the adult child who feels only he can take care of Mom because he is the special child, ameliorating guilt is particularly difficult. There is a conflict between the wish to feel special and the wish to not feel guilty. Unfortunately, they are linked—if you are the only one who is special enough to take care of Mom then you will feel guilty for allowing anyone else to care for her. Reducing guilt involves giving up feeling special and allowing or encouraging other family members to participate in caregiving.

Finally, for those who feel guilty because they always criticized other people for putting their parents in nursing homes and now want to do it themselves, let this be a lesson in humility and compassion. It's much easier to make judgments about people when you are not in the same position. People change and life situations change. Before you had children or worked full-time you might have felt you wanted your parents to live with you when they needed care. But now your situation may have changed; you may have changed. Forgive yourself.

Part II

RELATIONSHIPS THAT OFFER SUPPORT OR CREATE CONFLICT

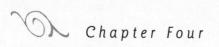

Chapter Four

SPOUSES

> My mother never liked my husband, and she was never
> nice to him, so he doesn't want to see her. I understand
> how he feels, but I am left with the burden by myself.
>
> —*A married caregiver*

AT SIXTY, my husband, Richard, still feels angry toward his mother because she invited his grandmother to move in when his grandfather died. The family of four lived in a house with three bedrooms and Grandma was put in Richard's room—when he was five years old. Grandma stayed there until he was ten. I was shocked that his parents put his grandmother in their son's rather than their seven-year-old daughter's room, but I am more surprised that Richard is not angry at his father—only his mother. Richard says his father did not want his mother-in-law to live with his family, but he never insisted that his wife and her brothers make other arrangements for their mother. Instead, he permitted Richard to share his room with his elderly grandmother.

Was Richard's father being a good husband or was he abnegating his responsibility as a husband and father? It's a difficult question to answer—we have to examine our assumptions about what it means to be a "good husband" and "good father." There is not one universally agreed-upon answer to these questions—and our perspective changes over time. In the 1950s, when Richard was growing up in an upper-middle-class family, a good father and husband was one who was a good economic provider. Fathers were not expected to be involved in child care—men were supposed to go out to work, and women were supposed to stay home and take care of the children. Sixty-three percent of families in 1950 were composed of a wage-earning dad, a stay-at-home mom, and one or more children.[1] Richard's family fit the dominant demographic perfectly: his mother stayed home in the suburbs and his father took the Long Island Rail Road to work in New York City. Now only 17 percent of all American families conform to the tradition of wage-earning dad, stay-at-home mom and one or more children.[2]

Expectations of what it means to be a good husband and father have changed as more women entered the workforce. Since more than 70 percent of all married women with children under eighteen participate in paid labor outside the home, we have come to expect married men to do more than bring home a check.[3] As the economic structure changed so did the division of labor within the family. Husbands, especially upper-middle-class ones like Richard's father, are expected to share in the domestic chores and play a larger role in the care of their children. Fathers are expected to play an emotional role in the family, not simply an economic one. So what does this mean about Richard's father?

From the traditional 1950s point of view Richard's father *was* being a good husband and father, but his son was left feeling unprotected. From my point of view as a psycho-therapist, Richard's father failed him in a fundamental way. In a good marriage a spouse can help a caregiver realize that her mother is not her primary relationship anymore. The caregiver is no longer dependent on her mother as she was as a child. She has a husband to depend upon and a husband and children who depend upon her. Richard's father did not per-form this important function as a husband/father. He com-plained about his mother-in-law, but he did not take action.

Husbands can also be helpful to a caregiver by helping her find a way to alleviate guilt. For example, Sara's husband was able to help her do what made her feel good about herself without losing herself.

> I met my husband on a blind date and told him I had to leave to buy clothes for my mother, who was in a nursing home. He said: "Oh, can I come with you?"

Sara's husband was immediately comfortable with her role as caregiver. He joined her in it in a way that allowed her to marry him and still take care of her mother in a way that was part of her core identity.

> When we got married, one of the decisions was whether we should get Mom from the nursing home and bring her to the wedding. I couldn't face putting her back in the nursing home after taking her out for a day. So my husband sug-gested: "Why don't we have a second wedding at the nurs-ing home?" It ended up being wonderful for everyone. The day of the wedding there was a family support group meet-ing. People came up to me and said: "We haven't had any joy in this nursing home. Thank you for bringing some joy."

THE SPOUSE WHO ENABLES
THE LACK OF LIMITS

Remember Rose, from Chapter 1, who had such difficulty setting limits with her mother? Like Richard's father, Rose's husband, John, failed to help his wife set limits with her mother. Rose's husband did not even complain like Richard's father. Rose felt grateful that her husband did not pressure her to separate from her mother.

> My husband is a wonder. He has a lot of patience. I call him and say I don't feel like cooking, you better bring something in.

But Rose is unhappy having her mother live in her house. She feels controlled by her mother. She gave up her social life with her husband, daughters and friends for her mother: "She won't let us leave her alone, but when I tell her we're going out she doesn't want to go . . ." Rose's mother is using emotional blackmail on her. She is using her suffering as a way of making Rose feel guilty and manipulating her. As Susan Forward points out: "Becoming a caretaker to a sufferer is a full-time job."[4]

Rose feels she has no choice but to give in to her mother's demands; she feels victimized by her. Once, when she went out for dinner with her husband, her mother called 911, so they never did it again. Her mother's message is clear: "If you leave me I will suffer so much that you will be sorry." It would have been helpful to Rose if her husband, John, said,

"This is a problem, Rose. We can't live this way. The kids need to have a mother who can take them shopping or out to lunch. We need time alone together and I need to have a wife who isn't constantly drained and angry."

John has never done that. Rather, John seems to join Rose in her definition of the situation—that is, we have no choice but to do what Mother wants. John has never set any limits with his mother-in-law. She is living in his house, but he has never talked to her about the way she behaves. Rose says:

> He's not going to disagree with my mother. So she loves to see him. He goes in and she complains to him about me and he says: "I'll have to get after her about that." [She laughs.] He comes into the kitchen and laughs and tells me. I say to him, "You see what it's like to take care of her." [She laughs.] He's good. He's really good.

Rose's laughing does not feel like it's a response to something funny. When she says, "You see what it's like . . ." she shrugs, and I sense what she means is, "It's hopeless." She feels there's nothing that can be done to make the situation with her mother any better. But that's not true—that sense of hopelessness is a symptom of depression. John unknowingly adds to Rose's sense of hopelessness by going along with his mother-in-law's unreasonable demands rather than explaining to her that if she wants to live with his family, she has to make some compromises so that the situation will be more livable for them.

Rose does not understand John's role in her difficulties with her mother. She views his passivity as "helping." When he goes along with his mother-in-law's outrageous insistence that Rose and John cannot go anywhere without her, Rose experiences it as support rather than collusion: "He has no qualms about helping me pack her up to take her somewhere. He's real, real good. I manage."

Is Rose's husband a concerned partner or did he allow his wife to sacrifice important aspects of their marital relationship and their daughters' development? I think John *was* a concerned partner, but he seemed to make the same assumption as Rose—that they had no choice.

THE SPOUSE WHO HELPS SET LIMITS

Elizabeth and her husband, Tom, seem to have been able to set up a much more livable situation than Rose and John— although they gave up their home to move in with Elizabeth's mother. Elizabeth and Tom felt that they *had* options, but *chose* to live with Elizabeth's mother and take care of her. Elizabeth is a very striking woman with short white hair and a rather formal manner. She is fifty-seven years old and her husband, Tom, is sixty; they have two grown daughters. Born in a small town in Massachusetts, Elizabeth went to the University of Texas and then got a master's in counseling at the University of Pennsylvania.

I've been far from home since I was eighteen years old. That's the irony of it. I loved living in New York for all those years after school. My husband and I lived in a lovely neighborhood and knew everyone. I started a shelter for battered women and ran it for fifteen years.

Elizabeth talks with nostalgia about the years she lived in New York and ran a shelter for battered women. Her voice gets sad at the end when she adds: "Then my father died and my mother has very bad arthritis."

Elizabeth and her husband were running back and forth from New York to Amherst, Massachusetts, to check in on her mother. Then Tom got a job at a school in Massachusetts and Elizabeth kept her job in New York. Tom was living with her mother during the week; Elizabeth would join them on the weekend.

> It's amazing, he never could have done that with my father or his own parents, but he always loved my mother and felt closer to her than to his own mother.

Tom's feelings for Elizabeth's mother were a key element in their caregiving. *He* wanted to care for her mother as much or more than Elizabeth did. In addition, Elizabeth did not like having a commuting marriage. She decided to give up her job and move to Amherst. She and Tom decided to buy her mother's house and live with her.

I asked Elizabeth what kinds of things she does for her mother.

> I bathe her every night and my husband gives her breakfast and lunch because he's off for the summer. Then I make dinner for the three of us. She has good days and bad days—it's mostly related to the weather. On good days she can do a lot of things for herself, but on bad days she needs a lot of help. The problem is that you

don't know when there will be a bad day. You can't plan in advance and you can't really be spontaneous either.

It sounds like a situation that could be quite dismal. But in contrast to Rose and John, Elizabeth and Tom manage to take care of themselves while taking care of her mother. Once a week a woman comes in and cleans the house and bathes her mother so that Elizabeth and Tom can go out.

> And then every once in a while I call my sister and say: "I can't take it anymore, please come." She comes and we go away. Or my brother in New Hampshire will take her for two weeks and then we can go out to dinner and go bike riding and hiking while she's gone.

There are other ways in which Elizabeth and Tom have made the situation more livable. They have made the relationship more reciprocal by asking her mother for rent— that helps pay the mortgage and makes them feel that they are getting something back for taking care of her. In contrast to John, Tom supports Elizabeth by being clear with her mother about what they can tolerate when it is difficult for Elizabeth to do it.

> She had cataracts and was losing her vision. The doctor said she needed an operation to have them removed, but she didn't want to do it. My husband and I felt that we could not live with her if she was blind—she'd have to go to a home. He told her that she had to have the operation.

She didn't want to and felt very resentful. But she had it and now she's fine.

Elizabeth talked about how painful it was to deal with her mother's resentment when she has made such a big sacrifice for her.

She complains to my sister and brothers about me. Of course, they understand the situation. Recently I increased my work hours to thirty-five hours a week. When I told her she said: "What's the difference? You never do anything for me anyway."

Although she didn't explicitly say it, I got the impression that Elizabeth was happy to work thirty-five hours a week. It's hard for her to be with her mother.

It's not easy. But sometimes I just say to my husband, I've had it. I'm going for a walk. You deal with her. And he does. It works because he does it with me; we do it together.

When Elizabeth says, "We do it together," she is not simply referring to the caregiving. What Elizabeth and Tom have been able to do is make the house *their* house—they bought the house rather than simply living in the house owned by her mother. As soon as they bought it, they ripped off the kitchen and built a new one. Elizabeth said that helped a great deal to allay the feeling that she was giving up her whole life and moving home with her mother.

But perhaps the most important element in allowing Elizabeth and Tom to take care of her mother and feel good about it is that Tom has helped Elizabeth set limits on her mother's control over their lives.

> She would tell me what to do in the garden or how to do it and I couldn't stand it. Finally, my husband said to her: "We can't live here if you tell us what to do. We're used to having our own house and our own garden." That really helped. She does it once in a while, but it's much better.

Elizabeth was getting angry at her mother's controlling behavior, but she could not talk to her about it. It was her husband who intervened on her behalf and made it possible for Elizabeth to tolerate living with her mother without being angry toward her all the time.

IN THE CASES I have described, the daughters were the caregivers and in both cases the husbands agreed to living with their mothers-in-law. Now let's turn to a situation in which the son is the caregiver and his wife resented his need to care for his mother.

THE ABANDONING SPOUSE

Tony counsels teenagers for a nonprofit community organization in Columbus, Ohio. The office is a tiny hole-in-the-wall with papers and books strewn everywhere. It's hard to find a place to sit. Tony is wearing a pair of wrinkled chinos and a short-sleeved shirt. He's a husky Italian-American man of forty-six. He is married with two children—a nineteen-year-old son and seventeen-year-old daughter.

Tony's mother has had lupus for over twenty years, but during the last five years of her life, it was debilitating and she was on oxygen and bedridden. Tony's stepfather was there, but Tony still felt that he had to be the primary care-giver for his mother.

It was really hard. I was working, trying to take care of my family and trying to be there for my mother. Especially because it was only a mile down the road, I passed her home every day and I felt I needed to be there. I tried to be there as much as possible—sometimes every other day. She lived with my stepfather, but we [he corrects himself], I took care of her.

Tony had a very special relationship with his mother be-cause of his childhood. His parents divorced when he was a baby and his mother was left with two boys. When Tony was about eight years old, his mother couldn't deal with working full-time and caring for her two sons.

I lived away from my mother for about seven years from third grade to eighth grade—five years . . . I went with one grandmother and my brother went with the other grand-mother. I didn't go visit my mother that often. You know, you get involved with your friends and stuff. Then I moved back with my mother and stepfather and we moved up here. It was hard that relationship at home—feeling like I should be in both places. It was difficult.

Tony tells me about his traumatic past very casually. He doesn't seem to think that being sent away by his mother, separated from his brother, taken out of one school and having to start at a new one, after he had already been abandoned by his father, had much of an effect on his life. Tony casts the story of being sent to live with his grandmother in an interesting way. He reverses the relationship between his mother (the adult at the time) and himself (the child at the time) when he says he didn't go to visit her very much because he was involved with his friends. He feels that even as a child it was his responsibility to take care of his mother; he is careful to hold his mother blameless for not visiting him! He seems to need to protect her.

Tony had a strong wish to be close to his mother once he was reunited with her as a result of her marrying his stepfather. When he married, Tony and his wife, Jan, bought a house down the road from his mother; he continued to feel a strong need to take care of her—perhaps as a result of his childhood experience as well as the tragic death of his older brother.

He got shot fifteen years ago and ended up in a traumatic brain injury hospital. That was kind of difficult. So I was the only son left. He was hanging out in an after-hours bar with people that were known not to be reputable and had an argument with a guy over my brother's girlfriend and the guy pulled out a gun and shot him in the head. He died two years before my mother did.

Tony's wish to be close to his mother was intensified by his feeling that he had to be a "good kid" because his brother's brain injury, twelve-year hospitalization and subsequent death were so painful for his mother on top of her own illness.

He was not a good kid. He was a drug addict. When she was sick, I was the only one left. I was always the good kid. Even if I did something a little wrong, I didn't want to be like my brother.

There was always a split in the image of the two brothers—Tony, "the good kid," and Joey, "the bad kid." Tony lived with the expectation that he had to make up for his brother's badness with his goodness. Unfortunately, Tony's wife did not understand the psychological importance of Tony's taking care of his mother.

One of the other situations that really affected me was my wife and two kids just stepped back, away from the whole process. I felt like I was really alone. It's two years later and it's still there. It really changed our relationship—more with my wife than the kids.

Tony felt very conflicted about his obligation to his wife and children and his need to take care of his mother. He wanted Jan to understand how much he needed to care for his mother, but she didn't. Perhaps she felt abandoned by Tony because of the intensity of his involvement with his mother.

Jan wouldn't go visit at all. When my mother was in the hospital, I'd run down to visit her. She'd say: "Oh, you're going *again* . . ." Little things like that made me feel bad. I'd say, "Do you want to take a ride?" Even if she didn't want to sit in the room, she could have come for a ride with me. I'd only stay half an hour or so. My mother couldn't talk a lot, but she knew you were there and she appreciated you coming. That was really hard. When my mother passed away, I was there by myself.

I asked Tony if he and Jan had gotten any help to sort out what happened between the two of them when his mother was sick: "No, once in a while we talk about it, it's just there. We don't argue. We don't ever argue. It's just the way it is." I asked him why he doesn't seek help since he seems to be in chronic pain: "Yeah, I am. I don't know. With whatever goes bad, I just try to put it aside. I'm involved with kids."

I asked him if he thought there was any connection between feeling abandoned by his wife when his mother was sick and his experience of being sent to live with his grandmother as a child. I sensed Tony's depression and went further with him than perhaps I should have. I pointed out that the way he described doing other things to avoid the feelings of hurt and anger at his wife sounded similar to the way he described coping with his mother sending him to live with his grandmother.

> That's kind of deep. I think of it as just one of those things. That may be. I don't know. The way I deal with things is I don't give myself a lot of time to think about stuff—just keep moving. Overall, I'm a happy-go-lucky kind of person. I'm always smiling. Of course there's always that lingering pain there.

There was hopelessness in his laugh. He seemed to reject any possibility of other ways to understand his experience. He felt stuck. Tony did not seem very happy-go-lucky to me. On the contrary, he seemed like a hurt little boy who felt abandoned by his mother at eight and abandoned by his wife when he needed her most. But Tony seems to cope by giving others what he did not get from them.

> When my wife's parents were sick, I wanted to see her take care of them. I wanted to make sure that she went down and visited. I said to her: "You'll be sorry later if you don't do it." She wound up being there when her mother died last fall, because I pushed her to do that. I felt good about it. Now her dad is ill and she seems to have a different attitude. So hopefully, little by little we'll build that whole thing back up.

Tony's view of his problems with Jan is that she did not understand the importance of caring for elderly parents— his or her own and that made him feel abandoned by her when he was caring for his mother. Tony seems to believe that by Jan caring for her dad in a way Tony deemed appropriate, the trust in the marriage will be rebuilt. However, Tony never talked to Jan about how he felt about what he experienced as her lack of support during the last years of his mother's life. He still doesn't talk to Jan about how he feels about that experience and how it has changed their relationship. Jan has never talked to Tony about how she felt about him spending so much time away from her and their children in order to care for his mother. Perhaps she felt that he was overly involved with his mother's care. But Tony says she never discussed that with him, she just made hostile remarks like: "Oh, you're going *again*."

From my experience as a psychotherapist, it seems unlikely that trust can be rebuilt without talking about the breach and understanding what each of them was going through at the time. Very likely both Tony and Jan are hurting. Just as Tony may have experienced Jan's lack of support as a repetition of his childhood experience of being sent away by his mother, Jan may have experienced Tony's absences as a repetition of an early experience in her life. Intractable marital problems often involve unconscious repetitions of childhood traumas. Unearthing the meaning of the empathic failures and the depth of the pain is difficult without the help of a therapist.

THE IMPORTANCE OF THE SPOUSE WHEN THE CAREGIVER IS AN ONLY CHILD

Jonathan is a fifty-year-old only child. He is married to Barbara, who is an accountant. Jonathan recently went back to school to fulfill a lifelong dream of becoming a social worker. I interviewed him twice over a period of two years of caregiving and I interviewed Barbara as well. When I first interviewed Jonathan he was living two hours from his parents' house. His mother, Betsy, who has bipolar disorder, was eighty years old at the time. She had had a knee replacement and needed another. His father had coronary heart disease and advanced cancer of the bladder which metastasized to his liver. His father needed oxygen, but his cancer was in remission.

Jonathan felt angry because he and his wife, Barbara, had been trying for years to get his parents to move into an assisted living facility in Brooklyn. That would make it easier for Jonathan to visit them and it would make the adjustment easier for the survivor when one of them died. Jonathan's

Dad thought it was a good idea. But Jonathan says: "My mother's the one who dug in her heels and said: 'No, I'm not doing it.' So I was really mad at her."

When Jonathan's father was diagnosed with cancer, his parents needed extensive help in the home. Jonathan kept trying to get his mother to take some responsibility and make decisions, but his mother *could not* do it. Jonathan felt she *would not* do it. That made him angry at her. He ended up making many decisions about hiring help, but he felt angry at his mother for not cooperating. Jonathan set up homecare for his father. He had a bathroom put in on the ground floor and set up a downstairs bedroom area for his father. He hired someone to shop, clean and cook.

Jonathan's father died a year and a half ago. Only then did Jonathan and his wife, Barbara, realize how much his father had been taking care of his mother. Despite all of Jonathan's efforts to create support for his mother, she had a major depressive episode a few months after his father's death and she had to be hospitalized. Jonathan devoted himself entirely to getting appropriate treatment for his mother. She was first put into the psychiatric ward of a general hospital near her home in New Jersey. Jonathan was driving back and forth from Brooklyn to the hospital in New Jersey on an almost daily basis or sometimes staying over at his mother's house. But Jonathan felt that she was not getting the appropriate combination of therapy and medication there and was able to get her transferred to a hospital that specialized in geriatric psychiatric disorders.

When Betsy was ready to leave the hospital, Jonathan had to face the problem of where his mother would live. Barbara has been helpful to him by pointing out that his mother is not capable of making any decisions. She explains to him that his mother is not willfully *refusing* to make a decision; she is simply overwhelmed by the prospect. It was probably that fear of being overwhelmed that made her reject the idea of moving to an assisted living facility before her husband died.

It was clear to Jonathan and Barbara that Betsy was not able to live on her own. Jonathan's mother needed help to ensure that she took her twice-daily medications; she needed meals provided and transportation to her doctors' appointments. Therefore, when his mother was getting shock treatments, while Jonathan was visiting her and dealing with the doctors, Barbara was looking at two possible assisted living facilities that are located near their house. Once the decision between the two facilities was made, Barbara made the arrangements for her mother-in-law to move.

Jonathan makes all the medical appointments, medical decisions, etc.

> Barbara has been phenomenal. We complement each other. I'm not interested in the financial aspects and she's not interested in the medical, psychological, social aspects. It's burdensome for Barbara, but she's not being asked to step out of her comfort zone in terms of her skills and her emotional makeup. We've worked well as a team.

Jonathan and Barbara's caregiving roles are an example of gender role reversal. Jonathan does the emotional nurturing, while Barbara takes care of the practical tasks like paying bills, estate management, etc.

Aside from her ongoing psychiatric problems and increasing dementia, Jonathan's mother eventually had a second knee replacement. So there have been many medical appointments and decisions. His mother doesn't understand what the doctor tells her, so Jonathan has to speak to the doctor. Barbara says Betsy is someone who can carry on a wonderful conversation and be quite charming. She *appears* to understand what the doctor is telling her, but she doesn't really process it. It is not clear whether her lack of comprehension is the result of intense anxiety or dementia, or some combination of the two. But Barbara says: "What that means is that even if she tries to convey what the doctor says to us it doesn't make any sense."

Barbara says that Jonathan can immediately tell when his mother isn't listening or doesn't know what is going on. He gets angry at her, trying to get her to focus on a problem or make a decision. Jonathan says that led to a confrontation in a restaurant. He kept asking his mother to answer his question about what she wanted and his mother finally said, "You're badgering me. Stop badgering me." Jonathan says:

> My mother took a lot of lumps in the beginning. We had one pretty heated scene in a restaurant one night where she was crying and I was crying. [Bursts out laughing.] One of the people in the next booth had an expression on her face as if she were wondering: "What are these crazy people doing?"

Jonathan knows that is not the right way to talk to his eighty-two-year-old mother. He chides himself for losing his temper, but also feels justified. "From a therapeutic standpoint it sucked. It was a dumb thing to do. But I had to get those things out."

Barbara offers Jonathan support by listening to him ventilate. But she also steps in to mediate between Jonathan and his mother. She says that Jonathan's mother's approach to life is to want problems to go away rather than confronting them. She does not want to make decisions.

> She will say "yes" to everybody without actually dealing with the issue at hand. When Jonathan hears that, he knows she is not paying attention or understanding what's happening, and it throws him into a tizzy. He will say: "Mom, you really *have* to understand."

Barbara explains to Jonathan that, at this point, his mother does not *have* to understand. He has to make the decision without her understanding.

> Jonathan tries to make her understand some fairly complicated things and then she gets more and more frustrated and breaks down in tears.

What makes it so hard for Jonathan to accept that his mother is not capable of understanding certain issues or making decisions for herself? He wants to feel his mother *could* be more independent because otherwise he has to face her total dependence on him. He has been worrying about his mother since he was a little boy. As a child, Jonathan had to deal with a mentally ill mother.

> I was ashamed to have my friends come to the house because my mom was in a bathrobe and a shower cap and all

the curtains were drawn in the house. She would get so depressed, that she could barely move. She'd get my father off to work and make us breakfast. Then she'd go upstairs, lock the door, draw the shades, lie on the floor, and she kept a bottle of whiskey under the desk. And when she'd wake up, she'd take a drink of alcohol. Just enough to get her into a semicomatose state and she would just lie on the floor.

Jonathan's mother was misdiagnosed as a schizophrenic and went through extensive hospitalizations. She was away for months at a time when he was a child. She tried to kill herself more than once. Jonathan says:

I saw the scars on her wrists. Fortunately, it was a cry for help. Meaning she didn't go real deep. They were fairly superficial cuts. She tried to drink lye. She *did* drink lye. Then she tried to do herself in with pills. She underwent extensive convulsive therapy; she was medicated improperly. It wasn't until the mid-seventies that she found a psychiatrist who understood bipolar disorder and prescribed lithium.

When Jonathan was nineteen, his mother tried to kill herself with an overdose of pills. He says:

I could tell when she was going into a depressive cycle. I could look at her and I could see it coming and I could predict it. One day I was looking for my mother and I knocked on the door, and I heard a little voice. The door was locked. I said: "Open the door!" And then I realized there was an empty pill bottle on the floor.

Jonathan has good reason to wish that his mother could take care of herself and let him focus on his own life. However, it has kept him constantly angry at his mother. Barbara mediates and sometimes intervenes to stop the escalation. She says:

> My mother-in-law, and my father-in-law when he was alive, have always seen me as more like them than Jonathan. They have always seen me as someone who was more on their wavelength than he is.

Barbara tries to use Betsy's sense of camaraderie with her to be a calming influence. She lets her vent her frustration with Jonathan as well as trying to get Jonathan to give up his fantasy that his mother can live independently.

Barbara's support role is particularly important for Jonathan because he is an only child. She says:

> There is no one else to help him out other than me. So I am a second caregiver. I pay all of Betsy's bills. I arranged the move from her house in New Jersey to the assisted living facility. I unpacked all of the cartons and set up the apartment for her and I take care of all the financial and administrative issues.

The facility is close to Barbara's office so she picks up Betsy's mail while she is at a rehabilitation hospital recuperating from knee surgery, and if there is a problem with anything at the assisted living facility, they call Barbara.

Barbara seems to be setting more limits on her participation in the caregiving process. For example, Betsy went into the rehabilitation hospital last Wednesday and Barbara has been there once, while Jonathan has been there four times. She says:

> One of the hardest things as a spouse is that you are being relied on in many ways, but you don't have any decision-making power. When it comes right down to it, I'm not the child. It's *his* mother. He has the final say.

She says that Jonathan is only now beginning to see that his mother "doesn't get it" and can't make decisions. Earlier Jonathan wanted to help his mother to become an independent woman and he got angry at her when she did not.

> He wanted to give her the opportunity to make a decision, but she goes into a panic if she has to make a decision. For example, while decorating her apartment, she had a manic episode because she had to make decisions about colors and fabrics. She called the decorator at 5:45 a.m. on a Friday to ask her if she were coming to her house in a little while. When the decorator told her she wasn't coming that day but on Monday, she got very argumentative with her.

Jonathan has been working on accepting that his mother cannot be more independent.

> I've come to realize that, although I want her to be more self-sufficient, it's not going to happen. It never was and is not going to be. I seem to be learning and relearning that lesson.

He is learning to accept who his mother is, and in many ways always has been, and to be more accepting of himself as well. When he says he's "learning and relearning that lesson," he seems to forgive himself for not responding perfectly to his mother every time. But he is proud of his progress.

> One of her friends called and said: "Your mother's coming home tomorrow and the refrigerator is empty. What should I buy?" I called my mom and told her about it. She said: "That's a good idea." But I could hear the hesitancy in her voice. I said: "Well, what should I tell her to buy?" I knew my mother was having an anxiety attack over this decision. I didn't get angry at her.

Another problem is that it is hard for Jonathan to distinguish between cries for help to which he needs to respond immediately and whimpers that do not require him to rush to his mother's house. Jonathan has had years of practice being attuned to nuances of his mother's voice. Barbara says Betsy often calls to complain to Jonathan and he feels he has to immediately drop everything and visit her. Barbara reminds him that his mother may *want* him to visit, but that is not the same as *needing* him to take care of something. Before his father died, Jonathan promised to care for his mother. So he has to struggle with his guilt and sense of obligation as well as his anxiety that his mother is capable of regressing very quickly. Barbara says that Jonathan is in a perpetual state of expecting the worst. Every time the phone rings and it's *not* his mother or *about* his mother, he takes a sigh of relief. Nevertheless, Barbara says Jonathan is getting more able to say no to his mother without getting angry at her.

With Barbara's help, Jonathan is accepting his mother's limitations. Accepting that his mother cannot take care of herself and cannot make decisions for herself has helped Jonathan forgive her for the pain she put him through when he was a child. He is coming to realize that she really didn't have any control over her behavior. She failed him, but not because she wasn't trying or didn't love him.

WE HAVE SEEN the important role the spouse can play, but often doesn't, in helping the caregiver negotiate the relationship with the elderly parent. Richard's father and Rose's husband stood by as their wives' inability to set limits intruded on their family's happiness. On the other hand, Elizabeth's husband, Tom, was extremely helpful to her because he was an equal partner in caring for her mother and helped Elizabeth set limits with her.

Tony and Jonathan are atypical caregivers because they are sons caring for their mothers. Tony's story illustrates the negative impact that caregiving can have on a marriage if the spouses do not have the same expectations about caring for their parents and do not negotiate their differences. In contrast to Tony, Jonathan's wife was willing to share the burden of caregiving. She never took it over, he remains the primary caregiver, but she offered support to Jonathan and was sympathetic to his being an only child.

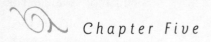 *Chapter Five*

SIBLINGS

"Hi Mom."

"Hi."

"Did you get the flowers for Mother's Day?"

"Yes, and Phil is so wonderful. He's so nice to everyone, and everyone talks about him. He's just so good to me."

I can feel my blood pressure going up. I feel the rage rising in my chest. I get off the phone quickly. I'm trying not to cry.

"I'll see you tomorrow, Mom."

"Oh good, great, I'll see you then."

The tears well up. I'm fifty-nine years old and I still feel unappreciated by my mother.

TAKING CARE OF YOUR PARENTS may strengthen the bonds with your siblings and intensify your sense that you can count on them. Our relationships with siblings are our longest, offering many opportunities to understand and work out unresolved issues that remain from childhood. This becomes critical in times of crisis, such as a parent's sudden illness or gradual decline. A group of siblings can become a team offering one another support and helping set limits. If there are only two siblings, they can be partners and divide the emotional and/or financial burden.

However, as Stephen P. Bank and Michael D. Kahn point out in *The Sibling Bond,* the early sibling relationship gets reactivated as elderly parents require extensive care.[1] In her book *Brothers and Sisters: How They Shape Our Lives,* Jane Mersky Leder describes the way that childhood relationships exert power over our adult sibling relationships.

> The quickness with which all the "stuff" from childhood can reduce adult siblings to kids again underscores the strong and complex connections between brothers and sisters. We can enter a family gathering as confident adults and exit feeling as unsettled as we did during childhood. Our siblings push buttons that cast us in roles we felt sure we had let go of long ago—the baby, the peacekeeper, the caretaker, the avoider.[2]

The most frequent conflicted sibling relationship that gets reawakened when elderly parents need help is sibling rivalry, and the most common brother-sister conflict relates to the splitting of responsibility and authority. The sister is the one most likely to have the day-to-day responsibility, while the brother is most likely to be seen as the authority (that is, the one who has the power of attorney, is executor of the will and makes the major financial decisions). In most families there is one primary caregiver who is responsible for the care of the parent. The vast majority of them receive little or no help from their siblings. For a female, having all male siblings greatly decreases the chances of getting help.[3] Thus, when

siblings are of different genders, there is an interplay of gender roles and psychodynamics.

You may assume that daughters were more likely to care
for their parents "in the old days" when fewer women were
employed outside the home. But research has shown that
college-educated women who have worked continuously
throughout their adulthood are more likely than homemakers
to become caregivers.[4] Just as most women add on a second
shift when they work outside the home, retaining their role as
primary parent and continuing to do the majority of the
housework, female caregivers who work outside the home
add on a third shift. While being employed reduces the average level of a son's caregiving by twenty hours a month, having a job does not reduce the level of his sister's assistance.[5]

Discussions comparing the way sisters and brothers care
for elderly parents parallel discussions of the gendered division of labor between husbands and wives. Husbands are
more likely to undertake tasks that have clear and identifiable
boundaries (for example, mowing the lawn) and tasks that
have greater discretion in how and when to complete them
(for example, minor household repairs). Wives, on the other
hand, are more likely to take responsibility for aspects of
family life that do not have clear and identifiable boundaries—keeping up relationships with family and friends,
making sure the children are happy in school, etc. They also
take primary responsibility for tasks that must be performed
on a regular basis such as shopping, cleaning, bathing the
children and cooking. Brothers and sisters divide caregiving
responsibilities along similar lines.[6]

In her book *Respecting Your Limits While Caring for Elderly
Parents,* Vivian Greenberg points out:

Over the years I have been struck by how much more difficult it is for daughters than for sons to set limits. As a result, caregiving is a more stressful experience for them than for their male counterparts. In an effort to be "good daughters" they place their needs secondary to those of their parents.[7]

Compared to sons, daughters use less replacement support and are more involved in their caregiving role.[8] Hence, sisters are more likely than brothers to experience caregiving as stressful. And the stress of the caregiver role tends to spill over to other aspects of the caregiver's life—for example, employment and family.[9] When compared to noncaregivers, female caregivers average three times as many stress symptoms, take more tranquilizers and antidepressants, and report substantially less participation in social and recreational activities.[10] Most important, daughters remain preoccupied with their parent's well-being even when not actually rendering instrumental assistance. In the daughter's eyes, caregiving (like mothering) is a boundless, all-encompassing activity rather than a clearly demarcated set of discrete tasks. For caregiver daughters, the dominant element (and burden) in their caregiving is not the particular chores they perform, but the continual sense of responsibility for their parents' emotional state. Women are simply more likely to *notice* a parent's emotional state. Sisters are much more likely than their brothers to be attuned to feelings and provide the emotional work of caring for elderly parents.[11]

When there are brothers and sisters, one of the sisters usually becomes the primary caregiver. Which sister becomes the primary caregiver is sometimes the result of geographic proximity. Frequently, adult offspring live far away from their parents. Only one-third of children aged forty-five to fifty-four live within fifty miles of their mothers (who might be married, divorced or widowed).[12] They may have moved away from where they grew up or their parents may have moved to another state in search of sun and leisure activities.

This makes it difficult for middle-aged children to manage their parents' care when they develop a chronic illness or become disabled. The burden usually falls on the sister living closest to the parents. Fifty percent of older parents live within five miles of their closest child—and the closest child is usually a daughter.[13] In these situations, the brother, often physically distant, tends to be given the authority in the parent's life, while his sister does the day-in and day-out caring for her parents.[14] The sister is left feeling unappreciated by her mother and angry toward her brother, who does little, but is idealized by their mother. For example, Gertrude is a seventy-two-year-old English teacher in a private school in Columbus, Ohio. She has a Ph.D. in English education and was chairperson of the English Department for many years. The day I interviewed her, her large dining room table was piled with term papers waiting to be graded. She describes her one-hundred-year-old mother's condition:

> My mother is physically very well, but she can't remember who I am. Sometimes she thinks I'm her sister—she asks me about Momma and Papa.

Gertrude's brother is five and a half years younger. The age and gender difference created a great deal of distance between them. Nevertheless, there is still competition. Gertrude told me that her brother is "a well-known professor" and when he is in town he visits his mother once a week and has lunch with her. However, he is rarely in town because he is often on leave, going to conferences and giving lectures. She feels that he assumes that his work is more important than hers.

Gertrude carries the emotional burden of caring for her mother.

> I pay the bills; go to the butcher; buy her underwear; pay the women who care for her. I call her every day. I would say he's involved minimally. He just went on an eight-month sabbatical. *They were away for eight months!* He came back three days after her stroke. I wrote him a note thanking him for the gift they brought me from their trip and telling him that I'm going to my college reunion next weekend. I got a message on my answering machine saying that he was going to Cleveland for the weekend. So he basically assumes I'm taking care of things.

When I asked Gertrude how it feels to be the one who takes care of things, at first she said what she feels is expected: "I don't mind doing it . . ." But then she added her feelings of resentment:

> I don't like the fact that he feels he can go and do whatever he wants and never tell me or ask me if it interferes with my plans. I don't think that if he knew what I was going to do that he would consider it when making his own plans. I happen to be a very loyal and conscientious person. I do what has to be done. Somebody has to do it.

Thus, it seems that overall the traditional expectations ascribed to male and female children are still intact for Gertrude and her brother. The experience of caring for her elderly mother has revived Gertrude's childhood feelings about differential expectations and treatment of her and her younger brother when they were children.

Gertrude and her brother are acting out their traditional roles in a family script in which every member has an internalized set of expectations. The current relationship is filtered through the internal one from the past. This is not limited to different gender-related expectations. For example, my friend Esther explained to me that her younger sister had always been sickly and her parents viewed everything she did in the context of overcoming adversity. Esther, on the other hand, was viewed as someone who had things easy and didn't exert herself. For Esther, these mental representations of herself and her sister continue into the stage of caregiving. Her sister views her professional work and family obligations as so taxing that finding time to care for her mother with Alzheimer's is almost impossible. On the other hand, she views Esther's professional work and family obligations as more flexible and less time consuming. Esther accepts this definition of herself, although it makes her angry. It feels "natural" to her. As a result, Esther spends much more time caring for her mother than her sister does and continues to feel a festering resentment at the inequity with which the burden is shared.

Esther and her sister illustrate that sibling relationships are not simply between the siblings, but they can also never be separate from the relationship to the parents. Sibling relationships take place in the context of a "family script" that involves a complex set of relationships between each child and each parent and each child in relation to the other children and each parent. We can see this more clearly when we look at the relationship between Karen and Robert.

CREATING A SIBLING CONNECTION THROUGH CAREGIVING: CHANGING OLD PATTERNS

Karen, Robert and Jane all live in the same small town where their mother lives, but until their mother got sick, they had very little to do with one another. I interviewed Karen and Robert. The social worker at the senior center suggested that I talk to them, but discouraged me when I suggested that I also call Jane; Robert and Karen similarly discouraged me from calling their sister. As a result, I can only include whatever I was able to glean about Jane's role in the family based on my interviews with Karen and Robert.

Karen is a forty-one-year-old married woman with two children. Although her older sister and brother are college graduates, Karen got married after high school and works part-time cleaning houses. She is a warm, pleasant woman who lives in a neat suburban house that is part of a subdivision.

Karen's mother had to organize her family's life around her husband's illness: Karen's father was diagnosed with cancer when she was a year old and he died when she was twelve.

Karen's mother cared for him all those years. Now, at seventy-three, her mother is dying.

The last six months have been very bad . . . She couldn't
get out of bed, couldn't eat, messes in the bathroom that I
had to clean up. She's in the hospital now. She has pneumonia.

Karen feels that she has to take care of her mother the way
her mother took care of her father.

I still feel like I'm supposed to take care of my mother. I
have this whole thing in my head. She took care of my father. She took care of my grandmother.

Karen strongly identifies with her mother as a caregiver to
her father and grandmother, and because Karen's father was
diagnosed with cancer when she was one, Karen's needs got
lost somewhere. Her mother must have been distraught; she
had already experienced two major losses and a trauma.

My mom lost two babies, a boy and a girl. She gave birth
and they died. One lived three hours and one lived three
days. When my sister came along she had a cleft palate, so
she needed extra care.

When Karen was born, Jane was two years old and Robert
was eight years old. In between, their mother had two still-
births and then gave birth to a baby with a cleft palate, Jane.
Very likely she was depressed and overwrought by the series
of traumas. Then within a year of Karen's birth, her father
was diagnosed with cancer. There was not much of a chance
for Karen to get her mother's focused attention. But what
made it even worse was that the other two siblings did not

nurture Karen either. They did not become a support system for one another as a result of their father's illness and mother's distraction. Rather, they remained emotionally isolated from each other, each one trying to get whatever they could from their parents and discounting one another.

> Recently, I'm finding out that Jane was Daddy's little girl. She's always hated my father, but now I realize she hated him for leaving. I was talking with my uncle about it . . . Robert was the apple of my mom's eye and Jane was the apple of my dad's eye.

If her sister was the apple of her father's eye and her brother was the apple of her mother's eye, and her mother was taken up with caring for her father, what happened to Karen? She was depressed. She describes symptoms of her childhood depression to me, although she doesn't name it as such.

> My sister says my mom yelled all the time when she was a child. I don't remember that. I slept all the time when I was a child. I don't know why.

Although she describes it to me, Karen does not seem to be in touch with how alone she felt as a child:

> When my mom knew that my dad was about to die, she sent my sister and I to my uncle's in Virginia for a couple of weeks. I remember my aunt coming into the little room where we were watching television and she said: "Your father passed away." I just went to my room and started crying. That was it really. I don't know how my sister and

brother reacted. My brother was twenty—he was in school.

Karen does not think it's strange that her mother sent her daughters away just before their father was about to die. None of the children were with him when he died. Karen was with her sister when she learned that her father died— but she went to her room in her uncle's house and cried alone. Her mother was not there to hug her and she could not emotionally connect with her sister, even at that moment. It made me teary to hear the story, but Karen told it matter-of-factly.

In *The Sibling Bond,* Stephen P. Bank and Michael D. Kahn point out that "sibling access" is a major determinant of the emotional bond between brothers and sisters. When siblings appear to have little emotional impact on one another, it's called "low access." Differences in age and sex diminish access by lessening the likelihood of common life experiences. Low-access siblings are often separated by more than eight or ten years, acting almost like members of different generations. In the case of Karen and Robert, they were six years apart. They had shared little time, space or personal history; they went to different schools and had different friends. They lacked a sense of shared history.

In addition, their parents discouraged them from creating an emotional bond and needing one another.[15] Sending Karen and Jane away and encouraging Robert to stay at college when their father was dying was a way of emotionally isolating the members of the family from one another. This kind of emotional isolation must have been typical for the family because Karen and Jane were only two years apart and they were physically together when they got the news of their father's death, but Karen went off and cried by herself and said she had no idea how Jane reacted. They did not feel that they needed each other.

In her loneliness, Karen turned to cleaning. Cleaning was a way of taking care of her mother and a way of feeling needed by her.

> My mother babied my sister and did everything for my sister. My sister never cleaned. She says she doesn't know how to clean. I always enjoyed cleaning. I would clean for my mother.

Karen defended against her aching by taking care of her mother and later in life it extended to other people. In fact, she told me that when her mother dies she is going to volunteer to clean the houses of old people. She said it made her feel good. Instead of experiencing her own wish to be taken care of, she helps others. And through her kindness, she can identify with the people she cares for so well.

Karen resisted setting limits on her caregiving even when it impinged upon her own children.

> I have an eight-year-old and a twelve-year-old. I could leave them home a little bit. But if I went to my mom's for fifteen minutes, it could be three hours later that I got home. I was over there all the time. When the kids were in school, I would drop them at school and go over there. I found this summer . . . was very hard—a real struggle. The guilt

of not being with my mom and having my kids . . . I was juggling all that.

The social worker at the senior center told Karen that she needed to take care of her husband and children.

Mom took care of my dad until the day he died. I said that to Bonnie [the social worker at the senior center] and she said: "Yes, that was her husband. But this is your husband. This is your mom but you have a family of your own."

Karen felt that Bonnie "gave her permission" to take care of her own family without feeling guilty about her mother. Bonnie represented the "good mother" who helped Karen set limits. Having a husband and two children was not enough for Karen to give herself permission to set limits caring for her mother. The event that enabled Karen to seek help from Bonnie was her husband's sickness. She became overwhelmed as a caregiver to both her mother and her husband. With Bonnie's help, Karen was able to transfer her identification with her mother as caregiver to her father, to her mother as caregiver to her own husband.

My husband just went through angioplasty. I took him to the emergency room at three o'clock in the morning. He woke me up and said: "I don't know, but I think I want to go to the hospital. I'm having these pains in my chest."

At that point in our conversation, Karen's eight-year-old son, Johnny, who had been listening intently for the last few minutes, corrected her.

No, Mom you took him to the hospital at three o'clock in the morning the first time, and then the second time, when he needed the angioplasty, it was just before I had to go to school.

Reflecting his anxiety about his father's health, Johnny knew every detail of his father's medical problems. Karen accepted his amendment to the story and continued:

The family doctor said to him that he couldn't keep putting off these tests. She scared him enough to take the test—an angiogram. When it was over the doctor came out and said we had two options—bypass surgery or angioplasty. He recommended angioplasty. I realized then that I'm needed here. I realized if my mom needs more care, we'll get it for her.

Despite her own childhood experience with a sick father, Karen did not seem to realize that her children would be deeply affected by their father's illness and Karen's over-involvement with her mother. Karen was unable to separate from her mother. She said: "I realized then that I'm needed here." She never realized that before because her mother was the center of her universe. Karen's desperate need to take care of her mother is rooted in her wish to be special to her mother in a way that she never was as a child. As a result, her son has his own separation problems. Johnny has developed a phobia about leaving the house because he has an insecure attachment to his mother as a result of her inability to separate from her mother. She whispered, so that her son could not overhear:

It helped me set my priorities. My son is having a very bad problem with everything going on. I explained to the pediatrician and she said she wants me to take him to a psychiatrist . . . He doesn't want to go to anyone's house. It's happened since Grandma went downhill and my husband has been sick.

Karen has been able to set limits on her mother's care, but only because she has transferred her need to be needed to her husband and her son. Unfortunately, instead of fostering a healthy sense of self and the confidence to move out into the world, the message to Karen's son is that the only way he can engage his mother is to stay home and need her to take care of him.

Karen's twelve-year-old daughter, Sarah, on the other hand, has developed a way of coping with her mother's absence that is based on her identification with her mother—she has become a caregiver. Her best friend has juvenile diabetes and she goes to the doctor with her and cares for her. When her friend went to an out-of-town hospital for medical tests she joined her for the trip. Unfortunately, Sarah and Johnny do not seem to have developed a supportive sibling bond. Sarah seems to spend most of her time away from home caring for her friend, while Johnny remains home suffering from intense anxiety.

One major reason for Karen's reluctance to turn to her brother for help is her internalized representation of Robert as distant and uninterested in her. Her complementary self-representation is as a needy child with nothing to offer her big brother. He is older, but he never took care of her. He stayed away from home as much as possible. Since he was the only boy and his mother's favorite child, Karen felt she could not compete with Robert; she could only clean in the hopes of getting her mother to love her. She has always seen Robert as powerful, distant and rejecting.

As a result of the consultation with Bonnie, Karen turned, for the first time, to her brother, Robert, for help. Robert is a forty-nine-year-old single man. He's tall and heavyset and seems uncomfortable and on edge. As I sat at the conference table in his office, I wondered why he volunteered to be interviewed. He seemed reluctant to talk, almost angry. He told me that he, Karen and Jane were never very close; he said they have nothing in common.

Although the three siblings were brought up in the same family and live within a mile of one another, Robert feels that they are all totally different—he "disidentifies" with both his sisters. In *The Sibling Bond,* Bank and Kahn point out that the disowning is usually the prerogative of the most favored child. It is unilateral—the privilege of the entitled child. Robert was the eldest child, the only son and his mother's favorite. He had the longest time with his father before he became ill. He monopolized the family's meager emotional riches and refused to protect his younger sisters. Instead, he felt superior to them and avoided uniting with them. He chose to stay at college when his father was about to die.[16]

Robert's interest in theater, which developed during the years of his father's illness, was another way of setting himself off from his sisters, and a way of distracting himself from what was going on at home. He went to school and stayed there for rehearsals after school, evenings and weekends. The "theater family" replaced his own family. Immersing himself in fantasy with a group of supportive teachers and friends must have been a welcome escape from his father's dying and his mother's depression. Although he did not make theater his career, he is still very active as an amateur. For Robert, the theater "is his life." He is not married, and until his mother got sick, he did not view his sisters as part of his life. At the end of the interview Robert said that he and Karen do love each other and they both love their mother and are trying to get the best care for her. Caring for their mother has given Robert more empathy for Karen.

I interviewed Robert when his mother was in the hospital—about two weeks before she entered a nursing home. He described his mother's condition:

> She went into the hospital because she had pneumonia, and broke her leg while she was there. She can't be left alone, and despite all of Karen's efforts and visiting nurses for the past year, there are periods when she's alone and in danger. She doesn't take her medicine properly, she loses her balance and falls, and her personal hygiene is getting worse.

Robert told me that his mother was going downhill and he convinced his sisters, despite Karen's reluctance, that she had to go into a nursing home when she got out of the hospital. He does not want Karen to be left with the burden of his mother any longer. He is worried about her, but knows that Jane will not offer her help and he feels that he cannot give the time that it would take to help Karen care for her if their mother went back home.

Jane lives in her mother's house. As Robert puts it: "She just never moved out." Robert said that Jane had epilepsy as a child and it affected her relationships with other children. He alluded to Jane's having other medical and psychological problems as well that might explain why she was living with her mother at forty-three, but he made it clear he was not going to explain it to me. Karen, on the other hand, seemed quite open about it as we sat in her kitchen a month later and talked about her family. She told me that Jane was born with a cleft palate and had gone through many operations. Despite the difference in their willingness to discuss Jane, both Karen and Robert accept that their sister cannot or will not help them in caring for their mother. Karen offered her understanding of why Jane is not interested in caring for her mother.

> Jane says that Mom's been yelling at her all her life. I don't remember that. I slept all the time as a child, I don't know why. When my mom is really bad she's really abusive. Jane says: "I'm used to this, she's yelled at me all my life."

Neither Robert nor Karen expressed any disappointment that Jane is not an equal partner in the process of caring for their mother. Their acceptance of Jane's refusal to participate in caring for their mother seems to be based on her traditional role in the family. She had medical issues, and so they seem to have learned not to expect anything from her. Indeed, this seems to have had secondary benefits for Jane. For example, although Jane is a college graduate and has a good job, Robert told me that he and Karen will give her the house that she shared with her mother when their mother dies.

Eventually, because of Robert's prodding, Karen agreed to put her mother in a nursing home. Before that, Robert told me he was afraid Karen was going to have a nervous breakdown because of the pressure of caring for her mother, her guilt about putting her in a nursing home and her responsibility for her sick husband.

Karen was cleaning my mother's house and taking her to doctors and doing everything she could. It was overburdening her. She has two kids and a sick husband.

Once Karen told Robert how overburdened she felt, the three siblings were able to share their experience of how difficult it was to deal with their mother. Before they put her in a nursing home, she needed twenty-four-hour care, but wanted to be at home, yet complained that there were too many people in the house. At that time Robert told me about how difficult it was to deal with his mother:

She's refusing help. We got someone from the Visiting Nurses Association aside from the nurse, but my mother started arguing by the second day. We can't get through to her that she's not helping herself. And if she goes into a nursing home, she'll probably not talk to anyone. But picking her up off the floor at 3 a.m. kills me. I'm a night person and I've only gone to bed at 2 a.m. and then I have to get up and go over there because she's fallen. It's difficult when someone just won't see what's right for them. The three of us got together and I said we just have to deal with the fact that we may have to force her to go into a nursing home.

Karen said that Robert didn't realize how much caregiving she had been doing. After her hospital stay, when it was clear that twenty-four-hour care was necessary, it was Robert that insisted that they had to put their mother in a nursing home despite her protestations.

These three siblings grew up so distant from one another, each trying to deal in his or her own way with a dying father and an overburdened mother, and they may never be emotional intimates. But the experience of caring for their mother brought them closer together. Robert says:

> The three of us have meetings now to talk about my mother. Before that we rarely saw one another and never got together with the three of us. I hope Karen gets over this and learns. She's got in-laws and her husband has only one brother, who is like my middle sister—pretty self-centered. Caring for her in-laws will fall on Karen, and knowing her she will feel the responsibility to do something.

Brothers and sisters draw on cultural definitions of gender that associate women with family work regardless of whether they are also employed outside the home. In most families in which there is a son and a daughter, gender is used as a taken-for-granted way to assign tasks.[17]

But that alone does not explain why Karen had so much trouble setting limits on her caregiving and why she did not turn to her sister and brother for help until she was desperate and felt out of control. That is not simply a function of gender, but the specific psychodynamic constellation in her family. Karen's father was very sick during her childhood;

her sister Jane had serious physical and emotional problems; and her mother was working to support the family and caring for her husband. Robert might have taken up the slack and been a nurturer to Karen, but he didn't. He turned away from the intense family problems and put his energy into school and theater productions. Instead of the children developing a support system for one another, they each existed in an isolated state, each developing their own adaptive strategies—cleaning for Karen, theater for Robert and being sick for Jane.

SIBLING RELATIONSHIPS can never be separate from the relationship to the parents. Hence, working out relationships among siblings involves working out feelings about parents as well. Sibling relationships occur in the context of a "family script" involving a complex set of relationships between each child and each parent and each child in relation to the other children and each parent.

Mutuality among adult siblings depends on feeling securely separate, which is based on having basic needs met early. Mutuality also means being able to see the other person as separate and having needs that are different from yours. It involves being able to feel that you are similar in certain ways, but different in others; it involves offering support and compassion, but not unquestioning loyalty. Mutuality allows for closeness that is not exclusive; it leaves room for other significant emotional relationships. If siblings had to band together because of a lack of parental involvement or they were alienated and polarized because of parental favoritism, mutuality is difficult to attain. In both cases, the identities of siblings remain entangled. Whether you remain tied to your brothers and sisters, or separate from them in ways that can never be bridged, the lifelong quest for a secure personal identity is inextricably woven into that of your brother or sister.

Robert, Karen and Jane did not get their own individual needs met enough to develop mutuality as children. Each one was too needy. Each one developed some way of trying to get their needs met. Now, with the crisis of their mother's illness, they are talking to one another on a regular basis. For the first time in their lives, these three siblings are sharing their experiences of their mother. They are beginning to partially identify with one another in a way that they were not able to as children, and they are developing mutuality which will benefit them all.

Part III

ETHNICITY
AND GENDER

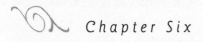

Chapter Six

CULTURAL SCRIPTS
FOR CAREGIVERS

Where I come from, in the islands—Jamaica—this is
what you do. A mother has a daughter to take care of her
when she gets old. This is our role; we grow up this way.

IN PREVIOUS CHAPTERS I have talked about the effects of
psychological and family dynamics on caregiving. However,
those dynamics play out within a social and cultural context.
The priority we give to our own needs as compared to our
children's or parents' needs is a combination of cultural and
psychological factors. Just as there are cultural scripts for
motherhood, there are cultural scripts for caregiving.

Though there is never a perfect correspondence between
individual behavior and cultural prescriptions for how and
what should take place, the script is like a map that guides
most people's choices.[1] Even if we don't follow the cultural
prescription, it impinges upon us. We feel we *should* be behaving in a particular way or we might imagine that other
people in our cultural group are critical of our choices—and

they *might* be. The interaction between the cultural and psychological scripts results in the particular constellation of caregiving in each family.

The dominant American cultural script for caregiving is that *a daughter* takes primary responsibility for caring for elderly parents.[2] Middle-aged daughters represent 77 percent of the children providing care for elderly parents.[3] However, in Chinese and Indian families the oldest son has primary responsibility for caring for his parents, though his wife does the work. In rural Ireland in the nineteenth century, when the eldest son inherited the family farm, the wife of the son who was going to inherit the farm was expected to look after her parents-in-law. But in urban America, women of Irish ancestry are expected to look after their own parents. Since Irish elderly are more likely to be born in the United States than Chinese elderly, for example, the cultural expectations of women of Irish ancestry are more congruous with those of the dominant American culture in contrast with women of Chinese ancestry.[4]

To some degree, the process of caregiver selection transcends cultural differences. Cultural values mediate the process primarily with respect to the gender of the child expected to assume the primary *responsibility*. Nevertheless it is usually a female who will take the primary caregiver role—either a daughter or a daughter-in-law.

Cultural differences not only affect *who* is deemed responsible for caring for elderly parents, but also *how*. For example, Latino-American and Caribbean-American caregivers tend to reject the idea of nursing homes—not just for financial reasons, but for moral reasons. They often feel that their parents *should* live with them and they should take care of them regardless of how they *feel* about them. During the waves of migration in the 1950s and '60s, Caribbean parents often migrated to the United States or to England without their children—leaving them behind with relatives for as long as five years. Despite their having been left behind, most of these now middle-aged daughters completely accept their role as caregiver to their aging parents and often care for the mother substitutes (that is, grandmothers, aunts, older sisters or cousins) who filled in while their mothers worked in the United States or England.

Italian-Americans also tend to reject institutional help and feel that they should personally care for their elderly parents even if they are incontinent and suffering from dementia. On the other hand, non-Orthodox Jews tend to feel that they have responsibility to see that their parents are cared for—but they don't necessarily have to *do it*.

The reality of different cultural scripts becomes clear when we look at the living situations of elderly members of different ethnic groups. For example, 28 percent of all Americans over sixty-five live alone, but only 12.9 percent of Asian-Americans and 18.2 percent of Latinos do. In contrast, 29.4 percent of non-Latino blacks over sixty-five live alone. Four percent of all Americans over sixty-five live with a child, but 22 percent of Asian-Americans do because of their strong feelings about honoring their parents. Almost 5 percent of the American population over sixty-five is institutionalized, but only 2.4 percent of the Latino elderly and 1.5 percent of Asians are. Asians, Latinos and blacks have strong cultural beliefs about family obligations and preferred living arrangements—they are much more likely to live with a demented parent than a white caregiver.[5]

At a recent conference, Ron Adelman, the cochief of the Division of Geriatric Medicine and Gerontology at the Weill Medical College of Cornell University, got a warm welcome from the gathering of social workers who had come to a panel titled "Can My Eighties Be Like My Fifties?" at the New York Academy of Medicine. Ron is a warm man who spoke about the need to train young physicians to speak to their elderly patients when they had a question rather than turning to their children as if the elderly person was invisible. He told a story about a patient he knew so well that he could tell that the patient had an infection because he was behaving differently in his office.

Then Ron told a story about his own father. When he lay in the hospital wanting to die, he said to his son: "Ron, don't do anything to help me that could get you in trouble." I'm not sure if he had tears in his eyes or if I was projecting because I had tears in my eyes. What a caring thing for his father to say to him; he wanted to protect his son to the very end. It was such a contrast to my father's words to me when he was dying: "Take care of your mother." I thought to myself that probably much of the reason Ron is such a caring doctor is because he had such a caring father. That must be why he feels so empathetic toward elderly people. Yet even though his father was so concerned with Ron's happiness and my father was not concerned with mine, we share the same cultural script. We were brought up with the expectation that when our parents got older, we would make sure they got the care they needed. But we never considered having them live with us. That is something we identify with the first generation of immigration from Europe. My grandmother lived with my aunt Hannah, but Hannah's children never considered the possibility of her living with them.

After Ron spoke, Michael Diaz, professor of medicine at Mount Sinai Medical Center, introduced himself. "Hi, I'm Mike," he said, immediately making it clear that he did not want to pull rank on a roomful of social workers. Mike told us that he was born in Puerto Rico and had come to East Harlem with his parents as a baby. He talked about how elderly Hispanic and black people come to the doctor's office with one or more family members. He seemed to be chiding those of us (like me) who sent an aide to the doctor's office with one of our parents when it was an inconvenient time for us—or worse yet let the parent go alone. He said that white doctors didn't even have enough chairs in their waiting rooms for relatives because they expect black and Hispanic families to behave like their own.

Mike takes pride in being Puerto Rican. He uses Spanish intermittently in his talk the way Jewish doctors sometimes use Yiddish expressions. He proudly told us that when he got married and he and his wife bought a house, they bought one that had an extra floor for the express purpose of having it available for their parents to live with them when they got older—and, indeed, his parents did live with him.

Here were two "good sons." Each one spoke lovingly of his parents. Each one feels great empathy for elderly people. Yet one, the Jewish doctor, never dreamed of having his parents live with him; while the other, a Puerto Rican doctor, would never have thought of his parents *not* living with him.

Even when the social class is the same (they are both doctors), having come from different ethnic backgrounds, their cultural scripts are different.

While it is true that the dominant American script for caregiving is that *a daughter* is supposed to take primary responsibility for caring for elderly parents, if there is no daughter, a son may end up being the caregiver—particularly if he is an only child or if he is Hispanic or Italian.

AN ITALIAN SON

At sixty-six years old, Vinny is a widower taking care of his ninety-four-year-old father. Vinny feels that he has no choice; he feels this is what he's "supposed" to do. He and his wife took care of her mother for eighteen years before she died at ninety-four.

> She came to live with us when I was forty-one, twenty-five years ago. We never went on vacation. We went out sometimes because my son lived upstairs, but we couldn't go away for any length of time.

According to Vinny's cultural script, like Mike Diaz's, elderly parents live with their children and it doesn't matter how the children feel about it or what condition the parents are in. Vinny described his mother-in-law's condition:

> We had to put a rope from her bedroom to the bathroom because she would stray. She'd go to the bathroom and end up in our bedroom turning the light on in the middle of the night.

"Did she have Alzheimer's?" I asked. Vinny didn't know. They never took her to a neurologist to find out. It didn't matter. Whatever it was, they would take care of her. His mother-in-law died in 1990 and then, in 1994, Vinny's mother died. "My father has macular degeneration. So he couldn't live alone, he had to come and live with us." Vinny could see no other options. In reality he had several choices: He could have found an assisted living facility for his father; he could have hired a visiting nurse to come to his house; or he could have insisted that his brother take more responsibility for his father.

"How did you feel about your father coming to live with you?" I asked.

"I had no choice, what could I do?"

My question reflects my cultural script: How you *feel* is a major consideration in making decisions. Vinny's answer ignores the issue of how he felt about it. It reflects the combination of his cultural script and his depression. In reality, Vinny had several choices, but he could not consider them. He had an internalized cultural script for what "a good son," an *Italian* son, is supposed to do, but he also has an insecure attachment to his father. He needs his father's approval and he cannot tolerate being separate from him. That would involve tolerating his father's anger and disappointment that Vinny will not give up his life for him. Vinny complains:

> He can't see and he depends on me for everything. But it's really hard. Like I could just have a cup of coffee and run out the door. But he wants breakfast and so I have to make him this big breakfast every morning. I met a woman, but

I can never see her. Taking care of my father is holding me back. I don't have a life. When I walk out of the house I feel guilty that he's alone. It's a lousy feeling that the only way out of it is my father dying.

I asked Vinny if he has thought about hiring some help. He said that he can't get an aide paid for by the state because his father has too much money. He owns too many houses—four of them. I asked him if he considered the possibility of paying for help. But he said that's impossible because his father won't spend the money. To underscore the point, he told me:

I go to Arizona with my father for the winter. But all I do is work when I get there. His houses need a lot of work and next to his house he bought this piece of property and planted this big garden. We call it a "Guinea garden." He's got lemon trees, olive trees, all kinds of trees, but they all have to be taken care of. When I went there with my wife she said: "You can't do this. This is ridiculous. You're retired."

Vinny's father's refusal to spend money keeps Vinny taking care of him. For example, Vinny recounted that he wanted to get him a Med Alert. He explained that his father could wear it around his neck so that Vinny would feel comfortable going out and leaving him alone. When Vinny explained this to his father he said: "How much is it?" Vinny told him the price and he said: "I don't need that." So Vinny feels he cannot leave his father alone. At sixty-six Vinny still feels that whatever his father says goes. He cannot stand up to his father or even his older brother.

Vinny's brother, Sal, is three and a half years older. Vinny said that Sal doesn't offer to help.

> Even when my wife was sick and I was caring for my wife *and* my father, Sal never offered to take my father. Everybody says, Why don't you tell your brother that you each have to take your father for six months? I can't do it. My father would feel like I was throwing him out.

Although Sal does not participate in the care of his father, it is Sal who has power of attorney. Vinny explained: "We're Italians—he's the oldest brother, so he has the authority."

Vinny is a good example of the interaction between cultural and psychological scripts. He is Italian, but he is also clinically depressed. He feels powerless and hopeless. He feels guilty because his only relief will come when his father dies. His normal activities are constricted by the kind of caregiving he feels obligated to perform. He is engulfed by his father's needs and demands and cannot separate enough to have a relationship with a woman. Since he is a retired widower, caring for his father is his only role and has probably intensified his feeling like a little boy who has to "obey" his father and older brother. His older brother is also Italian and, of course, has the same controlling and demanding father. But Sal seems to have been able to separate more. He does not need to show his father what a good son he is—perhaps because he feels more secure in his attachment to his father.

Vinny's brother seems to have cast off his responsibility as the older son in an Italian family. On the other hand, Vinny feels hog-tied by his cultural script. How can he have a life that is separate from his father without discarding heartfelt traditions? Vinny has to set limits so that he is able to take care of himself, and his father gets the care he needs. Of course, the care he *needs* is not necessarily the same as the care he *wants*. Once he makes that distinction, Vinny will have to tolerate his father's complaints and accept that his father may not appreciate him, even though he is striving to do the right thing.

AN AFRICAN-AMERICAN DAUGHTER

Traditionally, studies of ethnicity showed that elderly non-Hispanic blacks were less likely to be in nursing homes than non-Hispanic white elderly. However, the trend has been toward convergence in the last thirty years.[6] In 1990, 3.1 percent of black (non-Hispanic) Americans over sixty-five were institutionalized as compared to 3.3 percent of non-Hispanic whites. In 2000, 5.4 percent of non-Hispanic blacks over sixty-five lived in institutions. Indeed, the percentage of blacks over sixty-five in institutions was actually slightly higher than the percent of white (non-Hispanic) Americans. A recent study argues that young blacks have strong ideals of filial obligation and do not generally want to put their kin in nursing homes. Black caregivers report that they were brought up with the expectation of becoming caregivers—many have been caregivers from an early age. The authors of a study of black caregivers in Ohio point out that there is a "culture of caring."[7] Sixty-two percent of black nursing home residents as compared to 23.2 percent of other residents, for example, lived with children before entering nursing homes. In other words, living with children seems to be part of an elderly black person's trajectory into a nursing home much more commonly than it is for white elderly. However, the higher levels of impairment of the black elders may often make it impossible for their children to care for them at home despite their commitment to do so. Sally is trying to keep her mother out of a nursing home despite the high personal cost to her and her children and the protestations of her siblings.

Sally called the Senior Day Care Center to find out if I was coming to interview caregivers. She wanted to make sure that I would interview her. I called to tell her that I had reached my quota of interviews, but she pleaded with me. I told her I could only fit her in early on Saturday morning. She said that was fine; she wanted to talk to me. I wondered why she was so eager to tell me her story. When I arrived at the center, at 8 a.m., Sally was waiting for me. She is an attractive African-American woman wearing a stylish black suit. She greets me warmly as I come in apologizing for being a few minutes late because I got lost. She's eager to talk and seems excited about our interview.

She is a forty-one-year-old divorced mother of four. Her husband left her five years ago. She has three daughters, seven, ten, and fourteen years old and a nineteen-year-old son. Her ten-year-old daughter has cerebral palsy. When Sally's mother's friends called her and told her that her mother was incontinent and could not take care of herself, Sally took the three-hour drive to check on her. Her mother wasn't taking her medicines because she couldn't remember what to take or when. Initially, Sally hoped she could keep her mother in her apartment and visit her a couple of days a week. However, when Sally came back after each visit, her mother called every few minutes to ask her something.

Finally, Sally's five brothers and sisters decided their mother could no longer live alone. Sally describes her mother as a sixty-three-year-old in the body of an eighty-year-old. She has kidney failure as a result of diabetes, so she is required to be on dialysis three days each week, and her right leg has been amputated. She had a stroke and has dementia. Sally says her siblings all pointed to her as the one who should take care of her mother because she's not married and she is a nurse. They did not seem to consider that she is a working single mother with four children, one of whom is disabled.

> To be honest I really didn't want to take care of my mother. I was going through a divorce and it was too much. I was overwhelmed. But it's always been like that all my life. I was the one they called "the workhorse." They knew I didn't want my mom in a nursing home and if that was the alternative I would do it. My mom got really sick and my brother went to get her and just dropped her off at my house!

Sally was working 11 a.m. to 7 p.m. as well as caring for her children when her mother arrived at her doorstep. "It was unbelievable." Sally had not lived with her mother since she left home at seventeen to go to the state college. Since Sally's mother had never been willing to help care for her grandchildren, Sally's children did not know their grandmother very well. Her three daughters share a room and her son has a room so Sally gave her mother her bedroom.

> During that time my younger sister took my mom on weekends, but she and my mother never got along. My sis-

ter already had marital problems before my mother arrived, but then my mother was incontinent and would shit
all over the house and walk around naked in front of my
brother-in-law. My sister would call and tell me she was
going to throw my mother out the window. I would come
to the rescue. But after a while I just couldn't do it anymore. I'd go over to their house and my sister and brother-
in-law were fighting and I'd have to clean my mother and
get her dressed and take her home with me.

Why was Sally willing to take on the added responsibility
of caring for her mother when she was already overwhelmed
by her husband leaving her to support and care for four
children? She was not motivated by the hope of mutual
assistance because her mother had never cared for her
grandchildren when she was well and was now unable to
help in any way. Sally was not motivated by love and respect.
She did not feel that she owed her mother anything. I think
the answer is in Sally's identification as the "hero" of the
family.

Sally's mother and father separated when she was twelve—
her mother took the children and left. Sally says her father
didn't pay child support so her mom cleaned schools and
people's houses. Sally says she was the only one who could
sit down and talk to her father. He drank and was abusive to
her mother and the children. He worked in the steel mills
and was often laid off. He traveled to different places to get
work. She recalls watching him waiting for his check to come.

He smoked and he would smoke while he was eating.
Sometimes he didn't finish eating and he put his plate in

the refrigerator and he dropped ashes in the plate. Then he'd come home at 2 a.m. and wake us all up and line us up and scream that one of us is doing voodoo on him and we put ashes in his food. He'd beat us. Then we went to sleep and woke up the next morning and went to school. We knew it was going to happen. Then he'd give us "times off." He said our bottoms were getting too used to it so he'd give us "times off." Then it would start again.

I asked Sally if her father was drunk when he did this and she said no, she thinks he was psychotic.

He used to do this thing we called "fighting with the devil." My dad would go to the graveyard and bring dirt back to the house. He'd be yelling and hitting himself. When we got out of school, we knew we better have the house clean. We knew he'd beat us. We couldn't hear his car coming, hear his steps. We knew we had to get out of his way. If he were happy in the morning, he'd be abusive in the evening. If he were abusive in the evening, he'd be happy in the morning.

I asked Sally, "What did your mother do?" Her reply was that her mother did nothing. In fact, her father sexually abused her and her sister Lilly. She said he would make excuses to drive her somewhere and sexually abuse her in the car. She described her fantasy of screaming at the people passing by on the street: "Help me, help me." But she was silent.

She feels that her mother did not know he was abusing her, but she feels her mother knew he was abusing her sister.

My mother was very harsh with my younger sister. She was my father's favorite and my mother hated her. She would take an extension cord when Lilly was in the bath and hit her with it in the tub. Or other times my father was away and we'd all be scared and run to my mother's bedroom and she'd make Lilly leave and go upstairs alone. Lilly would be crying and yelling.

Sally said that once her sister showed her a story in the newspaper about a girl who accused her father of sexually abusing her and her mother threw her out of the house. They both smiled knowingly—they felt their mother would do the same thing.

Considering that her mother did not protect her from her father and was abusive toward her younger sister, it is hard to understand how it came to pass that Sally's mother lived with her for almost a year until Sally was able to put her mother in a low-income senior citizen apartment complex.

As I listened to Sally's story about her mother coming to stay with her, I thought to myself that it sounded like she was on the brink of a major depression during that time. She was suffering from chronic fatigue, anger and frustration. But then Sally's face changed. The anger and frustration were gone. To my surprise, she said:

I believe it was God that made a great difference. I was resistant to taking care of my mom. I respected her as my mom, but never had any deep love for her. But when I began to take care of her something in me began to happen. What has happened is that taking care of her made me start to [her face beaming] *fall in love with her*. I began to see things in her the way I see things in my children. All my energies turned to trying to make her survive and have a quality life. When she first came to my house I got a prognosis of two years and it's been three years.

As for so many African-American caregivers, her religious belief has been a major support for Sally. She feels a sense of personal enrichment and character building as a result of caring for her mother. Sally explained that she went to college to become a nurse, but she never graduated; she got pregnant and dropped out. Her mother was very disappointed in her.

So when my mother was at her worst, refusing to eat and wanting to die after her leg was amputated, I told her I was going to go back to school and she had to eat so that she could see me walk across the stage and get my diploma. My mother began to eat again. Last year I walked across the stage and she was there. That was the happiest moment of my life. It's made me a better person.

Sally went on to explain that: "This is life. Things happen and they don't happen the way we want, but then you have to be more organized." Sally had to deal with her mother's surgeries, her daughter's seizures and having finals all at the same time! To my amazement, she said:

It made me know what true love was all about. I never felt love for her, but when she was so tired and I would say: "Mom I need you to help, stand up." I could see her trying so hard. She would cry out for me: "Sally, Sally." It did something to me. I felt it's not all about me. You have to make sacrifices—I think my character has improved. I look at life differently.

Whereas Vinny's caregiving has led to a constriction of his social life and normal activities—living with his father has made him feel less and less like a man and more and more like a boy—Sally's caregiving has enhanced her sense of competence. It has increased her feeling of mastery and her self-esteem. She went back to finish college while caring for her mother. She was able to get low-cost housing for her mother and found a center where her mother can be cared for during the day. Sally goes to her mother's house every morning before she goes to work to wake her up, take her vital signs, give her medicine and get her dressed and ready to take the van to the day-care center. Then after work, Sally meets her mom at the van and stays for several hours. I asked her how she manages this with four children at home. Sally reassured me that she has raised them to take care of themselves. She told me that she prepares their meals ahead of time, but in an emergency her fourteen-year-old daughter and nineteen-year-old son know how to prepare meals. She casually explained that they have a pager so that if her ten-year-old daughter has a seizure, one of the older children pages her. Her sisters and brothers took a vote and decided their mother should be put in a nursing home, but Sally has the power of attorney and she refuses to do it.

Caring for her mother makes her feel like a hero—she is single-handedly saving her mother, and the gratification of that seems to outweigh the costs. Part of me is in awe of Sally. She has been able to turn her caregiving into a growth-promoting, transformative experience. But then, there is another part of me that has my own cultural script. My script says: Caring for your children takes precedence over caring for your parents. Clearly, her children are paying a price for their mother's heroism. Sally's two older children are left to care for themselves and their two younger sisters, one of whom is disabled. That does not seem to cause Sally any conflict. Perhaps this is due to her cultural script for mothering. Like so many African-American mothers, Sally feels that she needs to prepare her children to take care of themselves. Or perhaps it has more to do with her personal psychological script—her insecure attachment to her mother makes her need to feel close to her mother and appreciated by her. Wanting to be close to and appreciated by your mother can be a positive thing, but for Sally it is a driving force that keeps her focused so intensely on her mother that her children's needs become incidental. Hence, she has reproduced the same dynamic in the next generation. Her two older children are "heroes" in the making. They are doing the mothering while their mother is being a "good daughter."

A PUERTO RICAN DAUGHTER

Although the Latino population is composed of many diverse subgroups, extended family plays a salient role for all of them. Respect for elders is paramount, so it is no surprise that elderly Latinos are more likely to live with their children than in any other ethnic group.[8] While dementia greatly increases the chances that a non-Latino white elder will be put in a nursing home, Latino caregivers are less disturbed by memory loss and the inability to communicate.

Maria is a fifty-one-year-old single professor. Her seventy-nine-year-old mother has lived with her for the last six years, beginning soon after she was diagnosed with Alzheimer's disease. When Maria greeted me and escorted me into her office, she excused herself for a minute before we began our interview. When she returned Maria was beaming and handed me a picture of her mother wearing a graduation cap. The caption under her name said "Doctor of Philosophy, *honoris causa.*" Although her mother cannot speak or move, Maria was eager to have me meet her and gave me the picture because the venue for the interview was changed from her house to her office and I would not get to meet her.

Maria explained that her mother, Hortensia, was a well-educated woman. Hortensia's father was the mayor of their town and a political activist. When he had a stroke, Hortensia dropped out of college to care for him because she was the eldest daughter in the family and felt it was her obligation. Maria's father, on the other hand, was one of seventeen children born on a farm and only had an eighth-grade education. Indeed, her parents first met when her mother was teaching her father, Carlos, to speak English as a second language in preparation for his family moving to the mainland. Maria believes Hortensia saw Carlos as someone who would offer her adventure and take her away from her caregiving role with her father, but ironically she ended up taking care of Carlos—first by supporting his driving need to prove himself worthy of her and later by caring for him when he became ill.

Maria's parents married and moved to the South Bronx with his family in 1947. Maria says that although her mother loved her father, marrying a man of a lower social class had lifelong consequences for her. Her family remained in Puerto Rico and her mother never approved of the marriage. While Hortensia was able to be a teacher in Puerto Rico, in New York she could not teach without a college degree. She worked as a seamstress in a factory doing piecework, while her husband worked in a bodega. Maria remembers that there was never enough money, but there was always food. Her father dreamed of owning his own bodega (which he eventually did) and becoming middle class. He was driven. Maria describes him as a hardworking but macho man who was very controlling. She feels that her mother's identity faded away. In fact, Maria has her own theory about the etiology of Alzheimer's based on her feelings about her parents. She believes that people who lose their sense of self because of a controlling spouse or parent are more likely to develop the disease. So although Maria speaks lovingly of her father, she sees her mother's marriage to him as tragic in some way—her mother was never the same. I wondered, as I listened to her theory of how living with a controlling person can lead to losing your self and your mind, if that might be related to Maria's choice to remain single.

At first Maria told me that she is the primary caregiver because her sister, Victoria, has lupus, but as we talked more Maria said that there are deeper reasons. She explained that her mother always favored her sister.

My mother always paid more attention to my sister. She had more needs. She was always sick and they never figured out what was wrong with her. She had headaches. She was tired.

Maria tried to be the opposite. She developed a strong persona, she tried to look tough and not need anything. Her father worked twelve to fifteen hours a day, seven days a week, and since her mother was also working, Maria was often left in the care of her older sister, Victoria. While Maria says that Victoria made lunch and loved to clean the house, she was not very nurturing. Nevertheless, Maria says:

A lot of people say my mother has advanced Alzheimer's, she can't walk or talk. Why don't you put her in a nursing home?

Maria feels they just don't understand. First, they don't understand that Puerto Rican daughters don't put their mothers in nursing homes—no matter how poorly they might function. Moreover, Maria says they don't know her mother and that she still is attached despite the Alzheimer's disease. But, I think what they don't understand is Maria's attachment to her mother. They don't understand the gratification that Maria gets from caring for her mother. For example, when I first met her at her office she told me about losing her briefcase the day before. It contained student papers, her Palm Pilot and other irreplaceable items. I could feel the anxiety well up in me at the idea of losing mine. She found the briefcase after several hours of panic, and she turned to her vacant mother and said: "You knew I'd find it didn't you?" And when her mother smiled, probably understanding nothing of what had gone on in the previous several hours, Maria felt filled up and loved. Here is the key to Maria's pleasure in caring for her mother despite all the sacrifices it entails—financial and career sacrifices, getting up in the middle of the night to clean or otherwise care for her, and giving up a social life to make dinner and feed her mother every night. Maria's mother is a "good mother." Maria projects on her all the loving, accepting feelings that she did not feel from her as a child. When she was a child her mother turned away from her to Victoria. But now her mother's smile warms her heart in a way that she always wanted. Her mother isn't cooking for her father or taking care of her sister. Her mother belongs to her. Her mother is always there for her. Maria says she was always jealous of the relationship between her mother and her sister because her sister got all the attention. But she is the good daughter. She always was a good daughter, but now she is *the* good daughter. Her mother needs her and she takes care of her.

> Alzheimer's, I wonder how much of a blessing it is sometimes. When I don't feel well, she can pick it up. When I'm in a really good mood, she can pick that up. I think there are pieces that she can pick up and I feel really good when I can read her.

Maria feels that her mother is attuned to her moods and feelings. Maria experiences her as loving and concerned. In that sense the Alzheimer's has been a blessing for Maria, if not her mother. Indeed, when her mother was diagnosed with Alzheimer's she told Maria that she knew Maria would bear the burden of caring for her. She said: "Eventually I will know nothing and you will know everything." She held Maria as she sobbed and told her she was sorry for what she would have to bear. Maria had borne the burden of not being the chosen favorite for her entire life. Only when her mother developed Alzheimer's did she fully appreciate Maria.

VINNY, Sally and Maria are caregivers who have followed their cultural scripts. But, not everyone does. For example, Latinos may be *more likely* to have their elderly parents live with them, but not all of them do. In addition, siblings who have the same cultural scripts respond to them in different ways. Sally's siblings, Vinny's brother and Maria's sister did not follow their cultural scripts. However, it is possible to negotiate beyond one's cultural script without rejecting it entirely. For example, my friend Susan, whom I described earlier has become fluent in Italian and traveled to Italy to trace her family's history; she teaches a course on Italian-American writers. Susan is an Italian-American daughter who decided not to have her mother live with her, but arranged things so that her mother could live in her own house, as she requested, and not go to a nursing home. Adhering to your cultural script need not be an all-or-nothing choice. Susan is proud of her traditions and does not want to turn away from her mother. However, insisting on adhering to a cultural script when it is destructive to self and family is a psychological issue.

Is it a psychological *problem* for Vinny, Sally and Maria to care for their elderly parents? Or are they doing what is expected of them in their cultural context? How do we evaluate cultural norms that are different from our own? Is it *right* to have your parents live with you and make sacrifices for them or is it *wrong*? I don't think it is either right or wrong. I think the degree to which Vinny has given up his own life to care for his father has made him depressed and therefore it is a problem. He does not find it gratifying to care for his father. He does not feel, as Sally does, that it has made him a more competent person or given him a greater sense of mastery. On the contrary, it has made him regress to feeling like a boy who has to do what his father wants no matter what. On the other hand, Sally has followed her cultural script and found a way to make caring for her mother a gratifying experience. *But* her gratification has sometimes come at the cost of neglecting her children. Therefore, from my perspective, it remains a problem.

Finally, Maria has found caring for her mother a gratifying experience. Although Latinos are the most likely group to live with their elderly parents and care for them, research has shown they experience a high level of stress from doing so. Feeling a sense of filial obligation and stress from fulfilling it seem to go hand in hand for Latinos. But this is not the case with Maria. She is doing what Latinas are expected to do and her family in Puerto Rico is very supportive of her. She is also getting something from her mother that she has always yearned for—she feels she is the special daughter and is finally closer to her mother than her sister is. Maria does not have children, so caring for her mother has not impacted them. She has never married, but feels that she would not have done so anyway for reasons that are probably related to her early relationship with her mother, but not to her caregiving. Therefore, in Maria's case, there seems to be a perfect fit between her cultural script and her psychological needs.

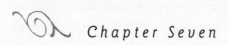

DAUGHTERS

> Do I love her? Yes, but not in the same way as those
> who say "I love my mother, I could never put her in a
> home." For loves are like people, each is different, and
> they are not just the same love which finds different
> objects to attach to.[1]

I FELT SO RELIEVED when I read Linda Grant's feelings
about her mother, quoted above; there are different kinds of
loving. It would be painful to feel that I don't love my
mother. No one wants to feel that. In some places, like Manhattan, many people have been in therapy and accept their
ambivalent feelings toward their parents. But in other places,
expressions of ambivalence are met with shock. People look
at you strangely if you don't visit your mother regularly or
talk frequently on the phone. I usually don't talk about my
mother in rural Connecticut where I have a weekend home
because, feeling so conflicted about her, talking to people
who don't express any ambivalence usually makes me feel
bad about myself. I ask myself: What's wrong with me that I
have so many angry feelings about my mother? So it was cu-

rious that when Patricia told me about her mother I didn't
feel bad about myself. I felt jealous of her admiration for her
mother; I felt envious of her awe. But I didn't feel bad about
myself.

Patricia is fifty-five and her mother, Charlotte, died six
years ago. She is a friend of the director of the senior center
where I was interviewing caregivers in Columbus, Ohio, and
heard about my study from her. She called to ask me if I
would *please* interview her, even though her mother died six
years ago, because she was eager to talk about her. I met
Patricia at her office in a Columbus hospital where she is
the director of the hospice program. She is an attractive
blonde, very well dressed, warm and eager to talk. Crammed
into a very small office with her employees right outside the
door, Patricia cried throughout our interview—and so did I.

Patricia's mother, a double amputee, had breast cancer five
years before she died and it recurred and spread the second
time. She refused any further treatment and chose to have
only palliative care. She remained at home throughout her illness and was up and about until three weeks before she died.

Patricia has an older sister and two younger brothers. She
also has two stepsisters whose mother died before they were
five. After her mother was diagnosed, although she did not
have any symptoms for several months, the out-of-town siblings began visiting New Hampshire more often. Charlotte
began having symptoms and became ill one day when Patricia
was at the house on one of her three- or four-day shifts. Her
mother went to bed that day and it was the beginning of a
three-week bedside vigil. All six siblings gathered at her
mother and stepfather's house. One brother came from Cal-

ifornia; her sister came from New Jersey; another sister came from Connecticut.

Patricia says they created their own hospice team at home. They made sure that someone was with her all the time. Patricia knew how to set up a hospice team because she had been working in a hospice program for thirteen years. She always felt her mother was very supportive of the kinds of things she was doing in hospice work, so it made good sense to her that her mother would choose to die that way. Her mother modeled what Patricia called "a beautiful death."

At the beginning of the first week, her mother directly discussed dying. But soon she didn't have the strength to talk. She could only whisper. She wrote everything down. She wrote logs about what she wanted to say. Patricia speaks in an awestruck tone about how her mother dealt with her death. She says:

> She brought each of us in to ask what we wanted of her belongings. For example, I always wanted her Wedgwood. She did this for each of her children. Then she did it for each of her grandchildren. She had one grandchild who was getting married. She talked to him about the woman he was marrying. She had another grandson who was college age. She talked to him about how he felt about different schools. She talked to a third grandson about the trip he just took to Africa. When she was talking to him she was on a respirator and she asked him to trace the trip on the map for her. She didn't want to miss anything.

Charlotte was able to be open and generous while she was dying. Patricia went on appreciatively about her mother:

Another day she asked to see each of the grandchildren again because she wanted to give them some direction. She told my son, in writing, he should stop using the word "like." She wrote that a thing "is" or "is not," it's not "like." He asked her if the bird at the feeder outside the window was a chickadee or a nut hen. She drew the beak of each one to illustrate the difference. She had so much knowledge and education and she wanted to share it to the end.

I was struck by how much Patricia respected and admired her mother. She felt she and her children could learn important things from her mother and that her mother was full of those important things—from grammar to a knowledge of birds to how to die. She admired the way her mother lived her life and the way she went about dying. I felt jealous of the twinkle in Patricia's eyes when she told me about her. I felt jealous of Patricia for having a mother whom she *wanted to be like*. She viewed her mother as strong and wise, but also brave. She began telling me how much suffering her mother overcame.

Patricia's father was a hematologist at a famous cancer hospital. At the top of his field and outwardly upstanding, he had a secret life. He was a bigamist—he married another woman because she was pregnant. He told Charlotte when Patricia was in the fifth grade. Her mother was devastated and decided to leave him and move to her parents' house in New Hampshire. Patricia's father drove the four children to the house, and her mother arrived soon afterward with Ethel, the babysitter. The same day they arrived, Patricia's grandmother had a stroke while driving with three of her grandchildren. Her grandmother died with Patricia's brothers and sister in the backseat. When Charlotte arrived eager to be comforted by her mother, she found out her mother was dead. Not surprisingly, she went into a major depression. She didn't get out of bed for over a year. She spoke to her psychiatrist in New York twice a week on the phone. Ethel took care of the children. Eventually, Charlotte got out of bed and went to secretarial school. She worked for a friend of the family who ran a tourism journal.

Then she started having trouble with her back and had a back operation. That was the beginning of another terrible experience.

> She had a rare back disease that was first diagnosed when she was forty. They were never sure what it came from. They thought it might have been that she had a spinal during the delivery of one of her children that was not completely sterile. It was an inflammation around the spinal cord. She had braces on her legs and then used a cane and then, finally, when her legs were amputated, a wheelchair. She stopped walking when she was fifty. She had been a tall, athletic woman—a tennis player. The first two years in the wheelchair she was very depressed, but eventually she adjusted and got around fine. At the end, she would get into the car and fold up her wheelchair by herself.

Charlotte modeled the ability to experience great pain and still be able to be autonomous and separate. She did not try to get her children to take care of her when she could not walk—she folded up the wheelchair and put it in the car. She valued doing things on her own as long as she was able.

Patricia wasn't with her mother when she died. She had left two days before. She doesn't seem to feel any guilt about it. Rather, she explains to me that her siblings who were there had never experienced death before. They all held hands and held their mother's hands when she died. She explains it as if her mother was so powerful that she planned it that way—another gift to her children.

> It's so amazing that my mother chose to die with the children who didn't know what it was like. She wanted to show them what a beautiful death could be like and not to be scared. We often run away from people who are dying because it's so frightening and she really shared with them a beautiful death. It was a wonderful experience for my brothers and sisters. They weren't scared. They didn't want to run away.

Physical caregiving and/or intimate conversations with an elderly mother evoke a complex array of feelings. For Patricia, caring for her mother in the last weeks of her life made her feel closer to and more admiring of her. Patricia said her mother taught her about dying—let her know how it felt as she went through it.

In contrast to Patricia, I cannot identify with my mother's emotional and intellectual experience of aging because we never talked about our internal experiences. Our conversations were, and are, limited to day-to-day experiences— where did you go; what did you do; how much did it cost? We have never talked about how anything *feels*.

Although I don't identify with my mother's feelings and I don't see her as a role model, I do identify with her physically. I look like her and I am built like her. My body is changing as hers did. I have that stomach that sticks out a bit and increasing numbers of brown spots on my face and hands. Arthritis and bunions do not mangle my hands and feet, but I have bursitis in my left arm and many mornings I have trouble hooking my bra, just like my mother does. I have wrinkles on my face in the same places as she did at my age and I know they will deepen into the crevices she has around her lips and chin. Patricia bathed her mother and helped her go to the bathroom and was not repulsed by her mother's legless body. But I have different feelings. Unlike Patricia, I have spent my life trying to be different than my mother. While Patricia admired her mother and wanted to be like her, I hate myself for all the ways that I am like her.

IT'S 91 DEGREES and I am sweating from walking one block from my air-conditioned car to Harbor View—my mother's assisted living facility. It's in Sheepshead Bay in Brooklyn and there's always a breeze, but nevertheless I'm sweating. I'm planning to take my mother for our usual walk over to the ice cream store where we empty her purse of the cookie-crusted pennies she collects and use them to buy her a chocolate Häagen-Dazs pop. My mother loves them. They have dark chocolate outside and milk chocolate ice cream inside. The Korean storeowner impatiently waits each time I count out all the pennies and wipe the cookie crumbs off. After that I'm looking forward to going on a new adventure—finding the Home Depot in Brooklyn. It's in a part of Brooklyn that I don't know and I've left plenty of time for getting lost. I'm relishing the challenge.

196 ♦ DOING THE RIGHT THING

When I find her in the large room where most of the elderly residents spend their day, she is sitting in her usual spot
wearing a black velvet jacket over a long-sleeved wool sweater
and a wool skirt. "Mom, aren't you hot?" I exclaim. She's
drinking hot tea! I kiss her hello and ask her if she'd rather
go have chocolate ice cream and leave the tea. She excitedly
agrees. I suggest she leave her jacket there since it's so hot
outside. An aide takes the jacket and whispers in my ear:
"She's put on some weight and she doesn't really have any
summer clothes she can wear." I feel guilty. I was in Europe
for two weeks and haven't seen my mother since she had her
cataract operation three weeks ago. While I was away there
was a terrible heat wave in New York. She must have been
sweltering. Forget Home Depot. I take her shopping for
summer clothes after we get the ice cream.

When we get to Loehmann's to buy her clothes, there's
not much to choose from—it's the end of July. I realize, also,
that I don't know her size anymore. She was a size 10 most
of her life, but I don't know what she is now. It's easy to buy
her tops—she needs a large. But I never bought slacks with
her and I have no idea what size will work. So I choose
all different sizes and we head for the dressing room. The
dressing room is upstairs. We'll take the elevator. No, they're
moving garbage on the elevator; we have to take the escala-
tor. Oh, no, I feel worried about my mother getting on an es-
calator. She doesn't see well and I'm afraid she will fall. But
we make it upstairs safely and head for the dressing room.
Suddenly, I feel this panic. Is she wearing a bra? She hasn't
been wearing a bra much in recent years. It's too hard for her
to hook it in the back. It's an open dressing room. I hate
Loehmann's dressing room; I'm always afraid I'll meet a pa-

tient when I'm in my underwear. But the prices are so cheap. Thank God, today she's wearing a bra. I don't want to look at her breasts, I don't like to see how they sag down and meet her stomach. It's so upsetting when I take her to doctors and they assume I'm going to go into the examination room with her. How can I not go with her? How can I not help her get undressed? But I don't want to see her undressed. When I took her to the gynecologist and his assistant assumed I was going into the examination room with her, I thought I might pass out. I waited until the doctor came to examine her, politely excused myself and left the room.

I don't want to think about my breasts sagging all the way to my stomach. I like my breasts. I've always taken pride in the fact that they don't sag. But my stomach reminds me of my mother's when she was my age. I cover it up with Eileen Fisher, but it's all there. Now she's all stomach. I don't want to look at her naked stomach. I fast walk; I play tennis; I do my time on the treadmill. I don't want to have that stomach.

The room is full of young Russian women with heavy accents and old Jewish women whose parents were born in Russia. We find a spot along the room-size mirror to hang all the clothes of different sizes that I've gathered. On one side of us, two of the old Jewish women are having an intense conversation about how one of them can't get her pants up. She's standing there in her panty hose with a stomach even larger than my mother's. I'm afraid to look at her. I don't want to see what she looks like without her pants. Her friend is telling her it's not worth buying the pants on sale if she has to put in a zipper. That will cost more than the pants would cost full price. But, she responds, I can't get *any* pants up. Her friend agrees that is a problem.

On the other side of us there's a young Russian woman wearing a pair of thong underpants. I'm facing her exposed behind. An older woman is telling her what a beautiful body she has and isn't it amazing that she has a child and still looks like that. I feel stuck in the middle, literally. On the one side is the body I'm afraid of having and on the other side is the body I never had!

It's time to try on the size 14 pants. My mother doesn't wear any underpants under her panty hose and I don't want to see her pubic hair. There's not much though and it's gray so it's kind of hard to see. It looks like she has none. I don't want to look closely to see if the hair's gray or gone. It's the same feeling as when I look at someone who is missing a limb and I can see the stump. It's a shock. I want to turn away. I've often wondered what that response is about.

The saleslady is Russian. She tells me it's pretty stupid to try those pants on. Don't I know my mother needs "petite"? Look how short she is! What a dope. I didn't think about petite. I sit my mother down and assure her I'll be back in a few minutes with some petite pants. I take the pile of wrong sizes out to the reject pile and set off to find the petite section. When I return, my mother is smiling and she's enjoying the banter in the dressing room. I help her step into each leg and pull up the pants. Bingo! We've got a light pair of pants and four sleeveless tops picked out for her. I have to help her put the wool skirt and long-sleeved sweater back on, but I console myself with the idea that in a little while I'll get her back to Harbor View and I'll get her out of that wool outfit and into something cool.

My mother is delighted when she changes into her cool new clothes. I feel like a good daughter. Now I can go to Home Depot.

At seventy-five, Lillian Rubin, sociologist and psychoanalyst, writes in her memoir, *Tangled Lives,* that she has also spent her life trying not to be like her mother. If you have an overly ambivalent relationship with your mother, you identify with her in a way that is not fully digested. Psychoanalysts call this type of identification an "introject." It is a part of you that is "not you"—a hated part of your self. When it emerges from you it feels excruciating.

A few days ago my younger son, Jason, twenty years old, sat down and told me that I make him feel guilty about spending money. He said every time I hand my charge card to a salesperson I have a grimace on my face. He told me that I still feel like I'm a poor kid from Brooklyn while the reality is that I'm an upper-middle-class professional woman from Manhattan. I cried. I felt pained. He is right.

Jason went on to say that I always use money as a reason for things—even when he knows that it's not about money. For example, there has been tension in our house for weeks because my husband and I want Jason to work as many weeks as possible during the summer before he goes off to Oxford for his junior year abroad. He has eighteen weeks off between finishing his sophomore year and going to Oxford. We want him to have money to travel while he is there. But, says Jason, we could give him enough money to travel. It is not that we *can't afford* to give him the money to travel while he is there. And, Jason goes on, why isn't working twelve weeks enough? Why do we insist he has to work sixteen weeks and only have two weeks off? "Why don't you talk about the real issue instead of making the issue money?" asks my very wise young son.

What *is* the real issue? What past reality am I bringing to this situation with my son? I remember the summer, as I described in the introduction, when I was five or six years old and my mother wouldn't buy me ice cream.

Oh God, am I doing the same thing to my son that my mother did to me? Am I saying: "You can't have six weeks of sleeping late and not working"? I even blurted out to him at one point: "*I* don't have six weeks' vacation." What nerve, I was telling him, to want two ice creams in one day. I was jealous of *my own son!* It makes me sick to my stomach to realize I did to him what my mother did to me. *More than anything else, I don't want to be like my mother.*

Lillian Rubin has spent her life trying to separate from her mother. She says:

> I've spent my life in a love-hate ambivalence with my mother, trying to reach her at the same time that I moved as far away as I could. There were periods, sometimes years, when I actually believed I had left her behind—that I had rooted her out of my inner life, that I had completed my lifetime project of disidentifying with her—only to find her popping back again at some unexpected moment.[2]

In her memoir, *Remind Me Who I Am, Again,* author and journalist Linda Grant writes:

> I was a feminist, I was a Marxist, I wanted the world turned upside down, but principally I wanted more than anything else not to be like my mother.[3]

Like Lillian Rubin, Linda Grant's mother constantly changed history. Both mothers refused to admit things that transpired earlier. This is very unsettling because it is both infuriating and undermining. "It was not a household which valued the truth . . . So I knew I came from a long line of accomplished liars." And like Lillian's mother, Linda's mother was angry and unloving. She says: "I was not a happy child."

> And this may have been because motherhood—at least of young children—was not one of my mother's talents. I grew up assuming that my mother did not particularly like children . . . I do not think she would have chosen motherhood if there had been any realistic alternative. She would, I think, have preferred to maintain her position as beloved child bride to a man fourteen years older than her.[4]

Nevertheless, the mother's terminal phase of life can offer an opportunity for reparation and growth. Understanding the childhood feelings that emerge during caregiving can transform the terminal period from simply a time of emotional pain and loss for a daughter into a final opportunity for her to develop as an autonomous woman.

When Linda Grant became the caregiver to her mother, who suffered from multi-infarct dementia, she looked at her mother in a new way:

> I see then that the mother in whose eyes I was a failed daughter is gone. That I am never going to win the great argument with her about the kind of daughter she expects me to be for my adversary has left the field.[5]

How does a daughter who never had an intimate relationship with her mother deal with taking care of her mother when she suffers from dementia? When asked if she loves her mother, she responds:

> But do I love my mother? I will collude in the public convention that children love their parents and none more reservedly than when they are cast into the role of "carer." But at least it's true that I care what happens to her.[6]

Ellen Gulden, the daughter who goes home to care for her dying mother in Anna Quindlen's novel *One True Thing,* only discovered who her mother was and what she meant to her during the months she cared for her. While Lillian Rubin and Linda Grant spent their lives trying to disidentify with their mothers and did so long after their mothers died, Ellen was finally able to identify with her mother after a lifetime of disidentifying with her because of her wish to identify with her idealized father instead. The months spent caring for her mother allowed Ellen to pare her father down to size and begin to appreciate the enormity of her mother's positive impact on her.[7]

Unlike the fictional Ellen Gulden, writer Louise DeSalvo was not able to work through her feelings about her mother before she died. In her memoir, *Vertigo,* DeSalvo describes her memory of the years she had with her mother while her father was off in the war and her sister was not yet born. When the men left, life took on an antic, festive, tribal quality.

> The women who were left behind . . . threw open all the doors to their apartments and children began to clatter up and down the five flights of stairs at all hours of the

day and night. Women and children wandered from one apartment to another without ceremony or invitation.[8]

DeSalvo says that although the women *said* they missed their men, they were far happier when the men were gone. Her idyllic time with her mother ends with her father's return. Her father did not represent pleasures separate from her mother. On the contrary, she experienced her father as an interloper and spoiler.

> Nighttime story hours were shortened or curtailed altogether. Snacks were forbidden. Mothers hushed their voices and hushed us, to listen with deference and awe to whatever the men had to say.[9]

Even after her mother dies, Louise still experiences her father as intruding on the intimacy she had with her mother. A few weeks after her mother's death, he gives Louise an envelope her mother left for her. But he makes it clear that he read it first.

Her sister, Jill, is another intruder—not so much in her life as in her suicidal death.

> In the years that have intervened since my sister's death, my mother's pain is clearly visible, ever present. She stops enjoying my children. She stops enjoying our family gatherings. She stops enjoying everything. Her mouth is permanently drawn downward into a frown. When we take family pictures, she forces a smile. She pushes herself, each day, through her routine, through her life. She isn't with us, though. She's with Jill.[10]

204 + DOING THE RIGHT THING

Louise suffered from depression her entire life—her mother's death is the *fourth* time she experienced losing her mother—when her father returned from the war; when Jill was born and completed the separation of "us wartime children from our mothers"; when Jill hung herself; and finally when her mother died. By the time her mother dies, she is so full of pent-up rage and depression that she cannot mourn her. Instead, she tries to hold on to her by identifying with her in the way that Freud described in *Mourning and Melancholia*. Freud says: "The ego wishes to incorporate this (lost) object into itself."[11] Louise says:

> I think my life is beginning to resemble my mother's. I don't go out of the house except to do my exercise walking or unless I have to. I stop seeing my friends. I cancel speaking engagements. I'm afraid to go anywhere, afraid . . . to live my mother's life, and in this way, I'm trying to keep her alive.[12]

Louise was not able to work through her anger at her mother at the end of her mother's life. Five years after her death, however, she asks: "How can a woman mother when she hasn't herself been mothered?" That is substantially different from what she told a friend the day her mother died: "I never had a mother, and now she's dead."

Louise's anger at her father and sister as the interlopers who took her mother away from her covers a deeper and even more painful reality—her mother's inability to mother. Louise's grandmother died in the influenza epidemic of 1918, when Louise's mother was two. Her grandfather farmed his daughter out to relatives and friends and finally married a woman who chided her stepdaughter with "You're not my blood." Louise's mother was depressed before Louise was born—she looks depressed in her honeymoon pictures.

WARDING OFF
A NEEDY MOTHER

Susan is a fifty-one-year-old marriage counselor. She and her husband and two daughters live in a large home in Brooklyn. When I arrived for our interview, she greeted me warmly and asked if I'd like a cup of tea. We talked in a sun-filled room with several couches with lots of pillows to lean on. She's a comfortable, low-keyed woman who seems very clear about who she is.

Susan grew up in California. Her mother, Sophie, had a chronic spinal condition as a result of whiplash from an auto accident when Susan was a young girl. During Susan's teen years, her mother suffered more and more neck pain. She had two surgeries, but the damage was never completely repaired. She was functional, but in pain, and then she got arthritis and it became more and more debilitating.

Susan says her mother's constant emotional pain preceded her physical problems. Sophie's mother died when she was eight years old. To compensate for her own wish to be mothered, she wanted to be "an ever-present, always-there mother"—the mother she never had: "But," Susan says, "I took care of her a lot emotionally. I was like *her mother*. She depended on me for that kind of closeness." Susan says her father was a kind and caring man, but he was not emotionally or physically there for her mother: "Her needs were enormous and my father's gratification was in his work." Susan's father was a physician who worked evenings and weekends. Susan's brother was not available to help Susan manage her mother's dependence on her either. They were never close as children because of their age difference—he went off to college when Susan was eight. Her father's absence and her brother's distance left Susan alone with her mother's neediness. She felt that she was drowning in it. Susan says:

> I needed to separate myself—to say, "I'm going to have my own life." Coming back to care for her made things complicated.

The pull to take care of her mother emerged again when her father died. Her parents moved from their house to a condo and her father started to slow down at work so that they could spend more time together. About a year later, he was taken to the hospital in severe pain three months after bypass surgery. After he died they realized that he had an infection in his tooth that had traveled to his aorta. Although this would have been terrible for any woman, for Susan's mother it was an even more severe trauma.

Susan says that before Sophie got cancer, she visited her mother twice a year and her mother visited her twice a year. Susan needed to keep her distance, across the country, so that she would not be overwhelmed by her mother's neediness.

> I wasn't angry at the end going to take care of her, but I was angry earlier, after my father died, when I felt she wanted me to take care of her. When I thought of her coming to live with us, I was frightened.

She says it was hard to leave her children and care for her mother when she was dying. But she explains:

> I wanted to do it. I wanted to comfort her. It felt like the right thing to do. At the end, when I was there, I was bathing her and emptying her bedpans. It's tough doing that for your mother. Seeing her so weak and deteriorated was painful. There was a piece of it that felt good, yes it was hard, but I could do it anyway.

Taking care of her mother emotionally was something that Susan was used to. The role reversal went all the way back to her childhood. Then she rebelled against it; she moved far away from her mother. She saw an ocean of neediness and turned and ran. However, when her mother was diagnosed with terminal cancer, there was something specifically wrong with her. And she was dying—it would not go on forever as Susan feared.

> When she got sick, I didn't felt guilty because then there was something definite wrong and I wanted to take care of her. At the end I was going every three weeks. It was after my father died and she was alone and lonely for twenty years that I didn't want to take care of her.

Once she was diagnosed with cancer, her mother's neediness had limits and Susan felt safe enough to respond. Indeed, she got in touch with her wish to take care of her mother.

A FATHER-DAUGHTER ROMANCE

While the child's relationship with the mother is originally a twosome and the triangular element (that is, mother, child and father) emerges later, the child's relationship with the father is a triangle from the beginning. For the girl, typically, her father is a deliciously intriguing person who is the first person outside the mother-daughter orbit. However, this was not the case for Louise DeSalvo, who experienced her father as disrupting the mother-child dyad. Fathers usually play an important role in helping daughters differentiate from their mothers and realize that being feminine doesn't mean being Mommy—there are ways of being feminine and yet different from Mommy. On the other hand, if the father demeans his wife to his daughter, the daughter grows up with ambivalent feelings about being a woman and a wife/mother.

Later, fathers become the center of a little girl's romantic fantasy and her competition with her mother. Optimally, the father is able to lovingly support and appreciate his daughter's emerging femininity, while making it clear that he has a special relationship to Mommy that is separate from her. With that kind of father, the girl is able to grow up feeling attractive and comfortable with herself—loving her father, but looking for another man to satisfy her adult needs. If her father is too gratifying (that is, makes her feel that he prefers her to her mother), it might be hard for the daughter to find any other man who can match him in her eyes—a recipe for disappointment.

Erica is an example of a daughter whose romance with her father made it difficult for her to invest her emotional energy in either of her two husbands.

Erica recounts:

My father took us on an ocean liner to Europe. They had a movie theater on the ship and I went with my sister to see *North by Northwest*. The man at the door asked how old I was and I said: "I'm eleven and a half." He said I couldn't go in. You had to be twelve. I was very upset and ran to get my father. He came down with me and said to the man: "It's true that my daughter is eleven and a half, but she is more mature than most twelve-and-a-half-year-olds. Please let her in."

Erica cries when she tells the story. Her father just died and no one will ever protect her, stand up for her and think she is as special as he did. I feel envious of her loss in a way. "My father wrote me a poem every night. He'd come into my room at bedtime and read me a book or talk to me about my day and then he would write a poem on my blackboard. It was this special thing between us." Erica felt her father was intensely interested in her—her friends, her day at school and her songs. Because my relationship with my father was so different, I was always surprised when Erica would tell me she invited her friends to dinner with her parents. I wondered to myself: Why would your parents want to spend the evening with your friends? It was unthinkable for me that my parents would want to spend time with my friends. My parents never remembered my friends' names; they never talked to them; they never asked me to tell them about my friends. I was shocked that she felt her father was interested in her friends and was delighted to see them and learn about them. She invited her friends to visit with her father in order to please him.

When her father had congestive heart failure and grew weary of his failing body, Erica sang to him, cooked for him, brought friends to cheer him and took him to a psychiatrist for antidepressants. Erica felt angry with her mother for not taking good enough care of him—for not loving him as much as she did. She also began to understand why there was a lack of intimacy in both her marriages. She remained "Daddy's girl." Erica feels that no other man took care of her the way her father did and no other man can make her feel as special as her father. In contrast to Erica's father, my father made it abundantly clear that his special relationship was with my mother.

MY FATHER had congestive heart failure for about fifteen years before he died in 1996. During that time he would go to the emergency room several times a year because his lungs filled with fluid, and a few times he had pneumonia. Several times when he thought he was dying he said to me or my sister or brother: "Take care of Mom." The first few times he said this to me I felt furious, although I didn't show it. I wanted to yell at him: "All you ever think about is taking care of her. You're my father and you're dying. Why can't you say: 'I love you' or 'Be good to yourself' or 'I'm proud of you'? Why is your last communication the same as it has always been: 'You're not on my mind, I'm only interested in your mother'?"

At seventy my father was the star part-time salesman at Nat Sherman, the tobacco shop. He loved to regale us with tales of selling fancy humidors to wealthy cigar smokers. He worked at Nat Sherman's until he had his first heart attack in the store—they were not interested in having him return. He had gotten the job there after retiring from Bayside Oil, where he was a salesman and owned one-seventh of the company (two trucks). He was at Bayside for about ten years before he retired. For over thirty years before he went to Bayside he worked for the Hunter Coal Company on Flat-bush Avenue in Brooklyn. But when people stopped heating their homes with coal the company went out of business. It was just before my parents' twenty-fifth anniversary trip to Fort Lauderdale, Florida. My father, as usual, wanted to pro-tect my mother; he did not want to upset her before the trip. He told my sixteen-year-old sister what happened, but he asked her to keep the secret from my mother. He did not seem to understand that he was asking my sister to bear the burden instead of my mother.

My father was a short, bald, paunchy Jewish man, and my mother constantly ignored his wishes, disregarded his opin-ions and insisted that he be subjugated to her mother and her sister Gus. Most of the time he silently acceded. There are a few memorable occasions, however, when he stood up to my mother or my aunt and seemed heroic in my eyes.

When Eisenhower ran against Stevenson, my father was probably the only Jew in Brooklyn who voted for Ike. When my mother's family gathered one Sunday night at Aunt Mitzi's house, Gus (knowing that my father was the Lone Ranger voting for Ike) went around the room asking people for whom they were voting. When she got to my father, he said, "I'm voting for Ike," and she started screaming at him. When my parents returned home that night in 1952, I remember my mother was not speaking to my father because he had gotten up and walked out when Gus started screaming at him. He had done the unspeakable—he stood up to Aunt Gus.

When my sister wanted to move out of the family apartment and share an apartment with a friend in Greenwich Village, my father stood up to my mother and supported my sister's moving on. And when I wanted to go to the University of California at Berkeley rather than Brooklyn College, my father once again stood up to my mother. But there were not many other times; most of the time my father sacrificed all of us (himself, my brother, my sister and me) to please my mother.

For many years I was enraged at my father for not protecting us (or himself) from my mother and Aunt Gus. He was a collaborator and the three of us were the Allies. Our war continued during the Vietnam years when I was in the antiwar movement, which began at Berkeley during my college years. My father supported the war with all his heart. Perhaps you heard us yelling at each other?

When I returned home from college I got an apartment in Greenwich Village (like my sister before me) and began psychoanalysis and graduate school. I remained rather distant from my father for many years—interspersed with conversations that increased the distance. For example, I wrote this poem about my father thirty years ago—before I met my husband.

MY FATHER LOVES ME

Yes, there is no doubt that my father loves me.
He worries when I sound down on the phone,
And tries to pick me up with kind words.
"Mrs. Sweeney is 68 and she met a man on a cruise . . .
If Mrs. Sweeney can get a guy so can you . . ."
I note the kindness in his voice
I know the reason why I'm crying isn't because I think he's
    mean.
I know my father loves me.
That's why he's telling me this.
After all, Mrs. Sweeney is 68. Mrs. Sweeney is a widow.
Mrs. Sweeney is fat and ugly. But, of course . . .
Mrs. Sweeney is rich. But men aren't interested in that any-
    more.
I didn't yell at my father.
I didn't even tell my mother to yell at my father.
I didn't want to be mean to my father because
He didn't mean to be mean.
I know my father loves me.

I felt angry that my father was so distant. I felt he never
saw me. He had no idea how pained I was about not being
able to find a man I could love. My father could not deal with
emotions; he used aphorisms instead, for example, "better
dead than red." I wanted him to understand what mattered
to me; I wanted him to see me as a woman and understand
my yearnings. But he never did.

In the last year of my father's life, he began to stand up to my mother and I began to understand why he could not do it when my sister, brother and I needed him to. My father's father died when he was a little boy—maybe four or five. I remember a picture of my father at about that age dressed in a cowboy outfit. He always said that was from the time they lived out west in Arizona or New Mexico briefly before my grandfather died of tuberculosis at thirty-two. My grand-mother, a beautiful woman of thirty, was left with two little boys, my father and his younger brother, Bob. My father never talked much about his childhood except to say that his mother married a nasty man who owned a grocery store and she used to steal from the till because he was so cheap. She never loved her second husband; she married him out of desperation when she returned to New York.

But at the end of his life, my father was able to share more about his early life. He told my sister that when his mother returned to New York as a widow, she almost put the boys in an orphanage. Instead she decided to marry a man she didn't love who could support her and her children. But she was not a warm or loving woman, and I guess my father grew up wanting to win her love. Instead, he married my mother and spent his life trying to get *her* to love him. He was willing to do whatever she wanted to win her love. He gave money to her family; he took insults from her sister Gus; he accepted her unwillingness to have anything to do with his mother; he stood by mutely when she screamed at us endlessly and slapped me across the face until her hand hurt.

By the end of his life, I could forgive him. A few months before he died, my parents went to Florida and my father slipped in the bathroom. He went to a rehabilitation hospital in Miami for six weeks, but they told us they could not keep him there longer. He needed to be transferred to a nursing home or a rehabilitation facility that worked with people on a long-term basis. My brother went to Florida and brought my parents back to New York. My sister and I met them at the rehabilitation hospital in Coney Island when the three of them arrived from the airport at midnight by ambulance.

My brother was distraught from the experience of dealing with my father's incontinence and my mother's neediness on the plane. So he left immediately and went on vacation. My sister and I took over arranging things for my father's care and consoling my mother. He was in that facility for about a month or so before he died of congestive heart disease. I visited him twice weekly before going to teach my classes at Brooklyn College. He was in a rehabilitation hospital, but he did not want to do any of the exercises. He did not want to get out of bed. When I visited him, my mother was often there. But she didn't hold his hand or stroke him. I don't think my mother has ever been able to offer comfort to any-one—I have never experienced or witnessed it. I wanted to comfort him. I was able to feel that he was grateful for the times I fed him in his hospital bed and put cream on his dried and irritated arms and legs. He was grateful that I held his hand and kissed his face. It makes me cry as I write this, but it feels good because it's loving and not angry.

DAUGHTERS CARING for mothers frequently reexperience anxieties about merging and losing themselves in their mothers' neediness—particularly the daughter who feels her mother was always needy. Susan worked hard to stay separate from her mother and resented her neediness. But when her mother was diagnosed with terminal cancer and Susan knew it would not go on forever, she was able to take care of her mother without being overwhelmed. On the other hand, daughters who devalued their mothers, like the fictional Ellen Gulden, often find caregiving an opportunity to connect with their mothers for the first time. Sometimes a woman, like Maria in Chapter 6, finds caring for her mother an opportunity to have the intimacy with her that she never was afforded as a child.

While issues of identification and separation are central to the mother-daughter relationship, oedipal issues are often at the heart of the father-daughter relationship. I wanted to be more special to my father than my mother was; I wanted him to reject her because she was not comforting and turn to me. I was competing with my mother for my father's love. That's why it felt so painful to me to hear my dying father say: "Take care of your mother" rather than "Take care of yourself."

Taking care of the parent of the opposite sex revives old passions and conflicts, just as parenting does. In order to neither be seductive nor turn away from your child's sexuality in a way that is experienced as rejecting, a parent has to accept his/her own attraction and desire for the child of the opposite sex and then find an appropriate way to express it. Similarly, when daughters care for their fathers they regress and early feelings for the father emerge. This is what happened to Erica. While other daughters might find the feelings too threatening and turn away, Erica was quite comfortable with her feelings about her father, perhaps too comfortable. But if you can accept the feelings and find an appropriate way to express them, the caregiver experience can feel healing and life-affirming.

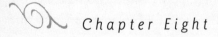 *Chapter Eight*

SONS

Whosoever knows the latitudes of his mother's body, whosoever has taken her into his arms and immersed her baptismally in the first-floor tub, lifting one of her alabaster legs and then the other over its lip . . . whosoever has kissed his mother on the part that separates the lobes of her white hair and has cooed her name while soaping underneath the breast where he was once fed . . . who has pushed her discarded bra and oversized panties (scattered on the tile floor behind him) to one side, who has lost footing on these panties, panties once dotted with blood of children unconceived, his siblings unconceived . . . to lift up his stick figure mother and to bathe her ass, where a sweet and infantile shit sometimes collects . . . whosoever slips his mother's panties up her legs and checks the dainty hairless passage into her vulva one more time, because he can't resist the opportunity here for knowledge . . . he shall never die.[1]

WHY DOES NOVELIST RICK MOODY follow these descriptions of son-mother intimacy and sexual connection and transgression with the phrase "he shall never die"? It seems to be the opposite of what we might expect—that a son would be struck dead for such inappropriateness.

Hex Raitliffe, the "hero" of *Purple America,* returns home to care for his paralyzed, incontinent, almost mute mother who is suffering from a degenerative neurological disease. In the one night in which the novel takes place, beginning with bathing his mother, we experience Hex's unsuccessful attempt to blot out his angry, sexualized relationship with his mother. Hex utters all the unspeakable thoughts and emotions that most men repress.

Moody describes Hex caring for his mother: "Her son tries to anticipate her needs, to preempt her need for words, to eliminate a language based on need, and thus to eliminate language." Hex feels so merged with his mother that words are unnecessary. Would being fully separate from his mother be the equivalent of dying?

Achieving manhood involves separating from the mother— the man must renounce his bond to his mother and enter into a new and independent social status recognized as different, even opposite, from hers. Thus the boy's development is, in many ways, more difficult than the girl's. The little boy has to differentiate himself and his maleness from his mother's femaleness even though she is the person on whom he is totally dependent. This process of differentiation or disidentification is a central part of a boy's inner life.

As a result of this essential need for the boy to disidentify with his mother, the movement away from the mother begins earlier in boys than girls. He has to extricate himself from the mother-infant oneness, but wants to know that his mother is still available to him if he needs her. The danger of merging with the mother is the boy's greatest anxiety; if he surrenders to his wish to return to that delicious infantile oneness with her, he fears both the loss of his identity as a separate self and the loss of his masculinity. If the boy's struggle to disengage from the mother is overly stressful, he may surrender and not develop a sense of masculinity and separateness or he may overcompensate and develop a macho veneer.

Adult sons are often more comfortable having physical contact with their fathers rather than their elderly mothers. Many sons, unlike Hex Raitliffe, are loathe to care for mothers because of the need to disidentify from the mother and defend against the wish to merge with her, as well as the need to disavow any sexual feelings toward her.

Although most adult children who are caregivers of elderly parents are female, the gender of the parent determines, in part, whether the daughter or son is the primary caregiver. While daughters are more likely to be caregivers than sons in general, when sons are primary caregivers, it is more likely to be for their fathers than their mothers.

A man who is the primary caregiver for his mother probably will have to confront challenges to his earliest and most fundamental concept of himself. Brought up to emphasize cognitive over emotional aspects of experience, socialized to provide and protect, he is now required to nurture. He is required to do "women's work." While all of the men in this chapter were nurturing as caregivers, Jonathan is the only one who feels comfortable talking about the emotional aspects of the experience. Repressing their emotional reactions seems to be part of the disidentification process. That is what makes Rick Moody's book so shocking—nothing is repressed.

Some sons become caregivers to their parents at a point in their life cycle when they are naturally more expressive and nurturing. As men approach middle-age they tend to integrate more of a range of feminine and masculine characteristics. They are less threatened by the feminine dimensions of their selves and feel less of a need to prove their masculinity.[2] Still, for a son to take responsibility for the physical care of his mother is fraught with the potential of having to deal with conflicts about his mother that, for some men, have remained unresolved since childhood. We can see, then, that for many sons being the primary caregiver to a mother is fraught with psychological danger.

CARING FOR MOM WHEN DAD WAS NEVER IN THE PICTURE

Ken is a fifty-four-year-old teacher. Gruff and heavyset, he was surprisingly willing to talk about his painful relationship with his mother, who had died fifteen years before. He told me he never talked to any of his friends about this, but he was eager to talk to me. Ken's parents were quite well-to-do. His father was a successful doctor and the family was financially comfortable until his parents separated when he was ten years old. Ken says his father was an alcoholic and "out of the picture" even when he was little. When I asked him about what he meant, it became clear that his father was never *in the picture with his mother*. His father was present, but there was no positive connection between his father and mother, so Ken felt that he had to take care of his mother. When his father got drunk, he hit her. Ken says: "I was left trying to protect my mother from my father. My brother was too young. I felt I had to take care of her."

When his parents separated, Ken's protectiveness toward his mother intensified. Ken explained that he could not separate from his mother. When he was a boy, he got so hysterical when she wasn't around that he was sent to a child psychiatrist. The treatment enabled him to separate enough to go off to college. But after college he came back to live with his mother for many years until he got an apartment in the same building.

Ken's younger brother, who was brought up by a nanny, moved to California when he went to college and never came back. In contrast, Ken says he always felt responsible for his mother. He recounts:

> She went through periods of tremendous anxiety. She couldn't cope. She'd be fine for a week or a month, but she was nervous and paranoid. She might have been manic-depressive. She was in therapy and on psychotropic drugs. It was extraordinarily difficult to care for her, but I didn't resent it. She'd call me twelve times a day.

Ken says he didn't resent it, but he was depressed and became alcoholic:

> The alcohol helped me deal with all the stress. I was dependent on it. But I only missed one day of work in all those years. It didn't hurt my functioning. I would drink a half a bottle of whiskey every night. I'd start drinking at 5:30 or 6 and drink until 10 and go to bed.

Ken had no relationships. He said he could not relate to women; he calls it "arrested development." His friends believed he would never get married, but they did not understand that his relationship with his mother was at the heart of the problem. All he did was work, drink and care for his mother. His mother would call him hysterically and he ran to her. Ken says meeting his wife was the turning point in his life: "I told her what was going on and she understood. I moved in with her right away." What his wife, Pam, "understood" was that Ken could not separate from his mother. He had a difficult time telling his mother that he was getting married. He said: "I think she was relieved and happy but also threatened."

Ken's mother killed herself three months after he got married. As insightful as he is, Ken attributes his mother's overdose to her feeling that he was happy and she "had no reason to hang in there anymore." He does not seem to want to know that she might have killed herself because she felt she had lost him and couldn't live without him. When he found her dead, he said, it was devastating, but a relief. He was finally free to have a life. But it was not so easy for him to have a separate life after all those years of being so intimately connected to his mother.

I wasn't sure I would be able to do it. I drank a lot. But five years ago the doctor said I can't drink anymore because I have a heart condition. I had to do it and so I did it. I stopped.

Had Ken's father been more available, Ken's separation problem with his mother might have been less extreme. The father plays a decisive role in the boy's struggle to disengage from the mother and be able to experience emotional and physical pleasures away from her. The father is a masculine alternative to the feminine mother, an other-than-mother figure. The boy can strive to be like his father and acquire his power. However, Ken's father did not help him disengage from his mother. On the contrary, his father put Ken in the position of having to take care of his mother (because of his absence) and protect her (because of his abuse). That prevented Ken from being able to separate from his mother and develop relationships with other women. The result was isolation, depression and alcoholism. The symbiosis between them was so extreme that when Ken was finally able to separate, with the help of his wife-to-be, his mother killed herself.

SHOWING APPRECIATION FOR A MOTHER WHO "WAS THERE"

Bob is an attractive sixty-five-year-old African-American man. He is married with two grown children, a son who is an attorney and a daughter who is a college professor. He is a retired technical training manager for a phone company. He has been retired for eleven years.

Bob's mother is eighty-eight and comes to the senior center five days a week. Physically, she is in good shape, but she has Alzheimer's disease. She was diagnosed eighteen years ago and his father cared for her at home for two years before he died.

Bob is the third of four brothers. After his father died, one of his brothers offered to oversee the mother's finances and have his son and his wife move into Bob's mother's house. They would care for her and live there rent-free. But the son and daughter-in-law could not cope with caring for an elderly woman with Alzheimer's. They moved out and Bob started getting calls from two of his brothers and the nephew who had lived with his mother telling him that the brother who was overseeing the finances was "not doing right." After the young couple moved out, Bob's brother was locking his mother in the house for the day and spending her pension money. He took all the knobs off the stove so she wouldn't start a fire, but she wasn't being fed, clothed or cleaned properly. Finally, Bob's other brothers and nephew asked Bob to take care of her. Bob says he had a conference with his wife and children and told them it would be a long haul—three to ten years. They all agreed to do it. Bob says the adjustment was not easy:

> It was hard for me to make the transition from child to parent. This is a child that doesn't get older, but younger. I had to wash her, clean her and take her to the bathroom. At the beginning she was conscious of being bare. It wasn't easy.

But Bob says it's a daily routine now.

> Monday to Friday my wife and I get her up, take her to the bathroom, get her washed, give her breakfast and get her out of the house between 9 and 10:30 a.m. My wife is a registered nurse and has experience with Alzheimer's patients. We take her to the center every day.

Bob's mother can't talk anymore. And he misses being able to go to events or travel. However, Bob says that it is hard to get respite care:

> Our biggest problem is we have no time for ourselves. Getting child-care is easy, but getting care for someone with Alzheimer's is not easy. People don't understand elderly people. It's harder to be with them. You can't play with them like you can play with a child. It's not fun. You can't just get a teenager from down the street.

I asked Bob if he ever thought about putting his mother in a nursing home. He said:

> I don't trust nursing homes. I've never seen an effective one. The staff in nursing homes is not compassionate. People have bedsores or don't eat. They put down the food and expect you to eat it, and if you don't they take the plate away. If I paid $40,000 a year we would find compassionate people, but I can't.

But the more we talked, the more it became clear that money is not the reason Bob does not put his mother in a nursing home. Although he doesn't say it, it seems obvious that caring for his mother had a great deal to do with his decision to retire so early. Bob wants to take care of his mother. His wife is willing to have his mother live with them and she does a lot of caregiving. But Bob says:

> It's *my* mother, so if my wife has a meeting to go to or wants to go to the movies with her sisters, she goes and I

stay with my mother. I cook, I clean, I wash clothes—we both do it.

I wondered why this sixty-five-year-old man is willing to bathe his mother and take her to the bathroom. Why is he willing to give up the benefits of being financially comfortable and fancy-free? Bob explained why he feels that he can't do enough for his mother.

I wasn't the best child. I was in trouble. I used to steal. I'd stay out late at night. I hung out with a bad crowd—a gang called the Casanovas. The thing that changed my life at sixteen was that the guys I was with robbed a store on a Saturday night and I was with them. On Monday, they all got arrested. Some got probation and some went to jail because they had prior records. I was afraid to go home. I told my parents I was there but I didn't do anything and they decided I should live at my aunt's house for a while. To this day I don't know why the police never came for me.

I was shocked. I could not imagine this warm, mild-mannered man with such an easy laugh being a juvenile delinquent! Clearly something important changed in him as a result of such a close call with the law. I could see that he was grateful to his parents for protecting him when he was so frightened. He told me that all of his neighborhood friends were either in prison or had been murdered. But was that enough to explain having his mute mother with Alzheimer's living with him for almost twenty years? Then Bob told me another story about his parents that made me understand how deeply he loves his mother and wants to care for her.

When I was eighteen I developed tuberculosis and I was in the hospital for two and a half years. It was like leprosy, no one came to visit me. People were too frightened. Only my mother and father came to visit me. Every day they came—they were always there. When I fell down they always picked me up.

Bob describes his parents as his "shield" and his "crutch." He said he could always lean on them. In return, he says:

I never borrowed money from them. I only gave to them and I could never give them enough. To this day I feel like I haven't given her enough.

At that point Bob asked me: "Did you meet her?" Since I had not, he took me out to the main room to meet his mother. "Isn't she pretty?" he asked. "Yes," I said, "she *is* a pretty woman." His mother was a petite woman dressed in a lovely outfit and her white hair was coiffed attractively. She smiled at me blankly, not having any idea who I was.

CARING FOR AN ADORED FATHER

When I entered the church looking for Tom's office, I was aware of a certain formality in the surroundings. I wasn't sure the interview would be useful because I imagined the minister I was about to meet would be a formal man who had the "right" feelings about his parents and would speak in aphorisms. Can a minister talk about ambivalence, I wondered to myself as I reached the door of his office? When I stepped into Tom's office, all those questions fell away. His office was messy with books and jazz CDs. He welcomed me warmly and seemed eager to talk. As we sat down to talk, Tom told me that yesterday would have been his father's ninety-ninth birthday.

Tom's caregiving began several years ago when his father, who had been caring for his mother, who had Alzheimer's, didn't answer the phone. Tom called the police and they broke into the apartment and took his father to the hospital. He had had a stroke. Tom rushed to New York to pick up his mother and bring her to his house in Connecticut. His mother lived with Tom, his wife and two children for a little while, but he and his wife felt caring for someone with Alzheimer's was overwhelming for the family, so they put her in a nursing home.

When his father got out of the hospital, Tom brought him to live with his family. After being with them for a short time his father developed a blood clot in his leg and needed an operation. When he got out of the hospital, Tom got him a room in the same nursing home as his mother. Tom says:

> He was never independent after that. I saw him every day for four years until he died. I can be pretty oblivious to un-pleasantness. I felt it was primal. If I hadn't done it, I would have missed out on one of life's essential duties. I felt it was my duty, but also my privilege. There's war, there's famine, there's pestilence and there's parents.

Tom's mom died two years before his father. He said she didn't know where she was or what was going on around her most of the time.

With my mother, the caregiving experience wasn't good. When she was out of it, it didn't bother her. I could walk past her room and feel like she didn't know the difference. When she knew how diminished she was, it was hard to bear.

But Tom had a different kind of experience caring for his father. Tom's father had been a professional football player— quite a famous one it seems. He played for eight years in the NFL, from 1926 to 1933. Tom felt very proud of his father and enjoyed how outgoing he was and how much people liked him: "Everybody loved my father. The nurses would bring him takeout food. They'd ask for his autograph." Tom told me that as a kid he adored his father. His favorite song was "Oh My Papa."

Tom idealizes his father. His eyes twinkle when he tells me about him. When he walked down the street, people knew him and they would call out, "Hi, Rob." When his father retired from football, he was a buyer for a large electric company. His father had contracts to buy millions of dollars of merchandise. As a result, he got very generous Christmas gifts from the companies from which he bought goods. There was cognac and scotch; hams and turkey; flowers and plants; cigars and cigarettes; wines and cheeses. Every New Year's Eve Tom's parents gave a party and all their neighbors and friends would come and indulge in the luxuries provided by his father. He says:

My father used to make a hell of a good drink before dinner and we would get blasted together when I was in college and graduate school. When he was at the nursing home, we'd sit and watch ball games and drink beer and it reminded me of those old days and it made me smile.

Tom felt his father was appreciative and it felt good to him. He told me life was chaotic, but it was convenient. The nursing home is down the block from the church. His wife would say, "Why do you have to go over there today?" But Tom wanted to see his father every day. The day his father died, he and his wife were going shopping at the mall and Tom wanted to stop and see him. His wife didn't want to and then finally said, "I'll wait in the car. Hurry up." His father died that night. I wondered if Tom felt guilty or upset that he wasn't there when his father died. He said, "I didn't feel I had to be there the moment he died. A lot of people put a lot of pressure on themselves. I didn't."

Suddenly, I realized why Tom, who seemed so unlike any expectation I had of a minister, *was* a minister—probably a wonderful minister. He said, "You have to forgive yourself. You can't worry about what you *can't do*." Tom accepts his own limitations. He forgives himself. He explains:

When this all started, I had a new job, two young children and my father and mother were both here needing care. There were three things tugging at me. I felt if I think about what I *can't* do, I will be overwhelmed, so I have to think about what I *can* do and not worry about the rest of it.

Tom's worldview is one of acceptance. For example, he talked about getting annoyed at his father.

My annoyance could be brought up with a phrase like: "Whatcha been doin'?" Which meant "Where have you been?"

Tom said he sees other people lose their temper with their parents and he is very calm and professional. But with his father it was different. He wasn't calm and professional—he was often annoyed or angry. For example, his father would say: "You said you'd be back in a minute and it's been five minutes."

> My biggest fear was my last encounter with him would be angry. But then again you're giving them dignity by being pissed off at them. It's real. There were stresses.

So Tom got angry and felt guilty about it: "Sometimes I was disappointed in myself that I couldn't get over that initial childhood reaction of being pissed off." But then he forgave himself. He told himself it was better to be emotional and attached and treat his father like a person who affected him, not an old man who was not worth getting angry at. He is humorously self-effacing, but underneath it is self-forgiveness:

> I can get into arguments all by myself. I can just go to the meat counter and argue about whether to get the pork chops or the chicken.

Tom's acceptance of himself applies to other people as well, like his brother, John. Tom's wife got angry when John visited. "Why didn't your brother offer to pay for half of the Chinese dinner?" "Why doesn't your brother get up and clear the dishes?" Tom says his brother was used to having his meals served to him and being viewed as an authority. Tom says he and John live in different worlds.

> We were on different sides of the Vietnam War and we had to come to an accommodation with each other about who we were. Sometimes his attitude would amaze me. He would come up to visit my parents and he would read the newspaper and not talk.

Tom is shocked that his brother described his childhood as being like the Harry Chapin song about a father who's always busy and the son keeps asking: "When are you coming home, Dad?" Then the son grows up and never has time for his father. Tom did not experience his father as unavailable and distant, but John did.

Tom explained that he and John grew up in different worlds. John was born in 1940 and Tom was born in 1947. His mother told him childrearing philosophy was turned on its head between 1940 and 1947. John was brought up on the advice of Dr. Spock: Feed the baby every four hours. Disregard the screaming. Don't comfort the baby or you will encourage him to keep crying in hopes of getting picked up. Let the baby cry until he gives up hope of comfort. The baby must learn to tolerate frustration and to wait for the next feeding.

As our interview was coming to an end, Tom showed me an article he wrote about his father after he died. Tom collected all the newspaper clippings and pictures of his father's football career and interviewed some of his surviving teammates. Tom said his father didn't talk much about his "glory days," but after his death Tom set out to get a full picture of his father's football career. In the article, Tom quotes a woman who wrote him a sympathy note when his father died. She was a cheerleader for a team his father coached in the years before World War II. She wrote: "He was an idol to the players. They were awed that they had this great star as their coach." He was an idol to his son Tom as well.

When I read Tom's article about his father, I thought about my writing about my parents. Both of us used writing as a way of pulling together fragments and seeing our parents as whole people. But I was struck by the difference between what I am writing about my parents and what Tom wrote. Tom's article was about the facts of his father's football career—the number of games, the number of passes, the number of yards. It was about his father. My writing is not simply about my mother and father, but my *relationship with my mother and father*. Our ways of putting our parents to rest seem not only to reflect the difference in our feelings about them, but also our genders. He wrote about the facts and I wrote about the feelings.

TRYING TO FORGIVE
AN ALCOHOLIC FATHER

Remember Jonathan from Chapter 4? Jonathan is an only child caring for his eighty-two-year-old mother, who has bi-polar disorder. Before his father died a year and a half ago, Jonathan was the primary caregiver for his father as well because his mother was unable to care for him. In order to do that, Jonathan had to confront his intense anger at his father for being sadistic to his mentally ill mother; for being critical and judgmental of him; for not taking care of him when he was a child and his mother was in mental hospitals; and for being an alcoholic.

Unlike Tom, who idealized his father and embraced his father's lifestyle and values, Jonathan feels contemptuous of his father's values and has spent his life trying not to be like him. He says:

> My parents were very much like the Cleavers—they wanted everything to be perfect. They wanted to wear the right clothes, have their kids go to the right school, belong to the right club, hang around with the right people and make the right connections. They were very much from that sort of Republican girl-boy network kind of a mold.

Jonathan sees his father as trying to please his grandfather. Jonathan's contempt is even more visceral when he talks about his grandfather, who he calls "Mr. Assimilation." Jonathan recalls:

> My father's father came from Switzerland. He was Roman Catholic, but when he came here he became Presbyterian. My grandfather was very successful in business and made a lot of money and he wanted to assimilate. He wanted my father to be the perfect American boy—go to Taft, go to a good college, work in New York, wear a dark suit and a white shirt and do everything by the book.

Jonathan feels that his father's need to please his grandfather led him to give up his own dreams and live the life his grandfather prescribed for him.

236 • DOING THE RIGHT THING

My father wanted to be a landscape architect, so he had to repress his interests to follow the paint-by-the-numbers lifestyle that his father demanded of him. My impression is that my father was totally programmed.

In contrast to his father, Jonathan gave up a job he never enjoyed and began studying social work at forty-eight. While that was a rebellion of sorts for Jonathan, it is not surprising that he chose a career of helping families in trouble considering his family's history.

Jonathan's father was severely wounded in World War II and spent two years in the hospital. He was one of the first patients in the United States to receive extensive reconstructive surgeries over a two-year period. He was listed for amputation, but his arm was saved. However, as a result, his physical skills were compromised. When Jonathan was a child, his father couldn't play ball. A lot of the physical things that a father wants to do with his son, he was not able to do. He had huge grafts taken out of his abdominal area, and his arm was deformed. Jonathan says that it also affected his father's body image.

In addition, Jonathan's father came home from the war with post-traumatic stress syndrome—he had flashbacks and nightmares.

I can remember waking up as a kid, on a number of occasions, where he was awake, his eyes were open, he was cradled in my mother's arms, screaming, "Medic, medic, I'm hit!" crying. Tears were streaming. I remember as a small child walking into the room, just thinking, "All right, he's not dreaming because his eyes are open." I had no expla-

nation; I had no frame of reference for it. My mother
would just say, "Your father's okay. Don't worry." She would
hold him the moment that he was hit by the mortar shell.

After the war, Jonathan's father became an alcoholic. He
never drank during the week, but was drunk all weekend.
Jonathan says that when his father drank, he was cruel and
verbally abusive.

One night we were in the kitchen and my father was
drunk. He said to my mother: [imitating his father in a
loud, raspy voice] "Go ahead, goddamn it, tell him. Tell
him you're a Jew!" You know, I wanted to kill my father.
Thank God there wasn't a gun in the house.

Jonathan felt enraged at his father's cruelty toward his
mother—particularly the way he used Jonathan against her.

I would say to my father, you know I'm really concerned
about Mom. He would then get her behind closed doors
and say, "See, see what's happening? Your son knows it.
Your son can see what's happening. Would you pull yourself together? Look what you're doing. Look what you're
doing to this family." That was the way my father was—he
thought depression was just a bad attitude. Just get rid of
the bad attitude and get on with life.

Jonathan says that his father was extremely judgmental
when he was a child. He used the same tone and language
with Jonathan that he did with his mother. Jonathan recalls
learning in psychology class that you are supposed to talk to

the person about their behavior. You don't want to erode the person's self-esteem. You want to help the person develop a mindset that will increase their self-esteem. But Jonathan says his father was the opposite. What he did was the antithesis of focusing on the behavior rather than the person. He describes his fear of his father.

> I remember I would get very poor grades in math. I would come home from school with my report card. And I would sit on the back porch. I would sit on the milk box, petrified. I'd sit there till it was dark, it'd be after dark, and I'd hear my parents in the kitchen: "Where is he? Do you think he's okay?" My mother would start making phone calls. Then, all of a sudden, someone might come to the window and see me, or I'd get up and walk in through the door. I'd show him the report card. It was never: "You know you're doing well in the other subjects." He'd say: "You're never gonna get into college."

Jonathan was alone with his father during the times his mother was hospitalized. He was drunk a lot of the time. In 1973, when Jonathan was a senior in college, his mother tried to kill herself with alcohol and pills—it was her second or third suicide attempt. His mother was hospitalized again and his father was drinking excessively. Jonathan says his father had been drunk, disruptive and verbally abusive on Christmas Eve. When Jonathan came downstairs on Christmas morning he confronted his father. He says:

> I said, "Okay, I'm having you committed." My grandfather's sitting there in his three-piece suit, just looking

shocked, speechless, looking at us. His eyes were going back and forth like he was watching a tennis match. I said, "You're out of control. I'm going back to school. My mother is in an institution. You're no good to anybody, including yourself, right now. I can't leave you like this because you're crazy, so I'm calling the state hospital." He said, "No, no, no. You can't do that, put down the phone, put down the phone. I'll go to Alcoholics Anonymous."

Jonathan called Alcoholics Anonymous and they sent somebody over that afternoon to meet with his father. They gave him a mentor and he got into the program. Jonathan went to Alcoholics Anonymous meetings with his father for three weeks during semester break. When he returned to college after his Christmas break, his father started drinking again and stopped going to meetings. Jonathan pleaded with him to go back to AA, but his father cried on the phone and told him: "You don't understand what it's like to be married to your mother and have to go through this."

Jonathan got teary at this point and told me that at the time he was in his last semester of college and they offered him an opportunity to graduate with honors, but he had to take comprehensive tests. He turned down the opportunity because he was so emotionally drained from dealing with his mother's suicide attempts and his father's alcoholism. He felt he could not sit for the tests.

I called my father back and I said, "All right, here's the deal: I don't need you anymore. I'm going to have a college degree. It's paid for. You can't stop payment on your check now. I'm going to get a job. If you ever want to see me

again you both have to stop drinking. That's my deal."
They both stopped drinking. That was 1974.

Ironically, Jonathan's father was diagnosed with cancer just as Jonathan was leaving his job and preparing to enter the social work program. He became afraid that once again he was going to have to sacrifice school because of his father. All his old fear and anger surfaced once again:

> I was so upset because I was taking a psychology course and I had to take a week off. I had to have somebody else get notes for me. I was afraid of failing. My fears turned out to be unfounded. But I guess I had a lot of pent-up emotions about that.

Jonathan feels his father's derogatory attitude toward him has had tremendous ramifications in his life. After college, Jonathan went to Harvard at night to take pre–social work classes. He recalls:

> There were no pressures, nobody knew about it. I was pay-ing for it. I got straight A's. But I still, to this day, question my ability. I'm petrified of getting a B. To me, a B is a failure. I put this huge pressure on myself to be a straight-A student.

But Jonathan did not go to social work school then. He took a job doing something that didn't interest him. He put his dreams aside—just like his father did. But now, he says:

> I'm making up for what I missed. I have a feeling that on the one hand, I'm very lucky to have this second chance at the

career I always wanted. On the other hand, because I have this second chance, I cannot screw up. I've got to be perfect.

Jonathan still struggles with trying to please the father he has internalized, an abusive and sadistic father—his alcoholic father. Jonathan has to be perfect and get all As to please that internal father. Jonathan also struggles with his identification with that father. He says he's gotten more control over it in recent years, but he is afraid of it reemerging under the pressure of caring for his mother.

I could be very volatile at times. I could be very cruel to people. I modeled my father's behavior. If I was depressed, if I was not feeling good about myself, which was a lot of the time, I could be really nasty to people. It was like Abbott and Costello, you know how Abbott was supposed to be his friend but he always used to turn on him and be nasty? I could never watch Abbott and Costello because it used to remind me of myself.

Jonathan's father turned over all his financial assets to Jonathan a year before he died. That vote of confidence from his father meant a great deal to him.

The fact that it was really a clear-cut decision that this was what he wanted to do and that it would be a relief to him to do it meant a lot. This wonderful change has occurred and it really changed the way that the family has dealt with one another. It gave him a feeling of relief and it gave me a feeling of relief because I wanted to have a little bit more control in order to help them.

Jonathan feels that he was able to work through his feelings about his father before he died. They talked a lot about what had gone on between them. When his father was dying Jonathan told me:

> I really squared things with my father. The air is clear. It has really improved. Do I love him? I always have. But I love him unconditionally now. And I forgive and I forget and I think he forgives and we have a wonderful relationship now.

While Jonathan was able to work through his angry feelings toward his father before he died, he still struggles with his identification with him—particularly in relation to his mother. His father blamed his mother for not being able to function. He made her feel that she was being selfish or spoiled when she was overcome by depression. Jonathan struggles with trying to accept that his mother is not capable of taking care of herself. He reverts back to trying to get her to make decisions and getting frustrated and angry at her when she cannot, but then he reminds himself that she is sick—and he isn't a little boy.

CARING FOR a mother brings up any unresolved conflicts about physical intimacy and separation a man might have. The fictional Hex Raitliffe struggled with his sexualized relationship to his mother. Like Hex, Ken struggled with his inability to separate from his mother. It made him depressed, alcoholic and unable to have a relationship with a woman until he was in his forties and met his wife. Bob, on the other hand, has cared for his mother for many years, but his relationship with his mother does not seem to be fraught with sexual or separation conflicts. He loves his mother, but he does not seem to be psychologically entangled with her. He and his wife of more than thirty years care for his mother together, and he seems to feel very warm and loving toward her.

Caring for a father can offer a man an opportunity to be close to his father in a way that he was not able to as a child. It can also evoke a different set of psychological conflicts than caring for a mother. For Tom, caring for his father was an opportunity to spend time with an adored father. Tom did not have to overcome intense anger at him or the wish to not be like him. Jonathan, on the other hand, had to work through intense anger at his father and confront his strong wish to disidentify with him.

Caregiving that goes beyond financial control or mowing the lawn can be more stressful for men than women because men are less likely to have friends or family with whom they discuss emotional issues. Ken never talked to his friends or his brother about what he was going through with his mother. His wife was the first person with whom he ever discussed it. For many men, the experience of being the primary caregiver is the first time they have thought about how they *feel* about their parents. For those who allow themselves to know what they are feeling, it can be a rich, if painful, experience.

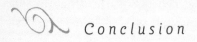 Conclusion

HOW CAN I HANDLE THIS BETTER?

C. WRIGHT MILLS WROTE: "Perhaps the most fruitful distinction with which the sociological imagination works is between the personal *troubles* of the milieu and the public *issues* of social structure."[1] "Troubles" occur within the character of the individual and his immediate relations with others. "Issues" transcend the individual and his inner life—they have to do with the organization of many milieus to form the larger structure of social and historical life.

Doing the Right Thing is about the connection between individual troubles and a major contemporary social issue. The social issue is the increase in the number of elderly people (13 percent of Americans). The troubles are the experiences of those of us who have to care for our elderly parents in a society in which there has not been provision for their care—only their longevity.

Taking care of an elderly parent is not like taking care of a child. Instead of fostering healthy growth and autonomy, you are witnessing slow or, in some cases, rapid deterioration. Instead of watching a child's world open up and expand, you are watching your parent's world contract. In contrast to a child's having his or her life ahead of them, an elderly parent is facing death ahead.

However, one important reason that parent care is like parenting is that it revives powerful elements of the original parent-child relationship. Caregiving reactivates daughters' feelings of dependency, needing to be understood and yearning for appreciation and approval. Caregiving evokes the vestiges of a daughter's oldest fantasies about her mother—it makes her regress. It awakens childhood feelings you didn't know you had or you thought you had left behind a long time ago.

You remain a child no matter how old you are because that old lady is *your mother*. For example, when my friend Alexandra visits her mother and she says, "Oh, I'm so happy to see you, I'm so glad you came," Alexandra doesn't feel like an adult. She told me, "I smile at her and give her a kiss on the cheek, but what I *feel* is: 'You never said that to me in all these years. You had to have lots of mini-strokes in order to express any positive feelings to me.'" After many years of psychoanalysis, finally getting her mother's appreciation still throws her back into the pool of rage she thought she left behind many years ago.

Most of the caregivers I interviewed did not experience taking care of their elderly parents as giving "payment" for services rendered. Indeed, many felt their parents had given them insufficient love and/or protection, neglected or abused them or entrusted their care to surrogates such as nannies. Only one caregiver, Bob, felt that he was paying his mother back for saving him from a life of crime and for the comfort she provided when he was hospitalized for tuberculosis as an adolescent. Why are people who feel they were not loved or adequately taken care of by their parent willing to take care of that parent? For many there's a deep yearning for appreciation. It's a final attempt to be recognized as a "good daughter" or "good son"—worthy of the love never given.

Author and social worker Vivian Greenberg calls the caregiving stage "the last dance." The last dance is unique because it symbolizes the end. Parents and children who have bungled earlier stages have a harder time with the last one—they are used to two solos. The last dance can be the final heart-wrenching disappointment or it can be a coming together in love and forgiveness.[2]

The child who is the primary caregiver is often *not* the child who was closest to the parent or has the best relationship with the parent. Often, the caregiver is the child who is still trying to work out an unresolved conflict about the parent. The caregiving period then becomes the stage for repeating old conflicts—or, as we have seen in some cases, an opportunity for finally working through those conflicts. Sometimes it is worked through with the parent, but, unfortunately and perhaps more often, it is worked through by the caregiver alone.

So how do we find meaning and comfort in this phase of our relationship with our parents? My philosophy is that there are no one-size-fits-all answers. But there is a way of thinking about the difficulties that caregiving brings that can help us find our own custom-made answers. Caregiving forces us to think about our relationship with our parents—the past one and the present one. It makes us examine our values and priorities; what makes us feel good about ourselves and what makes us angry; what makes us feel guilty and what makes us feel peaceful. In order to use the opportunity to know our selves and our parents better, we have to be willing to listen to our feelings even when they are ambivalent and even if we wish they were different.

We don't necessarily have to act on our feelings, because feelings and actions are separate. But knowing what we feel helps us decide whether we *want* to act. For example, you may want to have your mother live with your family, but you have to ask yourself some questions: How will I feel if I act on that wish (heroic, good about myself, angry and resentful)? What level of care will she need? Am I willing to provide that? What will I have to give up (time alone with my husband, friends, children or grandchildren or work responsibilities)? What will my husband and children have to give up (privacy, vacations and dinner out)? How will I feel about my mother as a result of her moving in?

After considering the answers to these questions and discussing them with family members, you may decide you do want to act on your wish to have your mother live with you. But you may realize you need to make provisions for private time, monetary compensation or out-of-home care. However, you may also decide not to act on that wish because you have a host of other feelings that militate against doing it. If you accept that you wish you could make the offer, it can soothe you to know that you want to help your mother. However, if you decide the negative consequences are too great, allowing yourself to feel both sides of the ambivalence can help you think of another option that will allow you to be as generous as you can without feeling stuck in an intolerable situation. You will be able to give yourself permission to look for an alternative that gets your mother the care she needs and also makes you feel comfortable. As one of my patients, who has a very difficult time tolerating her ambivalent feelings, said to herself: "Don't try to erase the ambivalence, weigh the valences."

Of course, no one likes to face the fact that a parent is dying. No matter how old you are, and how difficult your relationship with your parent might have been, facing their death means confronting that you don't have parents and you are soon to be the older generation. You will eventually have to come to grips with the issue of your own old age. But the last years of a parent's life can be a time when we can choose to work out conflicts that have plagued us for most of our lives. And perhaps, if we are lucky, we may develop a richer, deeper relationship with our parent before he or she dies and be able to remember our parent with love, warmth and acceptance.

In order to maximize the chances of making that happen, we have to first accept the fact that ambivalence is a natural and normal part of caregiving—for the caregiver as well as the elderly parent. The caregiver has to make personal sacrifices and struggle with anger and guilt, while the elderly parent has to give up their autonomy and allow themselves to depend on their children. With all the best intentions, caregiving is fraught with emotional conflict.

You also have to hold on to the reality that when you face your parent's ocean of neediness, the best you can do is bring a cup. Setting limits helps protect you from drowning as well as from feeling that you have to turn and run away. In that way it protects your parent as well because it *enables you* to help. It prevents you from getting stuck in a cycle of anger and guilt.

It is also important to pay attention to anger and guilt as signals that you have to understand, but not necessarily act upon. If you try to ignore those feelings and push on, they get worse. You may not express your anger directly, but forget to call your mother or meet her at the doctor. Or, worse yet, you may notice that you're getting headaches more often, yelling at your children or drinking excessively. If you are feeling angry or guilty, find someone to talk to about it. Angry feelings are a signal that you need to rethink your limits and/or that old, unresolved feelings are reemerging. Maybe you can talk to a friend or join a support group. If you find that you can't control your anger and/or guilt, it may help to find a therapist who can help you sort out the old feelings that are interfering in your caregiving.

It is important to remember that you have obligations and responsibilities in addition to any caregiving you take on. Those obligations cannot be abandoned for caregiving. You have obligations to your spouse, children, employer—and to yourself. Obligations have to be weighed against one another. An important meeting with your boss may trump your usual visit to your mother. Going to the mall to shop for college with your daughter may trump having your father to dinner.

You have to find a balance between being humane and not being self-destructive—your own personal way of bringing a cup. Not everyone will agree about what that involves. Some of your friends may feel it's terrible to put a parent in a nursing home, while others may feel that it is self-destructive to do anything else. Finding what you can comfortably give is something you have to find out for yourself because no one else can tell you what will make you feel good, angry or guilty.

However, I think there are some questions that you can ask yourself to help sort out whether your caregiving is destructive for you, your family or your parent.

1. Are you getting depressed, having anxiety attacks or getting physically ill from it?
2. If you are married or in a relationship, is that relationship suffering as a result of your caregiving? If you are not in a relationship, is the caregiving preventing you from having one?
3. Are your children being neglected (because of your absence or distraction) or abused (because you're in a bad temper) as a result of your caregiving?
4. Are you following a cultural script that is consistent with your own values? Or are you doing what you think other people expect or what you think you "should" do?
5. Does caring for your parent make you feel good or bad about yourself?
6. Are you giving something positive to your parent that he or she could not otherwise get? Or are you making a big sacrifice to do something that is only marginally important?
7. Are there options you are not considering out of hand or because of things you promised years ago that are no longer feasible?

As caregivers, we have to make peace with the reality that our parent is going to die. Despite our efforts, death is inevitable. All we can offer is comfort and support. We are limited in what we are able to do.

However, some of you also have to make peace with the fact that you have parents who will not accept your comfort and support—or will not acknowledge it. A difficult parent may have always been difficult and as he or she gets older those problems do not disappear. A father who was an alcoholic at forty may still be an alcoholic at eighty; a mother who had a personality disorder when she was thirty will most likely still have it at eighty-five. Illnesses and losses of later life can make a dependent personality more dependent; a controlling parent who feels out of control, more controlling; a self-centered parent even more focused on his or her own needs.[3]

On the other hand, your elderly parent's personality may have become difficult as a result of the death of a spouse or sibling, or a chronic illness. The latter case is easier to handle because there is hope that your parent can change with the help of medication, counseling or mourning. In the former case, however, when your parent has had these personality problems your whole life, you are most likely to repeat an interaction with him or her that was developed in childhood. For those of you who are struggling to care for a difficult parent, it is even more imperative to set limits that you and your family can live with and to pay attention to the warning signs that you are entangled in an old dynamic.

When our parents are old and soon going to die, we yearn for them to account for their lives. What do they feel good about and what do they wish they had done differently? Why did they treat us the way they did? What was going on in their lives that made them treat us that way? Some people are very lucky and get to have that life accounting with their parents. The bad news is that most of us are not so lucky. We have to do it ourselves or with the help of a therapist. The good news is that we can find peace. Peace may come from the satisfaction that you can have those conversations with your own children before your life is ending, even if you could not have them with your parents. Peace may come from understanding the historical and intergenerational context of our parents' way of treating us. Peace may come from knowing and accepting that you are separate.

NOTES

Introduction

1. Victoria Secunda, *When You and Your Mother Can't Be Friends* (New York: Delta, 1992), p. 4.

2. Arlie Russell Hochschild, "The Sociology of Feeling and Emotion: Selected Possibilities," in M. Millman and R. M. Kanter, eds., *Another Voice: Feminist Perspectives on Social Life and Social Science* (Garden City, NY: Anchor Press/Doubleday, 1975), pp. 280–307.

3. U.S. Department of Health and Human Services. 1999. *Health, United States, 1999: Health and Aging Chartbook.* DDHS Publication number (PHS)99-1232-1: 58. Also see Emily K. Abel, *Who Cares for the Elderly? Public Policy and the Experiences of Adult Daughters* (Philadelphia: Temple University Press, 1991).

4. Deborah M. Merrill, *Caring for Elderly Parents: Juggling Work, Family, and Caregiving in Middle and Working Class Families* (Westport, CT: Auburn House, 1997), p. 2.

5. Erik H. Erikson, *Identity, Youth and Crisis* (New York: W. W. Norton and Company, 1968).

6. In his famous essay about the life cycle, Erik Erickson posited eight stages in the life cycle—each one characterized by a central inner conflict. For example, the seventh stage, middle adulthood, spans the middle twenties to the fifties. Erikson says the central conflict is gen-

erativity vs. stagnation. Generativity is contributing to the welfare of future generations. It can take the form of having and raising children or it can take other forms—for example, teaching, writing or social activism. Stagnation, on the other hand, is being self-absorbed and not concerned about your legacy to future generations. Erikson's eighth and final stage is late adulthood, which begins in our sixties and lasts to old age. During this final stage of life the central conflict is ego integrity vs. despair. We either come to terms with our life and our impending death or we experience despair. Some people come to grips with their choices and mistakes and develop a sense of wholeness that Erikson calls "ego integrity." Other people become preoccupied with their failures and the losses that are part of aging—loss of friends, relatives and spouse. They feel despair.

7. Anna Quindlen, *One True Thing* (New York: Dell, 1994), p. 304.
8. http://www.thefamilycaregiver.org
9. U.S. Department of Health and Human Services. *Health, United States, 1999.*
10. Gail Sheehy, *The Silent Passage* (New York: Pocket Books, 1998), p. 247.
11. Abel, *Who Cares for the Elderly?*
12. http://www.thefamilycaregiver.org
13. Merrill, *Caring for Elderly Parents*, p. 3.
14. Psychoanalysts such as Margaret Mahler have talked about the process of "separation-individuation" in the first three years of life. "Individuation" is the process of developing psychological autonomy—perception, cognition and reality testing. "Separation" is the process of differentiating from the mother and developing boundaries. Margaret S. Mahler, Fred Pine, and Anni Bergman, *The Psychological Birth of the Human Infant* (New York: Basic Books, 1975).
15. The term "good-enough mother" was coined by D. W. Winnicott. Winnicott said the good-enough mother provides a "facilitating environment" for the infant to go through the maturational process. In contrast to Winnicott, I am using the term "mother" to refer to the person who is the primary caregiver—it could be a grandmother or a nanny or an aunt or a father. Similarly, I am referring to the mother as "she," because the primary caregiver is usually a woman, but it could be a man as well. D. W. Winnicott, *The Family and Individual Development* (London: Tavistock Publications, 1965).
16. Peter Blos, *On Adolescence* (New York: Free Press, 1962), p. 12.

17. Psychoanalyst Melanie Klein argued that all infants go through a stage in which they "split" the mother into an ideal, need-satisfying mother and a depriving, frustrating mother. Klein contended that adequate mothering allows the child to eventually put the two images of the mother together and be ambivalent. However, if the mothering is not adequate, the child needs to maintain the ideal image of the mother in order to keep it separate from the "bad mother." Hanna Segal, *Introduction to the Work of Melanie Klein* (New York: Basic Books, 1964).
18. Secunda, *When You and Your Mother Can't Be Friends,* p. 15.
19. Ibid.

Chapter One. Setting Limits

1. The term "attachment," which has been used loosely in caregiving literature, is based on John Bowlby's life-span attachment theory. Life-span attachment theory is based on the concept of infant attachment—the emotional bond between the infant and the mother or main caretaker. It is important to remember that attachment is an internal state within the individual. To the extent that the child finds comfort and security in the mother, the child forms a secure attachment and an internal feeling of the attachment figure as responsive and supportive. Although secondary attachments develop throughout life, the primary attachment colors the later ones. The primary attachment is maintained over distance and time; it is carried inside you. If it was a secure attachment, the adult continues to experience the feelings of comfort and security by symbolically representing the absent parent through memories, shared values and interests. John Bowlby, *Separation: Anxiety and Anger. Attachment and Loss Volume II* (New York: Basic Books, 1973).
2. Psychoanalysts call this phenomenon "transference."
3. Judith Viorst, *Necessary Losses* (New York: Simon and Schuster, 1986), p. 22.
4. Anne Wilson Schaef, *Co-Dependence: Misunderstood-Mistreated* (San Francisco: Harper, 1986).
5. Melody Beattie, *Codependent No More* (Center City, MN: Hazelden Information and Education Services, 1987).
6. Wendy Lustbader, *Counting on Kindness* (New York: Free Press, 1991).
7. Vivian E. Greenberg, *Respecting Your Limits When Caring for Aging Parents* (San Francisco: Jossey-Bass Publishers, 1989).

Chapter Two. Getting Angry and Getting Over It

1. Harriet Lerner, *The Dance of Anger: A Woman's Guide to Changing the Patterns of Intimate Relationships* (New York: HarperCollins, 1997), p. 112.
2. "Working through" is a process that is central in psychoanalysis and psychoanalytic psychotherapy. In psychoanalytic work the early experience is reexperienced with the analyst in a process called "transference." It's in the current experience with the analyst that the patient comes to understand and digest the early experience or trauma. The process of working through allows the patient to distinguish past and present and eventually move on without unknowingly repeating the early trauma over and over.
3. Lustbader, *Counting on Kindness.*

Chapter Three. Feeling Guilty and Forgiving Yourself

1. This desperate plea for help was posted on the discussion forum of Caregiver.com.

Chapter Four. Spouses

1. Roberta Satow, ed., *Gender and Social Life* (Needham Heights, MA: Allyn & Bacon. 2000).
2. Ibid.
3. Ibid.
4. Susan Forward. *Emotional Blackmail: When the People in Your Life Use Fear, Obligation and Guilt to Manipulate You* (New York: HarperCollins, 1997).

Chapter Five. Siblings

1. Stephen P. Bank and Michael D. Kahn, *The Sibling Bond* (New York: Basic Books, 1982), p. 16.
2. Jane Mersky Leder, *Brothers and Sisters: How They Shape Our Lives* (New York: Ballantine Books, 1991), p. 2.
3. Merrill, *Caring for Elderly Parents,* p. 101.
4. Julie Robison, Phyllis Moen, and Donna Dempster-McClain, "Women's Caregiving: Changing Profiles and Pathways," in *Journal of Gerontology: Social Sciences,* Vol. 50B, No. 6 (1995), S372.
5. Lenard W. Kaye and Jeffrey S. Applegate, *Men as Caregivers to the Elderly: Understanding and Aiding Unrecognized Family Support* (Lexington, MA: Lexington Books, 1990), p. 7.

6. Abel, *Who Cares for the Elderly?* p. 5.

7. Greenberg, *Respecting Your Limits When Caring for Aging Parents.*

8. Ada C. Mui, "Caring for Frail Elderly Parents: A Comparison of Adult Sons and Daughters," in *The Gerontologist,* Vol. 35, No. 1 (1995), pp. 86–93.

9. Mary Ann Parris Stephens, Melissa M. Franks, and Audie A. Atienza, "Where Two Roles Intersect: Spillover Between Parent Care and Employment," in *Psychology and Aging,* Vol. 12, No. 1 (1997), p. 35.

10. Abel, *Who Cares for the Elderly?* p. 107.

11. Sarah Fenstermaker Berk, "Women's Unpaid Labor: Home and Community," in *Women Working: Theories and Facts in Perspective,* 2nd ed., edited by Ann Helton Stromberg and Shirley Harkess (Mountain View, CA: Mayfield Publishing, 1988).

12. Karen L. Fingerman, *Aging Mothers and Their Adult Daughters: A Study in Mixed Emotions* (New York: Springer Publishing Company, 2001), p. xiii.

13. Ibid.

14. Mario Tonti, "Relationships Among Adult Siblings Who Care for Their Aged Parents," in *Siblings in Therapy: Life Span and Clinical Issues,* edited by Michael D. Kahn and Karen Gail Lewis (New York: W. W. Norton and Company, 1988), pp. 417–34.

15. Bank and Kahn, *The Sibling Bond.*

16. Ibid., p. 109.

17. Sarah H. Matthews, "Gender and the Division of Filial Responsibility Between Lone Sisters and Their Brothers," *In Journal of Gerontology: Social Sciences,* Vol. 50B, No. 5 (1995), S312–S320.

Chapter Six. Cultural Scripts for Caregivers

1. Ann Willard, "Cultural Scripts for Mothering," in *Mapping the Moral Domain: A Contribution of Women's Thinking to Psychological Theory and Education,* edited by Carol Gilligan (Cambridge, MA: Harvard University Press, 1988), pp. 225–43.

2. Although caregiving is predominantly women's work, care of the elderly is largely absent from the feminist agenda in the United States. Feminist scholars lavish attention on motherhood, but they continue to slight other forms of unpaid work, such as caring for elderly parents. Both forms of private domestic labors are undervalued because they are outside the economy. See Berk, "Women's Unpaid Labor: Home and Community."

3. Abel, *Who Cares for the Elderly?* p. 4.
4. Charlotte Ikels, "The Process of Caregiver Selection," in *Growing Old in America: New Perspectives on Old Age,"* edited by Beth B. Hess and Elizabeth Markson (New Brunswick, NJ: Transaction Books, 1985), pp. 136–50.
5. U.S. Bureau of the Census, 2000. "Relationship by Household Type (Including Living Alone) for the Population 65 Years and Over," Summary File 2, PCT 21.
6. Christine L. Himes, Dennis P. Hogan and David J. Eggebeen, "Living Arrangements of Minority Elders," in *Journal of Gerontology: Social Sciences,* Vol. 51B, No. 1 (1996), pp. 542–48.
7. Lisa Groger, Pamela S. Mayberry, Jane K. Straker and Shahla Hehdizadeh, "African-American Elders' Long-Term Care Preferences and Choices." Final Report, Award #90-AR-2034 (Washington, DC: Administration of Aging, Department of Health and Human Services, August 1997).
8. Carole Cox and Abraham Monk, "Strain Among Caregivers: Comparing the Experiences of African-American and Hispanic Caregivers of Alzheimer's Relatives," *International Journal of Aging and Human Development,* Vol. 43, No. 2 (1996), pp. 93–105.

Chapter Seven. Daughters

1. Linda Grant, *Remind Me Who I Am, Again* (London: Granta Books, 1998), p. 38.
2. Lillian B. Rubin, *Tangled Lives: Daughters, Mothers, and the Crucible of Aging* (Boston: Beacon Press, 2000), p. 49.
3. Grant, *Remind Me Who I Am, Again,* p. 46.
4. Ibid., p. 78.
5. Ibid., p. 166.
6. Ibid., p. 265.
7. Quindlen, *One True Thing,* p. 53.
8. Louise DeSalvo, *Vertigo: A Memoir* (New York: Dutton, 1996).
9. Ibid., p. 56.
10. Ibid., p. 245.
11. Sigmund Freud, "Mourning and Melancholia," in John Rickman, ed., *A General Selection from the Works of Sigmund Freud* (New York: Doubleday, 1957), p. 131.
12. DeSalvo, *Vertigo,* p. 252.

Chapter Eight. Sons

1. Rick Moody, *Purple America* (Boston: Little, Brown and Company, 1997), pp. 3–4.
2. Kaye and Applegate, *Men as Caregivers to the Elderly*, p. 14.

Conclusion. How Can I Handle This Better?

1. Mills, C. Wright, *The Sociological Imagination* (New York: Grove Press, 1959), p. 8.
2. Vivian E. Greenberg, *Children of a Certain Age: Adults and Their Aging Children* (New York: Lexington Books, 1994), p. 163.
3. Grace Lebow and Barbara Kane with Irwin Lebow, *Coping with Your Difficult Older Parent: A Guide for Stressed-Out Children* (New York: Avon Books, 1999), p. 8.

BIBLIOGRAPHY

Abel, Emily K. *Who Cares for the Elderly? Public Policy and the Experiences of Adult Daughters* (Philadelphia: Temple University Press, 1991).

Aranda, Maria P., and Bob G. Knight. "The Influence of Ethnicity and Culture on the Caregiver Stress and Coping Process: A Sociocultural Review and Analysis." *The Gerontologist* 37, 3 (1997): 342–54.

Bank, Stephen, P., and Michael D. Kahn, *The Sibling Bond* (New York: Basic Books, 1982).

Beattie, Melody. *Codependent No More* (Center City, MN: Hazelden Information and Education Services, 1987).

Berk, Sarah Fenstermaker. "Women's Unpaid Labor: Home and Community." In *Women Working: Theories and Facts in Perspective,* 2nd ed. Edited by Ann Helton Stromberg and Shirley Harkess (Mountain View, CA: Mayfield Publishing, 1988).

Berman, Claire. *Caring for Yourself While Caring for Your Aging Parents* (New York: Henry Holt and Company, 1996).

Biegel, David E., Esther Sales, and Richard Schulz. *Family Caregiving in Chronic Illness: Alzheimer's Disease, Cancer, Heart Disease, Mental Illness and Stroke* (Newbury Park, CA: Sage Publications, 1991).

Blos, Peter. *On Adolescence* (New York: Free Press, 1962).

Bowlby, John. *Separation: Anxiety and Anger. Attachment and Loss Volume II* (New York: Basic Books, 1973).

Cox, Carole, and Abraham Monk. "Strain Among Caregivers: Comparing the Experiences of African-American and Hispanic Caregivers of Alzheimer's Relatives." *International Journal of Aging and Human Development,* Vol. 43, (2) (1996), pp. 93–105.

DeSalvo, Louise. *Vertigo: A Memoir* (New York: Dutton, 1996).

Erikson, Erik H. *Identity, Youth and Crisis* (New York: W. W. Norton and Company, 1968).

Fingerman, Karen L. *Aging Mothers and Their Adult Daughters: A Study in Mixed Emotions* (New York: Springer Publishing Company, 2001).

Forward, Susan. *Emotional Blackmail: When the People in Your Life Use Fear, Obligation and Guilt to Manipulate You* (New York: HarperCollins, 1997).

Freud, Sigmund. "Mourning and Melancholia." In John Rickman, ed., *A General Selection from the Works of Sigmund Freud* (New York: Doubleday, 1957).

Grant, Linda. *Remind Me Who I Am, Again* (London: Granta Books, 1998).

Greenberg, Vivan E. *Children of a Certain Age: Adults and Their Aging Children* (Lexington, MA: Lexington Books, 1994).

———. *Respecting Your Limits When Caring for Aging Parents* (San Francisco: Jossey-Bass Publishers, 1989).

Groger, Lisa, Pamela S. Mayberry, Jane K. Straker and Shahla Hehdizadeh. "African-American Elders' Long-Term Care Preferences and Choices." Final Report, Award #90-AR-2034 (Washington, DC: Administration of Aging, Department of Health and Human Services, August 1997).

Groger, Lisa, and Pamela S. Mayberry. "Caring Too Much? Cultural Lag in African-Americans' Perceptions of Filial Responsibilities." In *Journal of Cross-Cultural Gerontology* 16 (2001), pp. 21–39.

Himes, Christine L., Dennis P. Hogan and David J. Eggebeen, "Living Arrangements of Minority Elders." In *Journal of Gerontology: Social Sciences,* Vol. 51B, No. 1 (1996), pp. 542–48.

Hochschild, Arlie Russell. "The Sociology of Feeling and Emotion: Selected Possiblities." In M. Millman and R. M. Kanter, eds., *Another Voice: Feminist Perspectives on Social Life and Social Science* (Garden City, NY: Anchor Press/Doubleday, 1975).

Ikels, Charlotte. "The Process of Caregiver Selection." In *Growing Old in America: New Perspectives on Old Age,"* ed. Beth B. Hess and Elizabeth Markson (New Brunswick, NJ: Transaction Books, 1985).

Kaye, Lenard W., and Jeffrey S. Applegate, *Men as Caregivers to the Elderly: Understanding and Aiding Unrecognized Family Support* (Lexington, MA: Lexington Books, 1990).

Lebow, Grace, and Barbara Kane with Irwin Lebow. *Coping with Your Difficult Older Parent: A Guide for Stressed-Out Children* (New York: Avon Books, 1999).

Leder, Jane Mersky. *Brothers and Sisters: How They Shape Our Lives* (New York: Ballantine Books, 1991).

Lerner, Harriet. *The Dance of Anger: A Woman's Guide to Changing the Patterns of Intimate Relationships* (New York: HarperCollins, 1997).

Lustbader, Wendy. *Counting on Kindness* (New York: Free Press, 1991).

Mahler, Margaret S., Fred Pine and Anni Bergman. *The Psychological Birth of the Human Infant* (New York: Basic Books, 1975).

Matthews, Sarah H. "Gender and the Division of Filial Responsibility Between Lone Sisters and Their Brothers." In *Journal of Gerontology: Social Sciences.* Vol. 50B, No. 5 (1995), S312–S320.

Merrill, Deborah M. *Caring for Elderly Parents: Juggling Work, Family, and Caregiving in Middle and Working Class Families* (Westport, CT: Auburn House, 1997).

Mills, C. Wright. *The Sociological Imagination* (New York: Grove Press, 1959).

Mui, Ada C. "Caring for Frail Elderly Parents: A Comparison of Adult Sons and Daughters." In *The Gerontologist,* Vol. 35, No. 1 (1995), pp. 86–93.

Moody, Rick. *Purple America* (Boston: Little, Brown and Company, 1997).

Olson, Laura Katz, ed. *Caring for the Elderly in a Multicultural Society* (Lanham, MD: Rowman and Littlefield Publishers, 2001).

Pyke, Karen. "The Micropolitics of Care in Relationships between Aging Parents and Adult Children: Individualism, Collectivism, and Power." In *Journal of Marriage and the Family,* 61, 3 (1999), pp. 661–72.

Quindlen, Anna. *One True Thing* (New York: Dell, 1994).

Robison, Julie, Phyllis Moen and Donna Dempster-McClain. "Women's Caregiving: Changing Profiles and Pathways." In *Journal of Gerontology: Social Sciences,* Vol. 50B, No. 6 (1995), S372.

Rubin, Lillian B. *Tangled Lives: Daugters, Mothers, and the Crucible of Aging* (Boston: Beacon Press, 2000).

Satow, Roberta, ed. *Gender and Social Life* (Needham Heights, MA: Allyn & Bacon, 2000).

Schaef, Anne Wilson. *Co-Dependence: Misunderstood-Mistreated* (San Francisco: Harper, 1986).

Secunda, Victoria. *When You and Your Mother Can't Be Friends* (New York: Delta, 1992).

Segal, Hanna. *Introduction to the Work of Melanie Klein.* (New York: Basic Books, 1964).

Seltzer, Marsha Mailick, and Lydia Wailing Li. "The Dynamics of Caregiving: Transitions During a Three-Year Prospective Study." *The Gerontologist,* Vol. 40, No. 2 (2000), 165–78.

Sheehy, Gail. *The Silent Passage* (New York: Pocket Books, 1998).

Stephens, Mary Ann Parris, Melissa M. Franks and Audie A. Atienza. "Where Two Roles Intersect: Spillover Between Parent Care and Employment." In *Psychology and Aging,* Vol. 12, No. 1 (1997), p. 35.

Tonti, Mario. "Relationships Among Adult Siblings Who Care for Their Aged Parents." In *Siblings in Therapy: Life Span and Clinical Issues,* ed. Michael D. Kahn and Karen Gail Lewis (New York: W. W. Norton and Company, 1988), pp. 417–34.

U.S. Bureau of the Census. "Relationship by Household Type (Including Living Alone) for the Population 65 Years and Over," Summary File 2 (2000), PCT 21.

U.S. Department of Health and Human Services. *Health, United States, 1999: Health and Aging Chartbook* (1999). DDHS Publication number (PHS)99-1232-1.

Viorst, Judith. *Necessary Losses* (New York: Simon and Schuster, 1986).

Willard, Ann. "Cultural Scripts for Mothering." In *Mapping the Moral Domain: A Contribution of Women's Thinking to Psychological Theory and Education,* ed. Carol Gilligan (Cambridge, MA: Harvard University Press, 1988), pp. 225–43.

Winnicott, D. W. *The Family and Individual Development* (London: Tavistock Publications, 1965).

INDEX

ABOUT THE AUTHOR

Roberta Satow, Ph.D., is a professor of sociology at Brooklyn College and a practicing psychotherapist in Manhattan. As a recognized authority on caregiving, Dr. Satow has been quoted in *The New York Times; O: The Oprah Magazine; Newsweek*'s Web edition; and other national publications. Excerpts of her book have been issued in *Today's Caregiver* and on Caregiver.com.

Dr. Satow has appeared on *The Diane Rehm Show,* AARP's *Prime Time Radio,* and several other NPR programs, and she has been featured in articles in *The Washington Post, The Charlotte Observer, The Tampa Tribune,* the Cleveland *Plain Dealer, The Dallas Morning News,* and *The Seattle Times.*

She delivered the keynote speech, "Caregiving and Mental Health: A Multi-Dimensional Issue," at a 2005 White House Conference on Aging held at Brooklyn College. Dr. Satow has given presentations at Mount Sinai Hospital in New York City, the National Caregivers Conference, the National Conference on Family

Relations, the New York City Alzheimer's Conference, the Joint Conference of the National Council on the Aging, and the American Society on Aging.

Additional information about Dr. Satow may be found on her website: http://www.robertasatow.com.

W9-BWV-064

HOOKED ON A FELINE

A MAGICAL CATS MYSTERY

SOFIE KELLY

BERKLEY PRIME CRIME
New York

BERKLEY PRIME CRIME
Published by Berkley
An imprint of Penguin Random House LLC
penguinrandomhouse.com

ISBN: 9780593199992

Berkley Prime Crime hardcover edition / September 2021
Berkley Prime Crime mass-market edition / August 2022

Printed in the United States of America
1 3 5 7 9 10 8 6 4 2

Book design by Kelly Lipovich

1

The stage set up at the end of the marina parking lot was in darkness, and there wasn't enough light from the stars and the sliver of gleaming moon overhead to make out anything, even though we were sitting just a few rows back. The crowd spread out across the pavement on lawn chairs and coolers had gone silent, so silent it seemed as though we were all holding our breath. But underneath that silence I could feel a faint buzz of anticipation, like the current of energy in the air just before a thunderstorm hits.

And then a clap of wood on wood, one drumstick hitting another, counting off the beat—*One! Two! Three! Four!*—cracked the quiet. And all at once there was music: the sound of a raucous electric guitar; and the crowd went wild. Beside me my friend Roma was grinning, bouncing on her canvas lawn chair, her dark eyes shining. She leaned sideways, bumping me with her shoulder. "That's Harry, Kathleen," she said in my ear, "which has to mean—"

She didn't get to finish the sentence because the smooth voice of the announcer boomed through the sound system, drowning out everything else. "Please welcome—after a very long absence—Johnny Rock . . ." He paused. I leaned forward, suddenly knowing what his next words had to be. And then they came: ". . . *and the Outlaws!*"

The stage lights came up and the crowd really went wild then, cheering, clapping, hooting and whistling. I couldn't take my eyes off the stage because that amazing electric guitar was in the hands of Harry Taylor— Harry, who mowed my lawn and kept just about everything running at the library for me. He was in his fifties with just a little hair left, his face lined from years of working outside in the sun. Harry looked like someone's dad, practical and dependable, which he was—not like some rock star guitar virtuoso—which it seemed he also was. I knew Harry played guitar. I knew he had been in a band, in *this* band, but I was dumbstruck that I had no idea he was so incredibly talented.

Roma was already moving to the music. "Close your mouth, Kath," she said, grinning as if she'd guessed what I'd been thinking. "I'm pretty sure you just swallowed a bug."

I didn't get a chance to answer because Johnny Rock had started to sing John Mellencamp's "R.O.C.K. in the U.S.A.," striding onto the stage from the left side. His voice was full and strong with just a hint of a raspy edge to it.

Johnny Rock, aka John Stone, looked like he could

have been actor Bradley Cooper's older brother—blue eyes, brown hair shot with a bit of gray waved back from his face, long legs and muscular arms in a tight black T-shirt and faded jeans. He had that same naughty-boy grin as the actor as well.

Harry was just behind Johnny's right shoulder, a few steps back. He, too, wore a black T-shirt and jeans, but not his ubiquitous Twins ball cap. I realized that he was playing the same solid-body Fender Stratocaster that he'd brought to Reading Buddies at the library, where he'd led the kids in an enthusiastic version of the Beatles' "Yellow Submarine." The song had been stuck in my head for days afterward.

Beside me Roma was already up and dancing. It seemed like the whole crowd was on its feet, spilling across the parking lot onto the grassy riverbank. Roma grabbed my hand and pulled me off my chair. "I can't believe they kept the whole band coming back together a secret."

"Me neither," I said, leaning sideways so she could hear me. Harry had been in the library just hours ago and there had been no hint from him that he'd be onstage tonight when I'd said I was looking forward to seeing Johnny in concert. I had no idea Harry was so good at keeping a secret. It seemed there were a lot of things I didn't know about Harry Taylor.

"Well, Mike checked my cracked tooth on Thursday and he didn't give anything away, either," Roma said, raising her voice over the crowd noise.

Mike Bishop, who had expertly completed a root canal on my upper-left molar just recently, was also

up onstage playing bass, standing behind and to the left of Johnny. Like Johnny and Harry, he was wearing jeans and a black shirt, along with a dark gray fedora over his gray curls. And he couldn't seem to stop grinning. He raised one arm in the air. "C'mon, people, you should be dancin'!" he shouted.

The outdoor concert was part of the Last Bash, a revival, after twenty-five years, of a summer festival celebrating food, music and small-town life. Mayville Heights was trying to bring back the celebration as a way to entice more tourists to our Minnesota town. The highlight of the event for just about everyone was the return to the stage of Johnny Rock, who had been a local celebrity in his teens and twenties, first as the lead singer of Johnny and the Outlaws and then as a solo performer. Johnny had gone on to become a very successful businessman. He had just sold his real estate development company and was going back to his first love, music.

I closed my eyes for a moment and just focused on Johnny's voice as the band segued into Boston's "More Than a Feeling." I draped my arm around Roma's shoulders and we swayed back and forth to the music, heads together like we were teenagers. The 1976 rock ballad showcased Johnny's vocal range. He was good—not just small-town-bar-band good—good enough to have had a career as a working musician, in my opinion. And I knew a little about the music business. My brother, Ethan, had his own band back in Boston, The Flaming Gerbils. I'd learned from watching his career develop how mercurial the music business could be,

how it took more than talent, how sometimes it seemed that talent was the least important factor. I couldn't help wondering what had derailed Johnny's long-ago musical aspirations.

Roma was singing, "It's more than a feeling," softly by my ear. I opened my eyes. Next to Roma, her husband, Eddie, and our friend Maggie were dancing. I knew Mags could dance but I hadn't known that Eddie could. I shouldn't have been surprised. Eddie Sweeney was a former NHL player. He was tall and fast and smooth on his feet, even without skates.

To my right Marcus—my Marcus—was dancing with Mary Lowe. Mary was easily a foot shorter than he was and several decades older, but she had some smooth moves herself. She caught my eye, raised her eyebrows and gave me a saucy grin.

I smiled back at her.

"Best night ever," Roma said.

It was one of her favorite expressions, but she was right. This was going to be one of those nights I knew I'd remember for a long time.

The band came to their last song way too soon. "You know, I could stay out here all night," Johnny began.

"Do it!" a voice yelled from somewhere on the edge of the riverbank. There were echoes of the words all through the crowd.

Johnny smiled. "Believe me, I'd like to, but like they say, all good things must come to an end." He gazed out over the crowd. "Thank you all for coming tonight and I hope you liked my"—he turned and looked over

his shoulder at the guys behind him—"our little surprise."

People started clapping again. I leaned back against Marcus's chest and he wrapped his arms around me. I wished the band *could* keep playing all night. I didn't want to be anywhere except where I was right now.

Johnny walked back to Mike and leaned an elbow on his friend's shoulder. Mike's hands were resting on his glossy black StingRay bass. He was about average height, with a stocky build and strong arms. He had a great mischievous grin, which he was giving to Johnny now.

"Mike and I met on the playground when we were what? Six years old?" Johnny asked.

"Seven," Mike said.

"Another kid, who I won't name"—Johnny coughed—"Thorsten." Everyone laughed. "Had just knocked out one of my front teeth with a swing. Mike looked all around and found the tooth in the grass. He gave it to me so the tooth fairy would come."

"Professional courtesy," Mike said, deadpan.

"We kinda lost touch for a while and then Mike came to audition for the band. And we've been friends ever since."

Mike looked up at Johnny. "You know, a good friend is like a good joc—" He stopped and held up one hand, a not-exactly-sincere expression of contrition on his face. "Sorry. This is a family venue. I'll start again. A good friend is like a good athletic supporter."

Johnny shook his head. "Really?" he said.

I wasn't sure if *he* knew the punch line to Mike's story but I knew there'd be one.

Mike nodded. "Absolutely. Not really very flashy." He raised an eyebrow. "No sequins. And sometimes makes you just a little uncomfortable." He held up a hand again. "But when life kicks you in the"—the drummer rolled a flourish on the cymbals—"you know you're always covered!"

Everyone laughed.

Mike pointed a finger at Johnny. "Love you, man."

"Friends to the end," Johnny said.

The two men fist-bumped and then Johnny moved toward the drummer. He ran a hand through his hair. "Paul and I met in detention," he began.

"We were set up," Paul called out.

More laughter.

Paul Whitewater was wiry with lean, strong arms in his black T-shirt and his bleached hair was cut very short.

"Now there are differing opinions on whether or not we deserved to be in detention," Johnny continued.

"That time," Mike added, deadpan.

Johnny narrowed his eyes at the bass player. "*That* time," he repeated. He turned his attention back to Paul. "My brief stint as a juvenile delinquent not withstanding, I couldn't have found a better drummer or a better friend."

"Back at you, brother," Paul said.

Ritchie Gonzalez was the band's keyboard player. He was stocky and solid with dark eyes, dark hair and

olive skin. He wore a black leather cuff on his right wrist and a silver skull bracelet on his left. The bottom of a tattoo peeked out from the edge of his T-shirt sleeve. "Hey, Johnny," he said with a smile.

Johnny smiled back at him. "Ritchie and I met in church."

"And the building *wasn't* struck by lightning," Mike interjected.

Johnny shot him a look but it was clear from his body language and the hint of a smile pulling at his face and eyes that he wasn't really mad. "You're going to get struck by something if you're not careful," he said.

Mike folded his arms over his instrument again and dropped his head but he couldn't completely rein in his grin, so once again his contrite act didn't quite work.

Johnny gave his head a little shake. "As I was saying, Ritchie and I met in church. It was during the music festival and there were about three classes' worth of kids down in the basement of St. Bartholomew's waiting for our turn to perform. Ritchie was fiddling around on this old organ he'd found down there."

"It was a Yamaha A55 Electone," Ritchie said. "Someone had probably donated it to the church."

"I'm sure they had no idea what they were starting." Johnny gestured at Ritchie. "So I'm standing there, looking oh so cool in my white shirt and bow tie." There was a ripple of laughter. "Thank you, Mom, for making me wear it to every music festival I was ever in. And Ritchie—who I'd like to point out was not

wearing a bow tie—started playing 'Light My Fire.' And I started singing."

Ritchie frowned. "Did you tell them we were in a church?"

Even from several rows back, I could see the gleam in Johnny's dark eyes. "And it was very shortly after our time at St. Bartholomew's that we met Paul. But you know that part of the story." His words got yet another big laugh. Next to me Eddie gave a two-fingered wolf whistle. Roma leaned against his side, her head on his shoulder and her arm draped across his back.

There was only one band member left. "Harry Taylor," Johnny said. Harry smiled at him. Johnny looked out over the crowd. "Do you want to know how long I've known this guy?" he asked.

"Yes," I called out. So did a lot of other people.

"When I met him, he had hair," Johnny said. "Lots of it."

Harry smoothed a hand over his almost bald head.

"The first time I heard this guy play, it was on a guitar he got from the S&H Green Stamps catalogue. And even then it was magic." Johnny clapped a hand on Harry's shoulder and they exchanged a look. They had the kind of easy connection that comes with old friends. "We've been friends longer than I sometimes want to admit to and I don't know a better person."

Johnny held out a hand, gesturing at the band. "These guys are more than just my friends: They're my brothers." He raised his arm in the air and Mike

began to run a bass line. Harry joined in on guitar followed by Ritchie and Paul and they moved into a song that I'd never heard before with Johnny covering every inch of the stage as he sang.

> *When you can't find the way,*
> *And you can't see the road,*
> *When your heart is too heavy*
> *To carry the load,*
> *When you can't find your voice,*
> *When the darkness won't go,*
> *When you're looking for somewhere*
> *to lay your weary head down*
> *I'll be your home.*

At the end of the song the other four members of the band joined Johnny at the edge of the stage to take a bow, arms around one another's shoulders. The crowd stayed on their feet, cheering and clapping, even after the men had all left the stage. I could see that they weren't going to let the band get away without another song.

The lights dimmed a little and Ritchie walked out from somewhere backstage. "Thank you," he said, waving at everyone as he slid behind his keyboard. He started to play a melody that I knew, but in the moment couldn't place.

Mike came out of the wings from the left side of the stage. He picked up his bass and put the strap over his head. "We love you!" he shouted to the crowd as he started to play.

Harry came out next, carrying his Martin twelve-

string. He raised one hand in recognition of the applause, which seemed like it was never going to end, before picking up the melody from Ritchie. Paul was right behind Harry, blowing a kiss to everyone before sitting down at his drum kit.

Johnny was singing before he was onstage—"I'll Stand by You," written by the Pretenders' Chrissie Hynde.

I swayed in time to the music and sang along softly with Johnny, wrapped in the warmth of Marcus's arms.

This time when the guys left the stage, everyone seemed to understand that they wouldn't be back again. Still, people seemed reluctant to leave as if, somehow, the spell the band had cast over the evening would be broken.

"Tired?" Marcus asked.

I shook my head. "No. I have all this energy I don't know what to do with. I know I couldn't sleep."

Roma cocked her head to one side, tucking a strand of dark hair behind her ear. "I know Eric was planning on staying open late," she said. "How about dessert? Or really, really early breakfast?" She turned and looked over her shoulder at Maggie.

Maggie's green eyes narrowed. "Do you think there might be more of that fruit cobbler we had the other day at lunch?"

Roma smiled. "There's only one way to find out for sure."

Brady Chapman was standing next to Maggie. I saw her reach for his hand and raise a questioning

eyebrow. The two of them were . . . I didn't really know what they were. Maggie insisted they weren't a couple but they spent all their free time together and neither of them was seeing anyone else. Mary Lowe liked to say they were "keeping company."

"It works for me," Brady said now.

Roma looked toward me again. I glanced up at Marcus, who nodded. "Let's go," I said.

Marcus grabbed our chairs. I looked around for Mary to say good night, but she'd already disappeared. We headed across the parking lot, all veering off in different directions because we'd all parked in different places. Roma and Eddie had gotten to the marina early to save a place for the rest of us and they'd managed to snag a spot close to the building. I'd parked my truck on a nearby side street. Based on the direction Brady and Maggie—who were already ahead of everyone else—were headed, they'd done the same thing.

When we got to Eric's Place, the café wasn't as busy as I'd expected. Nic, who generally worked nights, showed us to my favorite table in the front window. He was three or four inches taller than my five-six with a solid frame, deep brown eyes and light brown skin. "You just came from the Last Bash concert, didn't you?" he asked. Like Maggie, Nic was an artist. He created assemblages with metal and paper—things most of us recycled or threw away—and he was also a very talented photographer.

"It was incredible," Brady said.

"And it's true the whole band was there?"

Roma nodded. "You wouldn't believe how talented Harry Taylor is on guitar or Mike Bishop on bass."

Nic stared at her. "Dr. B. plays bass with the Outlaws? No way. You're kidding."

"Uh-uh," I said, taking one of the chairs closest to the window. "He's really good, too."

"He did my root canal last winter. Why didn't I know he'd played with Johnny Rock?"

Roma smiled. "Probably because the last time Johnny and the Outlaws played together you were a baby."

Nic grinned back at her. "Good point, but it doesn't mean I'm not a little jealous that I didn't get to see them tonight."

"So you'll get to see them next time," Maggie said, looking down at the dessert menu Nic had handed her when she sat down.

"Next time?" I turned to look at her. So did everyone else.

"Do you know something the rest of us don't?" Brady asked.

Maggie looked up at us. "What? No. No. It's just that everyone who was there tonight could see how much fun the guys were having. I can't believe they're just going to do that once and then walk away."

I thought about how often I'd noticed Harry smiling tonight and how Paul and Mike couldn't stop grinning. "You might be right," I said.

Nic was still smiling. "I hope you are." He gestured at the menu Maggie still held in one hand. "So what can I get for you?"

"Is there any more of that cobbler you had on Wednesday?" she asked.

"The strawberry rhubarb?"

Maggie nodded.

Nic's dark eyes sparkled. "Eric just took some out of the oven about twenty minutes ago. It's still warm."

"That would be perfect," Maggie said.

He looked around the table. "For everyone?"

We all nodded our agreement, looking a little like a collection of bobblehead dolls. "Please," I said.

Nic traced a circle in the air with one finger, working his way around the table. "Coffee, coffee, coffee, coffee, coffee and tea?" He ended the circuit at Maggie.

"I think I'll have tea, too," Roma said.

"I'll be right back," Nic said, heading for the kitchen.

Across the table from me, Roma was swaying from side to side, the motion so small, it was almost unnoticeable.

"Okay, so what song are you still hearing in your head?" I asked.

Her cheeks turned pink. "'Hold On,'" she said. "Hold On" was one of several songs the band had performed that had been written by Johnny and Mike. Johnny and the Outlaws had mostly been a cover band I knew, but they had performed some of their own songs as well. "I was remembering the first time I heard Johnny sing it. It was the very first time I saw them in concert. That was a long time ago."

Roma was older than the rest of us, although it wasn't something I ever thought about. I knew she'd

seen Johnny and the Outlaws in concert more than once before the band had broken up.

A smile pulled at her mouth and there was a far-away look in her eyes. "I was sixteen. They were play-ing at the high school in Red Wing—opening for some other group, and for the life of me, I can't remember who it was. What I do remember vividly is that Johnny had hair to his shoulders, Mike had a mullet and they were way better than the band they were opening for."

I tried to picture Mike Bishop with a mullet but couldn't get there. Then again, before tonight I would have never been able to picture him playing bass in a band, either.

"If they were that good, why did they break up?" Brady asked. Brady was a lawyer. He had a very prac-tical, logical streak.

Roma frowned. "I don't know. I just always as-sumed that real life got in the way. I don't imagine any of their parents thought being in a band would be a good career choice."

"I saw them in concert right before they broke up," Maggie said. "I was maybe six."

"What were you doing at a concert when you were six?" Roma asked.

She shrugged. "My dad was a big music fan. I don't mean it was at a club or anything close to that. The show was in the daytime. I know we were outside somewhere and Dad bought me a caramel apple. I have no idea what songs they did but I do remember that caramel apple. It was good."

Marcus leaned back in his chair. "I saw Johnny on his own in a little club in Minneapolis. I was eighteen. I had a fake ID. It was just Johnny and another guy playing guitar."

Eddie gave him an incredulous look. "You had a fake ID? You? Mr. Law and Order?"

Marcus was a detective with the Mayville Heights Police Department. Pretty much everyone in town would have described him as a straight arrow. "It was during my bad-boy phase."

Roma burst out laughing. She held up one hand and pressed the other against her chest. "I'm sorry, Marcus," she said. "I just . . . I just can't picture you having a bad-boy phase."

"Hey, I had long hair and a couple of days of scruff, and I wore Docs with everything . . . and okay, so I probably wasn't nearly as rebellious as I thought I was."

"No, you weren't," Brady said emphatically. "Ever spend the night in jail?"

"Yes," Marcus said. That got everyone's attention. "It was during training."

Brady shook his head. "Yeah. Doesn't count. Ever been chased by the police?"

"Oh! I have." Eddie waved one hand in the air.

Maggie didn't say anything, but I noticed she nodded her head ever so slightly. Had she been chased by the police at some point in her past? It seemed about as likely as Marcus ever having been a "bad boy."

"Who are you people?" Roma asked. "And why didn't I know my own husband seems to have had a run-in with the law?"

"I told you that story," Eddie said. "Back when I was playing. We were on the road in Chicago. Matts ended up naked. Remember?"

For a moment she still looked confused, then recognition dawned on her. "It was February. You were trying to snag the last playoff spot that year."

Eddie nodded, leaning back and resting both wrists on the top of his head. "Though technically that might not count as the only time I was chased by the police. It depends on how you define 'chased.'" He paused for a moment. "And 'police.'"

Eddie was saved from having to explain himself any further by Nic arriving at the table with our food. The strawberry-rhubarb cobbler was as delicious as it had been when Maggie, Roma and I had enjoyed it on Wednesday. It was still slightly warm from the oven, with a small dollop of vanilla-flavored whipped cream.

No one spoke until we'd all eaten pretty much half of our desserts. Then Maggie turned to Roma, holding up her spoon as though it were a magic wand that she was about to grant a wish with. "This was such a good idea," she said. "Thank you for suggesting we come here."

Roma smiled at her. "I can't believe Johnny got the band back together and no one figured it out."

Marcus shrugged. "Maybe there were people who did, but just didn't want to ruin the surprise."

I set down my spoon and reached for my coffee. "I can't get over how Harry didn't give himself away." I was pretty good at spotting subterfuge. My parents were actors and I'd learned a lot about the subtleties

of body language from them. "I told him how much I was looking forward to hearing Johnny perform and all he said was so was he."

"Which wasn't a lie," Roma said, licking whipped cream from the back of her spoon. "He just didn't say he'd be performing as well."

"Good point," I said. "And it was an incredible surprise. I'm glad everyone who knew kept the secret."

"You should tell Harry that," Maggie said. She scooped up a piece of rhubarb and swirled it through the whipped cream in Brady's bowl. She'd already eaten all of hers. His response was to nudge the dish a little closer to her without saying a word.

I took a sip of my coffee. "I will, the very next time I see him."

Mags lifted the lid of her little teapot and peered inside, then closed it again, seemingly satisfied with what she'd seen. She looked at me and gestured over her shoulder. "Just look over at the door," she said with a smile. "Harry just walked in."

2

Harry, Johnny and the rest of the Outlaws had just come in. Nic walked over to them, looking around the room as he did so. He said something to Johnny, who nodded, and the group started in our direction. Ritchie had his arm around a tiny, dark-haired woman. His wife, I guessed. Paul was holding hands with *his* wife, Sonja, whom I knew from the library.

There were two smaller tables to our left. Nic pushed them together and quickly rearranged the chairs, grabbing a couple extra from a nearby table.

Mike was still wearing his fedora. He dropped it on the nearest chair. Roma was already on her feet. Mike grinned, raising one eyebrow at her. His face was flushed. She hugged him and then pulled back and slugged his left arm. "You are such a sneak," she said. "I can't believe you kept a secret like that."

"Was it worth it?" Johnny asked.

Roma nodded. "Absolutely!"

"Your playing gave me goose bumps," I said to Harry.

He smiled. "Thank you," he said. He shifted from one foot to the other almost as though he was a bit uncomfortable hearing the praise.

Nic had come back with the coffeepot and was filling cups at the table.

"Do you think we could get breakfast sandwiches?" Johnny asked him.

Nic nodded. "Sure. Sourdough and fried tomatoes?"

"Sounds good," Johnny said. "Thanks."

Nic glanced at me and then dropped his gaze down to my mug for a moment. I nodded. He made his way over and topped up my cup and Brady's. "It shouldn't be too long," he said to Johnny as he headed back toward the kitchen.

Johnny turned to me. "So?" he asked, holding up both hands. Johnny was what my mother would have called "one of the good ones." It wasn't common knowledge, but he was a big supporter of the elementary school's brown-bag lunch program and Reading Buddies at the library.

"So 'wow' doesn't seem anywhere near adequate," I said.

He smiled. "Thank you. There was something magical about being up onstage with the guys again." He rolled his eyes. "I know it probably sounds silly, talking like that."

I shook my head. "Not to me. Both my parents are actors and I've seen firsthand that sometimes the whole really is more than the sum of its parts."

Mike joined us then. "Hi, Kathleen. How's your

tooth?" he asked. He couldn't seem to keep still. The fingers on his right hand were moving like they were still on the strings of his bass. He reminded me of my brother, Ethan.

"My tooth is fine and you were terrific," I said.

"Thank you," he said, giving me that little-boy grin.

"How did you manage to keep the reunion a secret?"

Johnny shifted from one foot to the other. Like Mike he still seemed to have that buzz of energy from the concert. "I still can't believe that we did. Mostly it was just dumb luck. I figured someone would mess up and it would get out."

"He means me," Mike said. "Hey, Kathleen, you know those old World War Two posters you have down at the library?"

I nodded.

Roma's husband, Eddie, had opened a hockey school in Mayville Heights. A cache of Second World War propaganda posters had been unearthed during renovations to the empty warehouse down by the river that was home to the school. Eddie had donated them to the library. I had an exhibit of the posters planned for November, and after that, they were going to be auctioned off with the proceeds going to our ongoing project to digitize all the old documents we had that were too fragile to be handled very often. The posters were in excellent shape and I was hoping they'd all sell.

Mike stuck out his lower lip and plucked at it several times with one finger like he was playing a guitar string. "'Loose lips sink ships,'" he said, quoting one

of the posters he'd seen in my office. Mike was work-ing on researching his family tree and he'd spent a lot of time at the library recently, going through old rec-ords and documents. "Everyone thought I'd never be able to keep quiet. And you were all wrong."

"I'm impressed by your secret-keeping skills," I said.

Mike put one hand on his chest and gave a slight bow. "Thank you," he said.

"Yeah, you did good," Johnny said. He looked at me. There was a gleam in his blue eyes. I had the feeling Johnny just might have used Mike's desire to prove everyone wrong to make sure their secret stayed secret.

Nic came from the kitchen then with a giant circular tray. I could smell Eric's signature breakfast sandwich and I almost wished I had ordered one instead of the cobbler.

I sat down again and picked up my coffee. Eddie had shifted in his seat and was deep in conversation with Paul Whitewater, who had turned his own chair sideways, and Brady, who was standing by the end of our table, hands jammed in his pockets. They had to be talking about hockey, I realized, based on the way Eddie was moving his hands almost as though he were holding a stick.

After more than one setback, the Sweeney Center was finally finished. The former warehouse space had an ice surface and a conditioning room. Eddie would start working with his first class of summer hockey students on Monday. Roma had told me that he was also donating coaching time and space to both the

boys' and girls' high school hockey teams. That didn't surprise me. That was the type of person Eddie was.

Sonja Whitewater was sitting beside her husband. She leaned sideways into my line of vision and waved. I waved back; then I stood up again and made my way over to her, carrying my coffee.

"So did you enjoy the concert?" Sonja asked. She had ice-blue eyes and blond hair cut to her collarbone.

"I don't know when I last had so much fun," I said.

She grinned. "I'm glad. I've always been more nervous than Paul is when he performs."

I nodded. "I know what you mean. My mom and dad are actors and Mom is always more anxious when Dad's performing than she is when she's the one onstage. And heaven help any critic who doesn't like his work."

Sonja laughed. "I think I'd like your mother. I'm exactly the same way. I'm glad you're here. I've been wanting to thank you for the book recommendations last time I was in. They were all a big hit, especially the series about the talking hamster named Einstein."

"It's one of my favorites," I said. "I'm glad you like it. And in case you're interested, we have multiple copies of all the books in the series so far."

"I can't tell you how glad I am to hear that," she said. "I would never complain about my kids reading but we go through books the way other families go through boxes of Cheerios."

"Kids who like to read," I said with a smile. "Music to my ears."

Sonja's phone buzzed then and she reached for it. "I'll see you Monday," she said.

Harry was seated on the other side of the two pushed-together tables from Sonja and Paul. Ritchie Gonzalez and his wife were on his left and there was an empty seat to his right. I made my way over to Harry. There was something I wanted to do.

"Harry, I owe you an apology," I said when I reached him.

He frowned. "Why? What did you do?" He indicated the chair beside him and I sat down.

"I kept you at the library, going on about my ideas for the cold frames this afternoon, and you had the concert to get to."

Harry was shaking his head before I finished speaking. "You don't have to apologize for anything. As I remember it, it was me who asked you to come out and show me where you want to put those boxes."

Harry had built several raised beds so the kids in our summer program at the library could grow their own vegetables. The project had turned out to be more successful than I'd hoped. We'd made salads with the first harvest of lettuce and radishes and not one child had complained about eating vegetables. A couple of days ago, we'd sent each child home with a small bag of tomatoes and yellow beans. I wanted to extend the growing season with cold frames so the Reading Buddies kids could have the same experience.

"Kathleen, you don't know Ritchie and Elena, do you?" Harry asked.

I shook my head. "I don't."

He gestured at his friend. "Kathleen Paulson. Ritchie and Elena Gonzalez."

I smiled. "It's nice to meet you both."

Elena had a mass of dark curls brushing her shoulders. She was wearing a black T-shirt with the words *I'm with the band* across the chest.

She looked familiar. I thought back to where I could possibly have met her before and then it hit me. "Are you a nurse?"

She smiled. "A nurse practitioner."

"You helped treat my broken wrist at the clinic about four years ago. I knew you looked familiar," I said.

"That's right." She tipped her head toward my arm. "May I?" she asked.

I nodded.

She reached over and gently fingered my left wrist. "It looks like you healed well," she said.

"I did, although I now have a better accuracy rate predicting rain than the meteorologist on Channel 4."

Ritchie smiled. "She never forgets a patient."

Elena shrugged. "I just have that kind of memory. I'm really good at trivia games, too."

"So am I," I said. "You know, we've been talking about doing a trivia tournament this winter at the library."

Ritchie looked at Harry. "You may have started something here."

Elena's dark eyes lit up. "We'll talk later," she said.

Ritchie leaned forward. "I think I saw you once in the library when I was meeting Mike. It's a gorgeous old building by the way."

"Thank you," I said. "It took a lot of work from a lot of people, including Harry."

Harry didn't say anything. He just gave his head a little shake. He was the most self-effacing person I had ever met.

"Kathleen, someone mentioned that Ethan Paulson is your brother," Ritchie said. Up close I could see some gray in his thick dark hair. "Is that right?"

"He is," I said. "How do you know Ethan?"

Ritchie smiled. Without a smile he looked more than a little imposing. With one he looked like a big teddy bear. "I don't really know him. I saw The Flaming Gerbils last winter in Red Wing and I got to talk to your brother between sets. Man, what a voice!"

I felt a rush of big-sister pride. I knew Ethan was enormously talented but it was always great to hear other people felt the same way.

"He would have loved tonight," I said. "You were all incredible."

"Thank you," Ritchie said. "It was a once-in-a-lifetime experience, getting out there again, all five of us together."

"Or maybe not."

I turned. Mike was standing behind me.

"Give it a rest," Ritchie said. He didn't seem annoyed by Mike's comment. I got the feeling he was mostly ignoring it.

Beside me Harry let out a breath. "Mike thinks we should all go out and do a few dates with Johnny," he said to me by way of explanation.

"You can't tell me you really don't want to do this again!" Mike exclaimed. "They loved us. You were there, Kathleen. Tell him!"

"Harry doesn't need me to tell him anything," I said, getting to my feet. "But I do need to tell you about a couple of resources I thought of that might be useful to help you finish your family tree." I tipped my head in the direction of the long counter at the other end of the diner and reached for my coffee. "I need a refill. Walk me over."

Mike rolled his eyes. "I know what you're doing," he said.

"I thought you would," I said. I smiled at Ritchie and Elena. "It was good to meet you."

"You too, Kathleen," Ritchie said. Elena nodded and smiled.

"So did you really come up with more ideas for me?" Mike asked as we made our way around the tables.

I nodded. "Actually the credit should go to Abigail. She remembered some documents that seem to be from some kind of accounting of people in this part of the state. We did a little digging and found them. They predate the first Minnesota Territorial Census of 1849 by a year. They might help you learn more about your great-great-grandfather's family."

"You're serious?"

I nodded. "The paper is very fragile and you'll need a magnifier and some patience to read the names."

"I thought I was at a dead end. This could be exactly what I've been looking for." Going on the road with Johnny seemed to be forgotten—at least for now. Mike gave me a saucy grin. "Kathleen, I would bow down and kiss your hand if your very large police-detective boyfriend weren't just over there talking to my cousin."

"How about you bring me coffee next time you come to the library instead?"

"Done!" he said. "And that will be Monday—probably afternoon if that's okay? I took the week off."

"It's fine with me. Abigail will be there and so will I."

Nic was behind the counter. He held out a hand and I gave him my mug. He refilled it and handed it back. "Thank you," I said.

Mike and I headed back to the others. "Hey, I really owe you a big thank-you for all the help you've given me while I've been researching the family," he said. "It turned out to be a much bigger project than I ever expected."

"It's part of my job," I said. "And I've found the whole thing fascinating." I took a sip of my coffee. "I had no idea your great-aunt, Leitha, went to college at sixteen, let alone learned to fly as part of the War Training Service. And she knew John Glenn."

"Yeah, that surprised me as well. She rarely talked about that part of her life." He pulled his fingers through his hair. "You know, Aunt Leitha is the reason I started researching the Finnamore family history."

I shook my head. "I didn't."

"Before she died she was taking part in a long-term study into heart disease."

"I *did* know that."

Leitha Finnamore Anderson had outlived her brother, her two nieces *and* a great-nephew. With the exception of the great-nephew, all had died from cardiac issues. Leitha herself had been ninety-three when her car went off the road this past spring. She had died

as a result of her injuries. Researchers wanted to know why Leitha—and people like her—lived so long and were physically and mentally in such good shape. Was it genetics? Was it lifestyle? Was it both? Or neither? And was there any connection with other traits such as eye color or height?

Mike made a face. "Like I said, there were things she never talked about, and once she was gone, I was sorry I didn't push more. I felt this urgency to learn about the family while there were still people left to talk to." He held up a finger as though something had just occurred to him. "That reminds me, Kathleen: At some point I'd like to have a family tree drawn out. Isn't there a guy at the artists' co-op who does that sort of thing?"

"You're probably thinking about Ray Nightingale," I said.

Ray was best known for his intricate pen-and-ink drawings, which each featured a tiny fedora-wearing duck named Bo somewhere in the design. Ray had also drawn several family trees for different people— in one case drawing a very detailed actual tree to showcase that family's connections.

Mike snapped his fingers. "Nightingale. Right. That's the guy I was thinking of."

"I'm sorry. Ray isn't in town anymore." I held up one hand before he could speak. "But I know someone who should be able to help you." I gestured at Maggie, who was deep in conversation with Johnny. "Do you know Maggie Adams?"

"The yoga teacher?"

"Uh-huh. And she's also a very talented artist."

Mike had already started to nod. "Wait a second. Did she make that mannequin thing of Eddie a few years back for Winterfest?"

I nodded. "Yes, she did." The "mannequin thing of Eddie" had been responsible for Eddie and Roma ending up together.

"You think she could make what I'm looking for?"

"I do. But if she couldn't, or if she doesn't have time in her schedule, Maggie could put you in touch with another artist who could help you. She used to be the president of the artists' co-op."

"Fantastic," Mike said. "Introduce me."

We joined Maggie and Johnny and I made the introductions, explaining to Mags what Mike was looking for.

"Off the top of my head, I can come up with a couple of ways to go," she said. "You could go very minimalist, with a clean, simple design, and focus on the fonts and the paper. Or you could take the completely opposite tack and do something very detailed. What were you thinking of?"

I knew that gleam in her eye. She was interested.

Mike shrugged. "I don't know. Something more than just names on a piece of paper. Something that could be framed and hung on the wall."

"You know that all you're going to find in the family tree are brigands and reprobates," a voice said behind us.

I turned to find Jonas Quinn—Mike's cousin—and Jonas's nephew, Lachlan, grinning at us. I knew Jonas from the library. He was an avid reader of military

history and "hard" science fiction and lately books on genetics, which made sense since Mike was digging into the family history. He was about the same height as Marcus, which meant he was just over six feet, and he had dark eyes and wavy dark hair cut much shorter than Mike's. Jonas was a college professor and Lachlan's guardian.

I knew Lachlan because he'd come to the library with Mike more than once. He was seventeen and a nice kid. He had the same thick hair as Mike and Jonas did, except his was long, pulled back into a ponytail. "A tangle of curls," I remembered Mary calling it.

"As you can probably tell, my cousin is not interested in our past," Mike said dryly.

"That's true." Jonas nudged his black brow-line glasses up his nose. "I'm looking to the future, which is Lachlan."

"Geez, no pressure," the teen said. I saw the gleam in his green eyes and knew he wasn't really feeling pressured.

"Lachlan wants to study music," Mike said.

"What's your dream school?" I asked.

Lachlan smiled. "Berklee," he said. "But I know how hard it is to get in, so I'm applying to other places as well. I want to be an audio engineer and music producer."

"He plays piano, guitar and bass," Jonas said.

I knew that Lachlan's father was Jonas Quinn's younger brother. Jonas had taken on raising the boy when his parents died as the result of a car accident. I could hear the parental pride in his voice.

"He's good," Johnny added. "I'm running out of things to teach him."

Lachlan ducked his head as a flush of color crept up his neck.

"I think you'd like Boston," I said as a way of changing the subject. "There's an incredible amount of music to see live. Whatever kind of music you like, someone somewhere in the city is playing it."

"That's where you grew up, right?" Lachlan asked.

I took a sip of my coffee. It had gotten cold. "For the most part. My family still lives there."

Maggie leaned into my line of vision. "Kath, you should connect him with Ethan," she said.

I nodded. "That's a good idea." I turned my attention to Lachlan again. "My younger brother, Ethan, is a musician. He could tell you all about the music scene in Boston, and a friend of his went to Berklee. Ethan teaches music and he has a band called The Flaming Gerbils."

Lachlan frowned. "Wait a sec. The lead singer? That's your brother? Ritchie played me a couple of their songs. They're really good. Man, I'd love to talk to him."

"Send me a text so I have your number and I'll pass it on to Ethan tomorrow," I said.

He pulled out his phone and I recited my number. He immediately sent me a text, then looked up smiling. "Seriously, thank you. There's so much stuff I'd like to ask him." The smile wavered. "You don't think he'll mind, do you?"

I laughed. "If Ethan's not making music, he's talking about music. He eats, sleeps and breathes it. He won't have any problem answering anything you ask him."

Maggie asked a question then about what other schools Lachlan was applying to. Watching him, I could see how much he resembled both Mike and Jonas. Like Mike he was very animated when he was talking, his hands flying everywhere, and he had the same way of tilting his head to the side while he was listening that Jonas did.

I pictured Ethan and Sarah, who didn't look that much alike even though they were twins, but who did share the same intensity about so many things. Ethan and I both had dark hair, but my eyes, like Sarah's, were brown and his were hazel. I felt a twinge of homesickness for my own family.

I could have stayed there talking all night. I saw Harry check his watch and Roma stifle a yawn.

Marcus came up behind me and put an arm around my shoulders. "Ready to go?" he asked.

I nodded. Across the room Johnny was at the counter getting the bill for his whole group, I realized. From the expression on Nic's face, he'd also added a very nice tip.

We gathered our things and said good night to Nic. Outside on the sidewalk I gave Roma a hug. "Thank you for suggesting this," I said, gesturing at the café behind us. "Best night ever."

"Absolutely," she said. She smiled, grabbed Eddie by the hand and they headed down the sidewalk.

Marcus was talking to Harry about something, their expressions serious. Maggie and Brady joined me. "Hey, thank you for suggesting me to Mike for his family tree," she said.

"So you're interested in designing it for him?" I asked.

She nodded. "I am. I got back into drawing when the bake-off was filming here and it's something I'd like to keep doing."

A failed attempt at resurrecting *The Great Northern Baking Showdown* had been filmed this past spring in Mayville Heights. Maggie had been hired to work with the show's illustrator.

"I can't wait to see what you come up with," I said. I turned to Brady. "A little bird told me your dad bought an air hockey table."

He gave his head a shake and smiled. "I'm guessing that bird's name is Rebecca."

"It is," I said.

"Doesn't surprise me," he said. "Rebecca is how Dad found out about it in the first place. She was at the office, they started talking and the next time I go out to the house, there's an air hockey table in the living room."

Rebecca was Rebecca Henderson. She was married to Everett Henderson. The office Brady had referred to was Everett's. Everett's assistant, Lita, and Brady's father, Burtis, were a couple. And to make things even more tangled, Rebecca and Everett were my backyard neighbors.

"I'll have to come out sometime for a game," I said.

"You know that's why he got the darn thing, don't you?" Brady said.

Brady had bought a pinball machine, which he kept out at his father's house. I was pretty good at pinball—as well as rod hockey, foosball and, yes, air hockey, the result of a lot of time spent hanging around while I was a kid and my parents did summer stock all up

and down the East Coast. When I mentioned my skill at pinball, Burtis had challenged me to prove it. I had. More than once.

I grinned. "Tell Burtis I'll be happy to take his money anytime." The last time we'd played pinball, Burtis had suggested a small wager on the outcome of the game. Double or nothing had netted the Reading Buddies snack fund fifty dollars.

Marcus joined me then. We said good night to Maggie and Brady and headed for the truck.

"I don't think I'm ever going to forget tonight," I said as I unlocked the passenger door for Marcus.

"Johnny's going to do a couple of shows in Minneapolis next month," Marcus said as he climbed into the truck. "Why don't we try to catch one?"

"I'd like that." I slid behind the wheel. "Mike is trying to get the others to commit to doing a few of Johnny's shows with him."

Marcus smiled and fastened his seat belt. "So maybe we'll get to see Johnny and the Outlaws again."

I held up one hand, my middle and index fingers crossed. "Let's hope."

Marcus and I enjoyed a quiet Sunday. We had pancakes with Owen and Hercules, which should have meant that Marcus and I had pancakes and the cats had cat food, but in reality meant that Marcus and I had pancakes and he snuck (forbidden) bites to them and I pretended not to notice.

I called Ethan, who said he'd be happy to talk to Lachlan and promised he'd text right after we hung up.

Then he spent ten minutes bombarding me with questions about the concert.

We walked down to the market at the community center after lunch and all anyone could talk about was the concert and the surprise reunion of Johnny and the Outlaws. I spotted Harrison Taylor Senior, Harry's father, with his lady friend, Peggy. He was carrying a canvas shopping bag in one hand. Peggy smiled when she caught sight of me and I left Marcus at the Jam Lady's stall, trying to decide between strawberry-rhubarb jam and pear butter, and walked over to join them.

"Your son was amazing last night," I said, giving the old man a hug. He had thick white hair, a white beard that he kept cropped shorter in the summertime and deep blue eyes.

"Yes, he was," Harrison said, a huge smile splitting his face.

"Did you know?" I asked, raising an eyebrow at him.

"I knew something was up. All of a sudden the boy was never around." Harrison gave a snort of laughter. "To tell the truth, I thought he was seeing someone and didn't want me to know."

Harrison had been pushing his son—who had been divorced for years—to, as he put it, get a mitt and get back in the game. If Harry had met someone, he probably *would* be pretty closemouthed about it.

"I had no idea Harry was that good," I said. "I knew he'd been in a band but . . ." I shrugged.

"Harry's not the kind of person to blow his own horn," Peggy said with a smile.

Harrison set the shopping bag on the ground

between his feet. "I remember when he got his first guitar and I'm kind of ashamed to say I told him it was a waste of money. He taught himself to play. Just sat there night after night in his room until the ends of his fingers cracked." He gave his head a little shake. "It's not a word of a lie. The dog wouldn't come in the house for six months. But that son of mine is stubborn."

"I wonder where that came from," Peggy said, almost under her breath.

Harrison shot her a look. "There's nothing wrong with my hearing, you know."

She leaned against his arm and smiled. "I know."

"Well, wherever his persistence came from, it paid off and I couldn't be prouder," the old man said. "I've been smiling since he started playin' and I don't think I'll be stopping anytime soon." His pride was evident in that smile and the sparkle in his blue eyes.

I spent a few more minutes catching up with Harrison and Peggy. Elizabeth, Harrison's youngest child, was coming for a visit in August and they were already planning a family barbecue.

"You're coming," he said. It wasn't a question. Harrison's definition of family was a wide one.

"I wouldn't miss it," I promised, standing on tiptoe to kiss his cheek.

I rejoined Marcus to discover that he'd bought the jam and the pear butter *and* a jar of the Jam Lady's marmalade, which was my favorite. We wandered around the market a while longer and then drove out to Marcus's house. I curled up on the swing on his back deck. Micah, Marcus's little ginger tabby, climbed up onto

my lap, swatting me twice with her tail as she got settled. Marcus set up the ice cream maker for peach ice cream and grilled spicy sausage and corn on the barbecue. It had been pretty much the perfect weekend.

Monday morning I set out the census documents I'd told Mike about in our workroom so everything would be ready when he arrived in the afternoon. Considering their age and the fact that for a long time they'd been stuffed, forgotten, in an old filing cabinet in the library basement, the pages weren't in awful shape. Like the rest of our old documents, they would eventually be scanned and added to our digital database.

I relocked the workroom door and went into the staff room for a cup of coffee, taking it back to my office, where I stood by the window looking out at the gazebo. It was another beautiful day. Marcus was bringing lunch later and I thought how nice it would be to eat outside. It was good to see things looking quiet out there. In the spring the gazebo had been targeted by a practical joker who had—among other things—left an inflatable pool full of Jell-O in it. Black raspberry to be specific. It had been several weeks since the last stunt and I was hoping our prankster had gotten bored and moved on. Both Mary and Harry were convinced this was just a temporary respite from Jell-O, stacks of hay bales and a full-sized Grim Reaper with a broom instead of a scythe.

"Get it? It's the Grim Sweeper!" Susan, who had worked at the library long enough to have seen her

share of stunts and pranks, had crowed with delight over that last one.

I was downstairs about an hour later, trying to fix a broken wheel on one of our book carts when Abigail called to me from the front desk.

"It's Marcus," she said, gesturing at the phone that I hadn't even heard ring.

"Thanks," I said as I got to my feet, brushing off the front of my flowered skirt. I walked over and picked up the receiver.

"Hi," Marcus said. He blew out a breath. "I'm not going to be able to make lunch." There was a flatness to his voice that told me he was in full police-detective mode.

"A case."

"Yes." He hesitated.

My stomach clutched. This was something bad.

"I'm sorry, Kathleen," he finally said. "There's no good way to say this. Mike Bishop is dead."

3

N o," I whispered. I closed my eyes for a moment and swallowed against the lump in my throat, which seemed to be stopping me from getting words out. "Are you . . . are you positive?"

"Yes. I wish I wasn't," Marcus said, "and I'm sorry but I have to go. I should make it for supper. I mean, if you still want to cook."

I nodded even though he couldn't see me. "I do." And because it suddenly seemed important, I added, "Stay safe."

"Always," he replied.

I hung up the phone and stood there, not moving, as Marcus's words began to sink in.

"Kathleen, what's wrong?" Abigail asked, coming around the side of the circulation desk. A frown creased her forehead and her eyes were narrowed in concern.

"It's, uh, it's Mike Bishop," I said slowly.

"What happened? Was he in some kind of accident?" She put a hand on my arm. Abigail had helped Mike with a lot of the research into his family tree. They'd gotten to be friends.

"I don't know what happened but . . ." I let the end of the sentence trail away. I didn't want to say the words out loud.

Abigail pressed her lips together and gave her head a little shake.

I swallowed again. It didn't seem to do anything for that lump in the back of my throat. "He's . . . dead."

A tear slid down her cheek and she swiped at it with one hand. "Are you sure?" she asked, looking away. "Maybe Marcus made a mistake. Maybe it was someone else."

I shook my head. "He doesn't make those kind of mistakes."

"I know," she said softly.

Neither one of us spoke for a moment. Then Abigail looked at me. "What do they give the dentist of the year?" she asked in a shaky voice.

I frowned at her, not really understanding the question. "I . . . I don't know."

"A little plaque." She laughed and then hiccupped. "Mike always had some awful dental joke to tell me when he came in and I'd always laugh because they were so bad." She wiped away another tear. "Why did the dental assistant refuse to date the dentist?"

I shook my head.

"He was already taking out a tooth."

I laughed then in spite of myself. "You're right," I said. "Those are terrible jokes."

"And remember how he hated it when someone called him a dentist?" Abigail asked. "Mary would do it just to tease him. He'd give her that look." She pushed her glasses down her nose and looked over the top of them at me. "And he'd say, 'Endodontist.' Then Mary would say something about how barbers used to do all that stuff *and* give you a shave and a haircut." She blinked away tears. "Oh, Kathleen, how can it be true?" Her shoulders sagged.

I didn't have an answer to her question. All I could do was give her a hug and blink back my own tears.

"You know Mike was genuinely excited about tracing his family tree," she said. "He told me that his cousin had warned him that he might find nothing but criminals and con men back there. He told me that he kind of hoped he would. That would be way more interesting than a family full of straitlaced rule followers."

"That sounds like Mike."

She gave me a small smile. "He looked like he was having so much fun being back onstage again. You could see it." She started to say something else and then stopped.

"What?" I asked.

"I was going to say that there's never going to be a night like that again, and then it hit me that now that Mike is . . . gone, there really isn't."

"We went to Eric's after the concert and they came in," I said. "Mike, Johnny, Harry—all of them. I told Mike

about those census documents you found. He was coming in this afternoon to take a look at them. I set everything out in the workroom. I should go put things away again."

"I'll take care of it," Abigail said. "I mean, if it's all right with you. I could use a couple of minutes by myself."

"It's fine with me," I said. "Give me a minute to get Levi to keep an eye on the desk."

She nodded. "Thanks." She glanced over at the books she'd been sorting. "So Marcus didn't say anything about what happened? If it was a car accident or a heart attack."

"All he said was Mike was gone. He had to go and he didn't give me any details." I looked around for Levi, our summer student. "I'll be right back," I said.

I headed for the stacks where Levi was shelving books. The fact that Marcus *hadn't* said what had happened to Mike Bishop bothered me and I hoped Abigail hadn't noticed my discomfort at her question. He could have easily said Mike had had a heart attack or been in a car accident if either of those things had occurred. But he hadn't and I couldn't shake the feeling that something a lot worse had happened. I hoped I was wrong.

When the library closed for the day, I drove out to Marcus's house to make supper. Rebecca was checking in on Owen and Hercules, who I knew would be fine, but who were also more than a little spoiled. Marcus and I had talked about introducing his Micah to the boys.

All three cats had been found out at Wisteria Hill—the old Henderson estate—and all three were far from typical cats, so I was hoping they'd get along.

Micah was waiting for me on the back deck. The little ginger tabby meowed hello and then jumped down to stand by the door and look expectantly at me. I let us both into the kitchen, set my bag on the table and dropped into one of the chairs.

Micah immediately launched herself onto my lap. She seemed to study me for a moment and then, as if sensing I was upset, she leaned her body against my chest with a soft "mrr." I stroked her fur and felt a little of the day's stress subsiding. The news about Mike had spread quickly and everyone who had come into the library seemed to want to talk about him. While it had been good to hear more stories about his sense of humor and quiet generosity, it had also been painful to realize that a good man was gone and wasn't coming back.

After a few minutes, I gave Micah one last scratch under her chin and set her on the floor. "Want to help me get supper?" I asked.

"Merow," she said, whiskers twitching.

That seemed to be a yes.

As I stood up, I realized that there were two physics textbooks on the chair next to mine. I leaned down and opened the cover of the top book. It had come from the library in Minneapolis. There was a piece of paper poking out from between two pages just beyond the midpoint of the text.

These two books were the fifth and sixth books on theoretical physics Marcus had requested via inter-

library loan. Since he had found out about the special "skills" that Owen and Hercules *and* Micah had, he'd been looking for some sort of logical explanation. I'd struggled with telling him that all three cats had abilities that seemed to violate the laws of physics, at least as we knew them at this point in time. I'd put it off longer than I should have. I knew it had been hard for him to accept that Hercules had the ability to walk through any solid object, while both Owen and Micah could literally disappear at will—and usually at the most inconvenient times. Even when Marcus actually saw it happen, it was hard to believe it wasn't some kind of trick. I understood how he felt. It had taken me a little time to accept that I wasn't hallucinating, that I didn't have a brain tumor.

The first time I'd seen Owen disappear, I'd been able to convince myself it was just a trick of the light and my own overtired brain. When Hercules walked through a closed door after hours at the library, I'd thought that maybe I'd had a stroke. I had long suspected Micah had the same skill as Owen, so it wasn't as much of a surprise the first time she vanished, although the knowledge had come with the added worry that now I had to stop putting off telling Marcus just exactly how smart all three cats were.

I closed the cover of the book and straightened up. Micah was watching me, her head cocked to one side in curiosity. "He's persistent," I said.

"Mrr," she agreed.

I didn't think Marcus was going to give up until he found something that explained how the cats could

do what they could do. That determined streak was one of the things that helped make him a good detective. Still, sometimes I thought he just needed to accept how things were and stop trying to find answers for questions that just might not have answers.

I washed my hands and set a pot of water on the stove to boil for the pasta. The cat watched and made little murping comments as I got out the rest of the ingredients for pasta salad.

"Should we eat in here or out on the deck?" I asked.

She immediately looked at the back door.

"Deck, it is," I said. "Excellent choice."

I moved the little round table Marcus kept out on the deck so it was in front of the swing and set it with place mats, napkins and silverware. While the pasta cooked, I put together a quick marinade for the chicken. Then I made the pasta salad, adding cucumber, celery, black olives and plump cherry tomatoes and radishes that Marcus had grown himself.

I'd just poured a glass of iced tea and stepped out onto the deck when Marcus came around the side of the house. "It's so good to see you," he said, wrapping his long arms around me and giving me a kiss.

"It's good to see you, too," I said. He looked tired. There was dark stubble on his chin, his pale yellow shirt was creased and I could see that he'd been raking his hands through his hair, something he did when he was stressed.

He reached up and brushed a stray bit of hair off my face. "Are you all right? I know the news about Mike was a shock."

"It's all anyone who came into the library was talking about. Do you know what happened yet?"

A shadow seemed to flit across his face. "Could I have a shower first?" He glanced over at the grill. "Do I have time?"

I nodded. "Go ahead. The salad's made and I'll start the chicken."

He blew out a breath. "Thanks," he said. He stopped to give Micah a scratch on the top of her head and went into the house.

The chicken was just about done when Marcus came out, wearing a pair of gray shorts and a red T-shirt, his hair damp from the shower. "Is that mine?" he asked, gesturing at the frosty glass of beer on the table.

"Yes, it is," I said. My iced tea was sitting to the left of the grill.

Micah was perched in the middle of the swing. "Get down," Marcus said, making a move-along gesture with one hand.

She wrinkled her whiskers at him and, instead of jumping down, moved to the left and then looked at him. It seemed to me there was a challenge in her eyes.

Marcus shook his head. "Fine. Close enough," he said. He sat down next to the cat and reached over to stroke her fur.

I took the plate of chicken over to the table and joined them on the swing. "That smells great," Marcus said as he reached for the tongs I'd set on the table. "What did you put on the chicken?"

"Eddie's marinade and Harry's barbecue sauce," I said. I shook my head and sighed. Saying Harry's

name made me realize how much he must be grieving right now.

Marcus put a hand on my shoulder. "I saw Harry a little while ago. He's okay. At least as okay as he can be under the circumstances."

"I can't believe Mike is dead," I said, dishing some of the salad onto my plate. "He was one of those people who just seemed so . . . alive." I looked at Marcus. "I know that doesn't make any sense."

"Yes, it does," he said.

I leaned back, balancing the plate on my lap as the swing began to gently move. "Marcus, what on earth happened? Mary said Mike died from a head injury. That doesn't sound like an accident."

Mary Lowe had come in to work at lunchtime. Her daughter, Bridget, was the publisher of the *Mayville Heights Chronicle*. Bridget always seemed to know the details of any police investigation long before they made any statements on a case.

Marcus swiped a hand over his face. "I don't know why I'm surprised to hear that," he said. "I swear, sometimes it seems like Bridget has the station bugged." Micah put a paw on his leg. He cut a sliver of chicken with the edge of his fork and gave it to her. She murped a thank-you. "It's way too soon for anyone to know the exact cause of death until the medical examiner finishes his work," he continued. "Bridget shouldn't speculate and spread rumors."

I noticed he hadn't said that what Mary had told me wasn't true. "Did someone break into his house?" I asked.

"Well, what's Bridget saying?" His voice was laced with sarcasm, which he seemed to realize the moment the words were out. "I'm sorry," he said. "It just . . . hasn't been a very good day."

I put my hand on his leg and gave it a squeeze. "I know," I said.

"At this point we don't know for certain what happened," he said after a brief silence. "Mike was found inside his house. If I had to guess, I'd say he died sometime Sunday night. Beyond that, I just don't know."

"Maybe it was an accident," I offered. "Maybe he tripped over something on the floor and hit his head. Maybe he had a seizure or a stroke."

"It's possible." Marcus didn't sound convinced.

"Could Mike have walked in on someone who broke into the house? I haven't heard of any break-ins in that area."

"There haven't been any. At least nothing that's been reported to us. I talked to Oren and the Kings. They haven't seen anything suspicious."

I folded one arm up over my head, my supper forgotten for the moment. "Do you think Mike was murdered?" I asked.

Marcus raked a hand back through his hair. "Don't ask me that, please," he said.

"Okay." I put a hand against his cheek for a moment. "Have something to eat," I said. "We don't have to talk about this right now."

He reached for the pasta salad and I picked up my fork even though my appetite was pretty much gone. I

realized from the way Marcus had dodged my questions that he suspected Mike Bishop had been murdered. I had a familiar sinking feeling in my stomach.

It was the end of the week before the medical examiner declared Mike Bishop's death a homicide. For once the newspaper didn't offer any opinion on what had happened before the official ruling. Marcus had shown up with the news and a quart of mocha fudge ice cream. We were sitting in my two big Adirondack chairs in the backyard. Hercules was perched on the wide arm of my chair, washing his face and sneaking looks at my dish, while pretending he wasn't the slightest bit interested in what was in it. Owen was sitting at Marcus's feet. He knew his chance of getting even a tiny taste was slim to none and there was no chance it would be coming from me.

"The news will be in tomorrow's paper," I said. It wasn't a question. Bridget would have been looking for the story in Mike's death.

"I'll be surprised if it's not," Marcus said. He and Bridget had a cool, slightly prickly relationship. He and Mary, on the other hand, were friends. They seemed to have an unspoken agreement not to talk about Bridget.

"There's no way it could have been an accident?" I asked. It wasn't that I doubted the skills of the medical examiner. I just hated the idea that someone—anyone—had deliberately ended Mike Bishop's life.

Marcus was shaking his head before I got the words

out. "I wish there was. I agree with the medical examiner, based on what I saw. Mike hit his head on the fireplace mantel and bled into his brain. Based on the location of the wound, there's no way it could have happened accidentally." His hand briefly touched the back of his head. "Between you and me, he was punched in the face right before he hit his head. I think he was moving away from the person who threw that punch. There was nothing on the floor he could have tripped over and nothing he could have slipped on."

Hercules looked at me, tipping his head to one side and narrowing his green eyes. "If Mike had tripped while he was moving away from whoever had hit him, wouldn't he have fallen forward, not backward?" I asked.

Hercules immediately looked at Marcus, as though he wanted to hear the answer to the question as well, as though I'd asked what he'd wanted to know—which wasn't as unlikely as it seemed.

Marcus shrugged. "He could have been backing up."

"So Mike fought or struggled with some unknown person, and that person hit him and then pushed him or hit him again, which sent him into the mantel."

"That's one of the possibilities."

Hercules looked expectantly at me again. Was there something else he wanted to know? "But that suggests what happened wasn't premeditated, that it was most likely an accident. So why didn't that person call for help? It doesn't make any sense."

"I know. Mike Bishop was universally liked. I don't

think you could find anyone in town—or in this part of the state for that matter—who had a bad word to say about the man."

"So why is he dead?" I said.

Marcus shrugged. "Right now I don't know."

It felt as though the entire town showed up for Mike Bishop's funeral on Saturday. That was one of the things I liked about living in a small town, this small town—everyone knew everyone else; everyone *cared* about everyone else.

It was more than four years now since I'd arrived in Mayville Heights. The head librarian position I'd come for was supposed to only be a temporary eighteen-month appointment, with the main part of the job being to supervise the refurbishment of the library in time for its centennial. I had applied on a whim, looking to get away from Boston after a relationship had fallen apart. The building had been beautifully restored, the collections had been reorganized and the computer system brought more or less into this century, but when the time was up, I found myself wanting to stay. I had Owen and Hercules. I had friends. I had a life I loved. I was lucky that the library board had wanted me to stay as well. As much as I sometimes missed my family back in Boston, Mayville Heights was my home now. Now I felt that sense of community very strongly.

Marcus and I sat with Eddie and Roma at the service. Roma had known Mike for years and she had taken his death hard. She had been pale but composed

when she and Eddie pulled into Gunnerson's parking lot, but when I'd hugged her, she'd held on a little tighter and a little longer than usual.

I had closed the library an hour early because all of the staff wanted to attend the funeral.

"I was leaving one night after my shift and Mike asked me what I was listening to," Levi had said to me when he'd asked for the time off to attend the service. "I told him ZZ Top. About a week later, he comes in and says he has something for me. It was a concert T-shirt from the band's *El Loco* tour. I said I couldn't take it and he laughed. He patted his gut and said it didn't fit his needs anymore, and if I didn't wear it, the shirt would just sit in a drawer."

The service was being held at Gunnerson's Funeral Home. Daniel Gunnerson Senior was at the front door, shaking hands and directing people. He was a short and solid man with deep blue eyes and a head of thick white hair. He wore a black suit with a crisp white shirt and a blue tie. The smaller rooms, which could accommodate several services, had been opened up to make one large space, and even so I wondered if there would be enough room for all the people I was expecting would come.

We took a seat about five rows back. Jonas and Lachlan were standing together at the front of the room with a bearded man I didn't recognize. Lachlan looked subdued. Jonas seemed even more serious than usual, his face pale. Their small family had gotten even smaller.

Roma looked around as though she was trying to find someone.

"What is it?" I whispered.

"I don't see Eloise," she said.

Eloise was the only other Finnamore cousin left. I'd met her when she'd come to town for her mother, Leitha's, funeral.

Marcus had heard our conversation and he leaned toward us. "She isn't coming. I spoke to her on Thursday. She had surgery on a broken leg a few days ago. She's not allowed to fly."

Roma nodded. "Thanks. I knew there had to be a good reason she wasn't here."

The man with the beard turned out to be a Unitarian minister and a college friend of Mike's. He led the service, sharing his own memories of Mike's sense of humor and his kind heart.

Jonas and Lachlan talked about how Mike had kept them together as a family. "He loved to cook, make music and bring people together," Jonas said. "He'd organize these Sunday meals, timed so that Eloise and the girls could join us from California over Zoom. We'd have dinner and they'd have lunch and the distance didn't matter because we were still all together like we'd been when we were kids."

I had to swallow back tears when Harry walked to the front of the room. He looked so somber in his dark suit. Roma was already holding Eddie's hand. She reached, wordlessly, for mine, squeezing it hard.

"Mike and I had been practicing for what turned out to be our last show for over a month," Harry said. "He loved the idea that we were going to surprise everyone. It was one of the best nights of his life, he

told me after the concert. And according to Mike, he had a lot of those." Harry raised an eyebrow. A lot of people were smiling. Mike had been a charmer.

Harry let out a slow breath. "When someone dies, we always talk about what a great person they were when a lot of the time they were really a jerk, but Michael Bishop was not one of those people. Everyone loved him and he was a dentist. How many people love their dentist?"

"Endodontist," Lachlan called out.

Across the aisle from me, I saw Mary wipe away a tear.

Harry smiled and nodded his head. "Right. Endodontist." He looked skyward. "Sorry, my friend." His expression grew serious again, and his gaze shifted to the pewter urn to the right of him under the photo of Mike playing his bass at the Last Bash concert. The polished container seemed too small to contain Mike's big personality. "The world was brighter with Mike Bishop in it and it's a little darker now that he's gone."

Johnny spoke last. "When Mike came to audition to join the Outlaws, he was dressed just like Sonny Crockett—Don Johnson—from the TV show *Miami Vice*: pleated pastel blue pants and a matching jacket with shoulder pads, a white T-shirt, loafers with no socks, shades and, because it was Mike, a mullet." He smiled at the memory. "I just knew from looking at him that he was the wrong fit for the band, so I asked him to play with Harry and do the bass line from Heart's 'Magic Man.' I figured there was no way he'd know the song. He was wearing a pastel suit for heaven's sake!"

There were a few ripples of laughter around the room.

"I was so sure he wouldn't be able to play it but he did and he played his part perfectly, in his own way, not a copy of anyone else. That was Mike."

Johnny had to pause for a moment and clear his throat. "People of a certain age will remember when Principal Haney canceled the senior class sleigh ride because he wasn't happy with the class average after Christmas exams. He got to school the next morning and his office was filled floor to ceiling with bales of hay." He glanced over at the urn and smiled. "He suspected Mike from the beginning but Mike had an alibi. He had spent the evening before calling bingo at the senior center like he did every Thursday night. Or so they all said."

There was more laughter.

"That was Mike."

Beside me Roma was nodding.

Johnny continued, "What most of you don't know is that when Mike was in college, he used to play stand-up bass for a Baptist church band, which meant he would be out playing at a bar with us until two a.m. and then he'd put on his white shirt, slick back his hair and be at the front of the church at nine thirty. He did that because the group's regular bass player—who also happened to be Mike's chemistry professor—was undergoing cancer treatment. That's also who Mike was."

He cleared his throat again. "Jonas and Lachlan asked us to sing something for Mike. We talked about

it and we just couldn't sing anything that was sad because it just didn't feel right."

Harry and Paul had gotten to their feet. They joined Johnny while Ritchie moved to the piano set off to one side.

"Mike learned this one from those Baptists, and when he wanted to get under my skin, he'd start pushing to make it our encore. Please join us if you know the words." Johnny looked over at the urn one last time. "Safe travels, my friend." He clasped his hands in front of him and began to sing the poignant words of the old hymn "I'll Fly Away."

Jonas and Lachlan stood up and everyone else rose as well. One by one, throughout the room, I heard voices begin to join in. It was profoundly sad and somehow uplifting at the same time.

Outside, a fine, soft rain was falling. As I stood under the umbrella Marcus held over us and watched Daniel Gunnerson carefully set all that was left of Mike Bishop into the hearse, I thought of something I'd heard my mother say: *Blessed are the dead that the rain falls on.*

I hoped it was true.

4

The interment at the Finnamore family crypt was private and would be taking place at a later time. At the beginning of the service, Daniel Gunnerson had made an announcement that there would be a reception immediately after and most people did stay to pay their respects and talk about Mike.

"It seems like half the town is here," I said to Marcus. I was hoping to tell Harry how sorry I was but hadn't seen him since the service ended.

Everett Henderson joined us. "Kathleen, may I steal Marcus from you for a moment?" he asked. He was wearing a perfectly tailored black suit with a patterned gray silk tie that I knew Rebecca had bought for him because I'd been with her when she had.

"Of course," I said.

Marcus caught my hand and gave it a squeeze as he moved past me. "I'll only be a minute." He and Everett moved to a spot closer to the windows where there were fewer people.

I felt a hand touch my shoulder and turned around to find Harrison Taylor standing there. His suit was gray, his shirt and tie blue. He'd trimmed his hair and his beard. I hugged him.

"You look nice," I said. It struck me that Mike would get a kick out of everyone all dressed up. I'd only ever seen him in scrubs or jeans.

"Thank you," he said. "I wish it was for a better reason."

I nodded. "How's Harry?" I asked.

"Pretty much how you'd expect. It's a damn sad day." He ran a hand over his beard. "I know it's late notice, but I was hoping you could come for supper tomorrow night."

"I could," I said. Marcus and I didn't have any plans. A couple of Eddie's hockey buddies from his NHL days were coming to spend a few days teaching at the hockey school and Eddie had invited Marcus to join them for dinner. "I don't want to put Harry out, though." Generally, when I had dinner with Harrison, it was his son who did most of the cooking.

"You won't be," the old man said.

I suspected he was going to ask me to see what I could learn about Mike Bishop's death. I'd gotten involved in that kind of thing before. People were more likely to talk to me than they were to the police. In that way being a librarian was a lot like being a bartender, I'd discovered.

We settled on a time and then Harrison excused himself to go speak to Daniel Gunnerson. I turned

around to look for Marcus, and Jonas Quinn caught my eye. He held up one hand, indicating that he wanted to talk to me. He said something to Lachlan, who was standing next to him, and then started across the room.

"Kathleen, thank you for coming," he said as he joined me.

"I'm so sorry," I said. "Mike was a good person. I'm glad I got to know him."

Jonas nodded. "Yes, he was. Him being dead is just so wrong and it should never have happened." He looked around. "You know, he would have liked this, all these people here in one place talking about him."

I smiled. "Mike was a people person. He'd come into the library and it would take him half an hour to get started on his research because he knew everyone and he kept stopping to talk."

"That research is why I wanted to talk to you," Jonas said. He adjusted his dark-framed glasses with both hands. "The last time I spoke to him, Mike mentioned that you had unearthed more information about the Finnamore family."

"Some census information for this area," I said. "Mike was trying to close a gap in the family tree. I thought it might help."

"Would it be possible to get a copy of it?" he asked. "I think Mike's research on the family is something Lachlan—and maybe Eloise for that matter—might want at some point. Not just because it's their family heritage, but because it was something Mike was

working on. I don't want everything to get lost in the shuffle. There's a lot to take care of right now."

"I understand," I said. "I can make copies of the census records for you and you can come in next week and get them. There's also a copy of a map showing land grants for this part of the state that's coming from another library in our system. Would you like that as well?"

He nodded. "Yes, I would."

I told Jonas I'd call when the map arrived so he could make just one trip to pick up everything.

He thanked me again. "I need to get back to Lachlan," he said. "I'll talk to you soon."

I watched him make his way over to his nephew and put one arm around the boy's shoulders. I knew from some of the things Mike had talked about that there was a lot of tragedy in the Finnamore family history. I hated that Mike himself was now part of that.

I looked for Marcus. He was still talking to Everett. I was guessing their conversation had something to do with the girls' hockey team. There had been rumblings that their funding might be reduced.

The room suddenly felt closed in and clammy. I was only a few steps away from a set of French doors that led out to the overflow parking lot. No one would notice if I stepped outside, so that was what I did.

The rain had stopped. The air was fresh and a little cooler. I remembered that there was a teak bench next to a small flower bed at the end of the building. I'd sit there for a couple of minutes and then go back inside, I decided.

I turned the corner to discover someone was already sitting on the bench. And she was crying.

She looked up at me. Her eyes were red and her makeup had smudged. I pulled a couple of tissues from my bag and handed them to her. She wiped her face. "Thank you," she said in a shaky voice.

"Can I get you anything?" I asked. "A cup of tea, maybe?"

She shook her head. "I don't think I could swallow it."

"I know what you mean," I said. "I was carrying around a cup inside just so people would stop offering me a drink."

She almost managed a smile. "You must have been a friend of Mike's."

I nodded. "I like to think so. I'm Kathleen Paulson."

"You're the librarian. Mike mentioned you. He said you'd been helping him with the family tree."

I nodded.

"I'm Tracy," she said. "I'm Mike's ex-wife." She held up a finger. "The first one."

"It's nice to meet you," I said.

She moved sideways on the bench. "Please, sit."

"I didn't mean to intrude."

She shook her head. "You're not. I was in there listening to people talk about him and I thought what a kick he'd get out of this—everyone dressed up, sharing stories. You know, I think the only time I ever saw him in a suit was actually at a funeral."

She'd had just the same thought as me. "You didn't have a fancy wedding?" I asked.

Tracy's lips twitched. She seemed to think my question was funny. Mirth gleamed in her dark eyes. It was better than sadness. "Good grief, no!" she said. "We were nineteen and madly in love. We eloped. Turns out, we were really just madly in lust. The marriage didn't last six months but the friendship did."

"That sounds like the Mike I knew."

"Every few months he'd call me or I'd call him, just to catch up. It was nice, having that connection back to when I was a dumb kid." She smiled. "I just talked to him a couple of weeks ago. He told me all about the research he was doing into his family's past. He was trying to work out when the so-called Finnamore green eyes entered the family tree. I teach high school biology. I told him he was wasting his time. There are too many factors that influence eye color. It's not as simple as something like hair texture or whether or not someone thinks cilantro tastes like soap."

"It does," I said.

She nodded. "I know."

We sat in silence for a moment. "I'm going to miss talking to him," she finally said.

I reached over and gave her hand a quick squeeze. "I should get back inside."

"Me too," Tracy said. "It was very nice to meet you."

"You too," I said.

"Do you want to go over to Fern's for supper?" Marcus asked as we pulled out of the parking lot about half an hour later. The sky was low and gray and it was

raining again. He was dropping me off and then going in to the station for a little while. "A case that's coming up in court soon," he'd offered by way of explanation.

"I have spaghetti sauce," I said.

He shot me a quick sideways glance. "Does one somehow negate the other?"

I shook my head. "No. I can have it tomorrow—Wait. I can't. I'll eat it Monday."

"Is there some rule that says you can't eat spaghetti on Sundays because I'm pretty sure I've broken it more than once?"

I smiled. "No, there isn't. It's just that I'm going out to have supper with Harrison tomorrow."

Marcus didn't say anything for a moment and he kept his eyes fixed to the road. I let the silence sit between us. "You know why he invited you," he finally said.

"Yes," I said. "He likes my company."

"He thinks you can figure out who killed Mike Bishop."

"He probably does."

"What are you going to say?"

I looked over at him. His blue eyes were still looking straight ahead. "I don't know," I said.

And I didn't. I adored Harrison. I considered Harry a friend. I wanted to help them if I could. This wasn't the first time I'd gotten mixed up with one of Marcus's cases, so I wasn't sure why I was so uncertain. Why this time felt different. Maybe it was because Mike and

I were friends or close to it. His death felt so personal. I wasn't sure I could be objective.

Marcus sighed softly. "I'm not going to tell you what to do, Kathleen."

I reached over and touched his arm. "I appreciate that."

"But I am going to *ask* you to think carefully about whatever choice you make. This case is deeply personal for a lot of people, including you and me. It's harder to be objective. It's harder to set your own feelings to one side. It's harder not to pick up other people's pain." He glanced briefly at me then. "That last part you're going to have to deal with no matter whether you say yes or no to Harrison."

We were at the house by then. Marcus pulled into the driveway and put the SUV in park. I undid my seat belt, leaned over and kissed his cheek. "I promise I'll think carefully about whatever choice I make," I said.

"I know you will." He kissed the side of my mouth and smiled at me. "You didn't give me a yes or no about Fern's."

"Yes." Fern's meat loaf and mashed potatoes were the ultimate comfort food and that sounded pretty good right about now.

"I'll call when I'm leaving," Marcus said. He kissed me a second time.

I got out, opened my umbrella and watched him back out of the driveway before I headed around the side of the house to the back door. Hercules was sitting on the bench in the sunporch. He made a face as

I held my half-open umbrella out the door and gave it a shake. I propped it in the corner and sat down next to him.

"Mrr," he said, cocking his head to one side almost as though he was asking if I was okay.

"I'm all right," I said, kicking off my shoes. "It was a nice service. Very sad."

Hercules moved closer, putting his two front paws on my leg. I stroked his fur. I had no idea how much of what I said to them either cat understood—a lot more than the average cat, I was certain. Given what else they could do, it didn't seem that implausible.

"I think Harrison is going to ask me to try to figure out who killed Mike Bishop." The cat wrinkled his nose at me as though considering what I'd just said.

Hercules and I had been listening to whatever songs by Johnny and the Outlaws I could find online. Even Owen seemed to like the band's music. He didn't always share my taste in music the way Hercules did. Whenever I had gotten involved in one of Marcus's cases, so had the boys, as far-fetched as that seemed. More than once, Owen's ability to disappear and Herc's to walk through walls had helped me learn something I wouldn't otherwise have figured out. I hadn't been able to convince Marcus of that, though.

Hercules seemed to have come to some sort of conclusion. He jumped down from the bench and went into the kitchen without waiting for me to unlock the back door. I sighed, picked up my shoes and followed him, stopping to open the door first. Hercules was

already halfway across the kitchen, headed for the living room. He was a cat with a purpose. I had no idea what he was up to.

He made his way across the room and launched himself into the big wing chair. I folded my arms and glared at him. "Excuse me. That's a people seat not a cat seat," I said.

His response was to stare pointedly at my laptop, which was sitting on the footstool.

I shook my head. "No."

Hercules looked over at me and blinked his green eyes a couple of times.

"Yes, I get that you think I should say yes to Harrison," I said.

He continued to look at me.

"I'm still thinking about it."

Hercules was as motionless as a statue. I knew better than to get into a staring contest with him. I wouldn't win.

"I need to get out of these clothes first *and* I'd like a cup of coffee," I said.

He meowed softly and began to wash his face. It was easy to be magnanimous when you'd won, especially when you were a cat.

I put the laptop on the kitchen table, started the coffeepot, then went upstairs and changed into a red-striped T-shirt dress that was comfortable for sitting around in but would also be okay to wear to Fern's later.

I had just poured my coffee when Hercules poked his head around the living room doorway and meowed inquiringly at me.

"I'm ready," I said. I snagged the nearest chair with one foot, pulled it closer and sat down. The cat padded over to the table and launched himself onto my lap.

"So what should we look for?" I asked. I talked to Hercules and his brother, Owen, a lot. Saying out loud what was running through my mind helped me make sense of things. At least that was how I rationalized it.

Hercules gave me a blank look. Okay, it seemed where to start was my department.

"By the way, where's your brother?"

"Mrr," he said with what looked to me like a shrug. Translation: *I don't know.*

Given the fact that Owen could become invisible anytime he wanted to, it was possible he was here in the kitchen right now. Possible but not very likely. Owen was very good at disappearing. Hiding the fact that he was "hiding," not so much. My guess was that he was either in his basement "lair," where he stashed things he'd swiped from around the house, or upstairs on the bed in the spare room—somewhere he knew he wasn't supposed to be.

"Maybe we should poke around on social media," I said to Hercules. "If Mike surprised someone who had broken into his house, maybe it wasn't the first time they'd done something like that. Marcus said there hadn't been any break-ins reported, but people don't always call the police if nothing's been stolen." I raised an eyebrow at him. "What do you think?"

"Merow!" he said. Hercules was almost always enthusiastic about helping me do some online research. He'd peer at the screen and move his head as though

he were reading an article or checking out a photograph. Oddly enough, more than once, a seemingly stray tap of his paw at the keyboard had landed me on just the piece of information I was looking for.

I thought about who lived in the same area as Mike had, working my way along the closest streets in my mind. Just about everyone used some form of social media, it seemed. A lot of people were talking about Mike's death and about the reunion of Johnny and the Outlaws. I couldn't find any mention of any break-ins in the area.

Hercules stayed perched on my lap, green eyes glued to the laptop screen, one paw on the table edge. When I leaned back and reached for my coffee, he tapped a paw on the touch pad, then turned and looked at me.

"Okay, what did you do?" I asked, leaning around him so I could see the screen.

He looked from the computer to me. If he could have raised an eyebrow and said, *Duh*, he probably would have.

We seemed to have somehow landed on the Facebook page for Keith King's storage business. I'd seen Keith a lot more frequently at the library in the past few months. He was one of the newest members of the library board, and like Mike, he had been researching his family history after receiving one of those DNA test kits.

I read a few of his posts but didn't find anything useful. I was about to give up and move on when I

spotted it. About three weeks ago, Keith had offered a deal on renting a medium-sized storage unit: rent for twelve months and get one month free. *Keep your snowblower and winter gear safe from anyone with sticky fingers who might walk through your yard.*

I leaned back in the chair, putting one hand on Hercules so I wouldn't knock him off my lap.

"That could just be a promotional line," I said. "It doesn't mean there's been someone wandering around people's yards out where Keith lives."

"Mrr," Hercules said without moving his gaze from the laptop's screen.

"Yes, I know. It doesn't mean there hasn't been, either." I could call Keith, but I wasn't sure how to ask him without explaining why I wanted to know.

I looked at the computer again. There were comments under Keith's post, I noticed. I scrolled through them slowly. The third-to-the-last one gave me what I was looking for. It had been made by one of the Reading Buddies moms. She had jokingly asked if Keith had a unit large enough for her car because she'd had some change and a set of AirPods swiped from it while the family was on their back deck eating supper. Another commenter had commiserated with her, saying that unfortunately you had to keep your car locked all the time these days, even in Mayville Heights. Someone had sprayed whipped cream all over her front and back car windows.

It wasn't exactly a smoking gun, and there was a big difference between grabbing a pair of AirPods

from an unlocked car and killing a man in his own living room. Still, I couldn't help thinking that I might be onto something. At the same time, I was uncomfortably aware that I was already digging into a murder I wasn't sure I wanted to get involved in—or even should.

5

Marcus picked me up just before six and we drove over to Fern's. It seemed I wasn't the only one who was looking for comfort food. The diner was busy but I was glad Marcus had suggested we eat out. It had been such a sad day, I was glad to be around other people.

Peggy was just coming out of the kitchen when we walked into the diner. She was still wearing the navy dress she had worn to Mike's service. She smiled, grabbed a couple of menus and showed us to a booth by the windows.

"How's Harrison?" I asked Peggy. "He didn't find the service too much?"

"I asked him that very question and he said he's not feeble yet, thank you very much." She shook her head. "That man is stubborn to the bone. On the other hand, it's a quality he passed down to all three of his children. I told him that was karma in action."

I smiled. Larry was actually the most easygoing of

all the Taylors. Harry, and especially Elizabeth, were just like their father.

"I almost forgot," Peggy said. "Eugenie says hello."

Eugenie Bowles-Hamilton was a cookbook author who owned a very popular bakery in Vancouver, Canada. We'd met when the revival of the *Great Northern Baking Showdown* was filming in Mayville Heights back in the spring. Eugenie was one of the two cohosts of the show, straight woman to Russell Perry, the lead singer for The Flying Wallbangers. I'd been hired, part-time, to research and provide background information for the hosts—primarily Eugenie—that fit with whatever each particular week's focus happened to be.

"You were talking to her?" I asked.

"I saw her in person. I was in Chicago for a couple of days last week to film a small part on another baking show."

"That's wonderful," I said.

Peggy had ended up stepping in at the last minute for one of the baking showdown's judges. She turned out to be great on camera, and even though the show ended up not airing, word of her warm personality and rapport with the other judge and the contestants had gotten around.

"Would you believe Richard suggested me?" she asked.

Richard Kent had been the other judge on the *Great Northern Baking Showdown*.

I nodded. "I would. The two of you had great chemistry."

"We work well together, and while I don't want to make a career out of this, it was more fun to be back in front of the camera than I'd expected." She smiled. "Your waiter will be right over."

After we'd given the waiter our orders, I spotted Mariah Taylor, Harry's daughter, clearing two booths at the far end of the diner. She was working at Fern's part-time for the summer and helping her father as well.

"I just want to go speak to Mariah for a second," I said to Marcus. "I'll be right back."

It had occurred to me that swiping a set of AirPods and spraying whipped cream all over someone's windshield sounded like the kinds of things a group of teenagers might do.

Mariah was stacking glasses in a large plastic bin. She noticed me and smiled. "Hey, Kathleen," she said.

"How's the job going?" I asked.

"Don't tell my dad, but I think I like working for him a lot better." She gestured at the table. "People are pigs sometimes."

"I know," I said. "I had this same job when I was your age. How many times have you found gum stuck to the back of a booth?"

She made a face. "Twice. One time I put my hand on it."

I nodded in sympathy. "I kneeled on a big wad of grape bubble gum once."

Mariah brushed a stray strand of hair back off her face. "This is where you're supposed to tell me to stay in school so I won't have to clear tables for the rest of my life."

I smiled. "First of all, there are worse jobs than this, and second, you're smart enough to know the value of staying in school."

"Yeah, well, could you tell my dad that last part?" Mariah said.

I laughed. "Bugging you about that kind of thing is part of his job description."

That got a smile out of her.

"Mariah, do you know anything about some cars being vandalized out near where you live?"

She flushed and her gaze slipped away from mine. "Sorry. I don't."

I tipped my head to one side and studied her. "You're a crappy liar, you know."

She stared down at the table for a moment. "You can't tell my dad."

"As long as you're not doing anything dangerous," I said.

Mariah shook her head. "I wasn't doing anything dangerous and it was a onetime thing, believe me."

I nodded. "Okay. What did you do?"

She dropped her gaze again. "I went to this party with a girl from my class. There was a lot of drinking and I heard a couple of other girls talking about spraying whipped cream all over someone's car because the owner had complained about this dog getting loose and doing you know what all over her flowers."

"Did you know the girls?"

Mariah looked at me then. "One is a year behind me and I didn't know the other one." She blew the stray hair off her face again. "The whole thing turned out to

be a stupid waste of time. The girl I went with hooked up with some summer guy and ditched me and I didn't have any way to get home."

"But you did get home okay?" I asked. I thought about how many times Ethan and Sarah had done something like that and then called me so Mom and Dad wouldn't find out. Not that I'd ever thought Mom and Dad were that oblivious.

"Yeah," she said, dropping a handful of forks into her bin. "I called Peggy and she rescued me. And she didn't rat me out to Dad. And before you say I could have called him, Peggy already said that."

I struggled to keep from smiling. "She's right you know," I said. "And you can always call me if you get into another situation like that."

"Really?"

"Really."

She smiled. "Thank you," she said. She looked over at Marcus. "You want me to tell him all of this?"

"Just the part about the whipped cream and the dog."

"Okay." She dipped her head in the direction of the booth. "You'd better go. Your food is ready."

On Sunday, Marcus and I decided to go to the flea market out on the highway. I had been making a half-hearted effort to find a couple of Adirondack chairs for his backyard.

"What about those benches instead?" he asked, pointing at a pair at a stall just up ahead.

"Maybe," I said. "Or maybe benches and a pair of Adirondacks."

He laughed. "You're not going to give up on those chairs, are you?"

"The arms are perfect for holding a glass of lemonade or a cup of coffee."

"Or a cat," Marcus said with a grin.

I smiled back at him. "That too."

We walked over to check out the benches and discovered that Burtis and Lita were doing the same thing. Burtis and Lita seemed like an unlikely couple on paper. He was rough-and-tumble and as a young man had worked for the town bootlegger. Lita had been Everett Henderson's right hand for as long as anyone could remember. I had no idea how Burtis and Lita had gotten together—as far as I knew, no one did—but they were good for each other and the way they sometimes looked at each other made my heart happy.

"You thinking of buying those for your backyard?" Burtis said to me.

I tipped my head toward Marcus, who was already walking around one of the benches, checking it out. "Marcus's yard," I said.

The ends of the bench were cast iron and the back and the seat were made of wood. Both pieces looked to be in good shape. The only issue was the fact that all the wood on both pieces had been painted a vibrant fluorescent orange, the same shade as a highway safety sign.

"I'm thinking that with a little elbow grease and some paint they'd look pretty good in my backyard," Brady's father said. He was strong and solid with

thick, muscular arms and a face lined and weathered from so much time spent outdoors. Burtis had lost most of his hair, just a few white tufts poked out from under his ubiquitous Twins ball cap.

Marcus tipped the bench forward with one hand so he could look at the underside of the seat. "Funny. I was thinking the same thing," he said.

"You should show a little respect for your elders and let me have them," Burtis said.

Marcus gave a snort of laughter as he set the bench down. "You're far from old. Nice try, though."

Burtis pointed a finger at him. "That sounds like something your father would say."

"I take that as a compliment," Marcus said.

Burtis smiled. "How is the old man?" he asked. Burtis and Marcus's father, Elliot, had been friends from the time they were teenagers.

"He's good. I talked to him a couple of nights ago. He says he's coming for a visit in a couple of weeks."

"Let me know if Elly May commits to a time," Burtis said. "We haven't been on a tear in a while." He grinned.

Lita shook her head. "One of us had better have bail money," she said to me.

I laughed. The last time Elliot Gordon had been in town, he and Burtis had taken a walk down memory lane with a few too many Jäger Bombs. The evening had ended with them serenading patrons in the lounge at the St. James Hotel with their version of "Sweet Home Alabama." The crowd had actually seemed to enjoy the music. Management, not so much.

Burtis and Marcus were haggling about the benches now.

"I saw the two of you at the service," Lita said. "Mike and I are . . . were cousins about four times removed."

Lita was related in one way or another to pretty much everyone in Mayville Heights. Her mother's family and her father's family were among the first non–Native American settlers in the area. As Rebecca had once explained it to me, "Half the town is cousin to Lita on her father's side and the other half is related through her mother."

"So you're connected to the Finnamores?" I asked.

She nodded. "If you go back far enough, some of the branches of our family trees intertwine." She glanced over at the men still debating who should get the benches. "Does Marcus have any suspects yet?"

I shook my head. "He wouldn't tell me if he did, but I don't think so."

"I hate the thought that someone broke into the house to rob it and then killed Mike. We like to think something like that would only happen in a big city, not in Mayville Heights, but past events show that's not true."

She gave me a knowing look, probably because I'd gotten tied up in more than one suspicious death since I'd arrived in town. I let it pass without comment.

"It's almost like that family is cursed."

"What do you mean?" I asked.

"It's only been a few months since Leitha died."

I remembered how Mike had explained that the

older woman was his great-aunt the first time he'd come into the library to start digging into the family's history.

"The Finnamores tend to die too soon," she continued. "That's why there's so little of the family left now. Leitha hated that there were so few children. She was proud of being a Finnamore. The thought that the line could die out gave her a lot of grief."

"She always introduced herself as Leitha Finnamore Anderson," I said.

"She claimed the Finnamores could trace their ancestry back to the *Mayflower*."

I nodded. "I'm not giving away any secrets because Mike was telling everyone. It appears from what he unearthed that that much is true, but instead of being on the ship for religious reasons, it seemed their ancestor was in fact just a hired hand who eventually ended up with a family in England and one here in the colonies."

Lita gave a wry smile. "That would have burned Leitha's biscuits if she'd known. That family line meant everything to her. She hated that Mike had been married and divorced twice and hadn't had any children. He used to try to get a rise out of her by saying he didn't have any kids that he knew of."

That sounded like Mike. "And Jonas has no children, either," I said.

"Well, Jonas is not a biological Finnamore," Lita said. "He's the child of Nathan St. James Quinn from his first marriage, although Mary-Margaret Finnamore Quinn was his mother in every way."

"St. James like the hotel?"

Lita nodded. "Yes. Nathan's family owned it for years until it was sold. The family built the hotel." She glanced over at Marcus and Burtis, who still seemed to be debating who was going to end up with the benches.

"This is going to be a while," Lita said. "There's a guy at the end of this row selling donuts. I'm going to go get half a dozen. Do you want to come with me?"

"Absolutely," I said.

The donuts were cinnamon spice, with and without sugar. I got half a dozen to take to work with me on Monday. When Lita and I got back, Marcus and Burtis were each buying one of the benches from the owner of the stall.

I smiled at Lita. "As Shakespeare would say, 'All's well that ends well.'"

We managed to get the bench onto the truck, off the truck and around into the backyard with a little physics (me) and a lot of muscle (Marcus). Those cast-iron ends were much heavier than I'd expected. Micah jumped up on the slatted seat, seemed to frown at the garish color and then, after she'd sniffed it and walked the length of the bench, meowed her approval.

I headed out to Harrison's for supper a couple of hours later, taking along some tomatoes from my garden and some cheese-and-ham biscuits that Rebecca had given me the recipe for. The old man lived in a small house on his son's property. He must have been watching for me because he and Boris, his dog, were standing

at the door when I climbed out of the truck. Boris, with his chocolate velvet eyes, came over to meet me. I bent down to talk to him before walking over to join Harrison. I knew no matter how well I washed my hands when I got home, the cats would smell Boris on me and I'd be in the doghouse, so to speak. The dog actually belonged to Harry but spent a lot of time with Harrison. He was gentle and quiet and I didn't like to think about what one of them would do without the other.

"I'm glad you made it," Harrison said.

"I'm glad you invited me." I gave him a hug and handed over the tomatoes and biscuits.

"Which are these?" he asked, eyeing the container of cherry tomatoes.

I'd been growing several varieties of heirloom tomatoes this year, letting Harrison try each one.

"These are sungold," I said. "They have a lovely sweet flavor. There are way, way more of them than I expected. And the biscuits are ham and cheese." I smiled. "Rebecca's mother's recipe."

He smiled. "Thank you. This will be my lunch tomorrow. Or maybe my breakfast. A man can eat only so much oatmeal and flaxseeds." I knew Peggy had been trying to get Harrison to eat healthier. He grumbled about it, but she'd had more success than his sons or Elizabeth.

We moved inside, Boris leading the way.

"We're dining alfresco," Harrison said.

"Does that mean I get to see the screened porch?" I asked. Harry and his younger brother, Larry, had

been working on the addition to the house in their spare time.

The old man smiled and nodded. "You're my first guest."

I smiled back at him. "I'm honored."

We moved through the house to the screened porch at the back. It was beautifully built—no surprise. The boys had their father's talent for carpentry. A set of wide steps led down to a small stone patio and Harry was there at the grill. He raised a hand in hello and I waved back.

"When he heard you were coming out, he insisted on grilling and you know what my boy's like when he makes up his mind," Harrison said.

"I have a little experience with the Taylor family stubbornness."

His blue eyes twinkled. "Are you suggesting he gets that from me?"

"Apples and trees, Harrison," I said. "Apples and trees."

There was a small table set for three. I knew Harry often ate with his dad when his kids were off with their friends or their mother, his ex-wife. I was glad he was joining us. I also knew there was a possibility I'd get tag-teamed by the two of them about Mike Bishop's death.

Harrison pointed to a couple of wicker chairs with deep green seats and back cushions. "Have a seat," he said. "Peggy picked those chairs, so I promise you they're comfortable. She said the two I wanted to use out here were older than Moses."

The chair was very comfortable. Maybe a couple of them would work in Marcus's backyard. I made a mental note to ask Peggy about them. Boris came over, leaned against my leg and set his head in my lap.

Harrison frowned at the dog. "Just give him a push," he said to me as he sat down in the other chair.

"He's fine," I said, reaching to scratch behind Boris's left ear. "He can sit by me whenever he wants." As if he'd understood my words, the dog turned to look at the old man as if to gloat.

"You're spoiled," he told the dog. Boris closed his eyes and gave a contented sigh.

"What's been going on at the library?" Harrison asked.

He was going to wait until after we'd eaten to talk about Mike Bishop, I realized, assuming I was right about why I'd been invited for supper.

I told him about the Summer Reading Club, the plans for a Money Week in the fall and about the library participating in World Mental Health Day in October.

"Sounds like you're keeping busy," he said.

I grinned at him. "It keeps me out of trouble. Tell me more about Elizabeth. You said she's coming next month?"

He nodded. "Before she goes back to college. It's taken a while for her to find her niche, but she's been making noise about medical school or biomedical engineering. I'm hoping one of those sticks. I have to say I'd love to have a doctor in the family."

I could hear the pride in his voice. Elizabeth had been placed for adoption when she was born. Harrison

and her biological mother had had a relationship when Harrison's wife was in a nursing home, something he still carried some shame about. It had taken some time for the two of them to get to know each other, but he had answered every question she'd had without dodging the messy ones and that had gone a long way to helping them build a close relationship.

Harry came in from outside then.

"You did a wonderful job on this porch," I said, gesturing with one hand.

"Thanks," he said. He cleared his throat. "I saw you and Marcus at the service. I wanted to thank you both for coming. I'm sorry I didn't get a chance to talk to you there."

"I liked Mike," I said. "I wish I'd had the time to get to know him better. He'd come in to work on the family tree, and first thing I knew, he'd be in one of the meeting rooms charming the seniors."

Harry laughed. "That sounds like him."

"What can I do to help?" I asked.

Before Harry could answer, his father spoke up. "You're a guest and you don't have to work for your supper."

Harry smiled. "Thank you for the offer, Kathleen, but I have everything under control. We'll eat in about five minutes."

As usual, the food was delicious: barbecued steak, chopped salad and sourdough bread. I recognized the bread as Rebecca's honey-sunny recipe. Harry confirmed that I was right.

"Peggy made it," he said.

"I'll remember to thank her next time I see her," I said.

During supper we talked about Harry's garden—his cucumbers were doing better than mine—and the fact that the prankster who had been leaving things in the library's gazebo seemed to have given up.

"Whoever it is will be back. You just watch," Harry said.

"Mary certainly agrees with you," I said. "I'm hoping that finding the camera that you and Larry put up might have made whoever has been pulling these stunts realize this whole thing really isn't funny."

Harry just shrugged. "We'll see."

For dessert there was orange-banana frozen yogurt that the old man had made in his son's ice cream maker.

"This is so good," I exclaimed. I fought the urge to use my finger to get the last creamy bit out of my bowl. The yogurt was the perfect combination of citrus and sweet.

"I still have a few tricks left up my sleeve," Harrison said with a mischievous grin.

Harry rolled his eyes. "And that's what worries me."

Harrison still had the grin. "You need to blow a little of the carbon out of your spark plugs, if you get my drift." He had a naughty-boy gleam in his blue eyes and I thought once again what a charmer he must have been when he was a young man. He was certainly charming enough now.

"And on that note." Harry got to his feet. He gathered our bowls. "I have a couple of things to do."

"Thank you for supper," I said.

He smiled. "You're welcome here anytime. It's the least I can do since you keep my father in muffins and reading material."

Boris was sitting next to my chair. Harry patted his leg. "Let's go," he said to the dog.

"Leave him be," Harrison said. "I'll bring him over later."

Harry gave his head a little shake. "All right," he said. "Don't feed him any of that frozen yogurt." He headed into the house.

"Do you want to stay out here or move inside?" I asked Harrison.

"There's a nice breeze coming in through those screens and no bugs," he said. "Are you up for staying out here?"

"Absolutely," I said.

We moved over into Peggy's new chairs. I looked out over the back of Harry's property. "This is a beautiful spot," I said.

"That it is," he agreed. He stroked his beard with his thumb and index finger.

I turned and looked at him, narrowing my eyes.

"I know that look," he said. "You think I had an ulterior motive for inviting you out here."

"Didn't you?" I countered. "You want me to dig into Mike Bishop's death."

"I wouldn't want to risk our friendship by asking

you to do that and putting you in a bad spot with Detective Gordon." He actually managed a little self-righteousness in his tone.

I got up and went over to hug him. "Because if I'm a true and loyal friend, I'll do it without you asking me. Am I right?"

He laughed and I knew I was. The old man wasn't just charming. He was crafty as well.

"Kathleen, what do you know about dowsing?" he asked.

I was surprised by the sudden change in the conversation. "Not a lot," I said. "I know it's been used to find groundwater among other things. The practice dates back centuries. Traditionally the dowser uses a forked branch from a tree or a bush—quite often willow or witch hazel—although some prefer using two metal rods. And dowsing is no more effective than just random chance."

He nodded. "I know it shouldn't work. I know there's no science, but there are some things in life that science just can't explain."

I thought about Owen and Hercules and their skills.

"I've seen a dowser find water when no one else could. It's like they have some kind of sixth sense or instinct that comes into play, and you have the same thing when it comes to getting to the truth. Just rely on your instincts and everything will be just fine."

I stayed for another half an hour and we talked about the increase in tourists the town had seen this

summer. Harrison told me more about the original Last Bash and how he hoped this revival wouldn't be just a onetime thing.

I finally got to my feet. Boris was in between our chairs and I reached down to scratch his head.

"Stay where you are," I said, leaning down to give Harrison a hug. "I should have a couple of books for you by the end of the week. I'll call you and one of the boys can pick them up."

"Thank you, my dear," he said. "You always do the right thing by me."

I knew he was referring to Mike's death but I let the comment go.

I went out the porch door and walked around the side of the house. As I headed toward the truck, Harry came out of his house and started toward me. I wondered if he'd been watching for me.

"You're heading out," he said when we met by the back bumper of the truck.

"I am," I said. "Thanks again for supper."

He let out a breath. "Kathleen, I'm not going to dance all around the farm. You know Mike and I go way back."

I nodded.

"I haven't known you nearly as long, but I consider you a friend as well. And without you, well, who knows if we would ever have found Elizabeth."

"I feel the same way about you, about all of you," I said.

He shifted uncomfortably from one foot to the other. "I'm sorry to presume on that friendship, but I

need you to look into what happened to Mike. I'm not trying to say that Marcus isn't good at his job, but people talk to you because you're not the police. You can find out things Marcus can't."

I wanted to remind him of all the reasons it wasn't a good idea. Instead all I said was "No promises."

He nodded. "That's more than enough."

We said good night and I got in the truck. I hadn't made any promises or actually agreed to anything. Harry might have said that was more than enough, but I wasn't so sure it was.

6

I had a restless night. I woke up before my alarm went off, even before Owen had the chance to poke me with a paw. I got to the library early and spent a couple of minutes walking around outside, checking the gazebo at the back—no hay bales or swimming pools—and the vegetables and flowers that the summer camp kids were growing in Harry's raised beds. Harry had already begun clearing a space next to the far end of the building for the cold frames. It was just another example of how kind and conscientious he was. I'd meant every word I'd said to him: I did think of him as a friend. Even though I wasn't sure what I could uncover about Mike's death, I knew I had to try.

I spent some time on my laptop at lunchtime but I didn't learn much more about Mike. He had been the top-rated endodontist in the state on Rate My Dentist. I didn't see how his killer could have been a disgruntled patient.

It was a quiet day, maybe because it wasn't raining,

and I got the chance to work on my presentation for the library board about the new library computers. They had approved the idea in theory. Now that we had started fund-raising it was time for more details.

As I drove up the hill at the end of the day, I decided I would go talk to Rebecca to see what she could tell me about Mike Bishop and his family. She had grown up in Mayville Heights and she often knew where the bodies were buried, so to speak.

Before I had supper, I pulled some radishes from my little backyard garden and gathered a few more sun-gold tomatoes to take over to Rebecca after I'd eaten. Hercules sat at one corner of the raised bed watching me—and keeping his feet dry—while Owen walked around the edge, lifting one paw a couple of times as if telling me which tomatoes to pick. I wasn't really sure what I was hoping to learn from Rebecca. Mike's life seemed like an open book. Most of us had at least one person in our lives who wasn't really a fan, but no one had a bad word to say about Mike. He didn't seem like the kind of person to have any skeletons in his closet, but if they were there, Rebecca would probably know about them.

"I'm not sure there's anything I can do to figure this out," I said to the boys as I chopped three of the tomatoes for my own supper. "Harry said people tell me things, things that they don't tell Marcus, but I'm not sure it matters this time."

"Mrr," Hercules said.

I wasn't sure if he was agreeing, disagreeing or wondering when we were going to eat.

Marcus had said very little about the investigation but I didn't think he had any suspects at this point. "What if Mike was just the victim of a random crime? What if someone broke in intending to steal whatever they could find and things just went wrong?"

Hercules seemed to consider the idea for a moment.

"Harrison and Harry think I can do something, but maybe I can't. I know that most victims of violent crime know their attacker, but sometimes things are just random."

I was talking out loud mainly just to work things out for myself. I didn't expect either cat to offer any theories on Mike Bishop's death, so I wasn't surprised to look over my shoulder and see that Owen didn't seem to be paying attention at all. He was peering under the re-frigerator at something.

"What are you doing?" I said.

One ear twitched but that was the only indication I got that he was listening. He swiped one paw under the fridge and sent a small refrigerator magnet skit-tering across the floor to stop by my feet. I bent down to pick it up.

It was one that Maggie had given to me. I hadn't been able to find it for a while and I had suspected it might have ended up in the stash of things Owen kept hidden—more or less—in the basement. Owen loved Maggie and had swiped her scarf and one of her mit-tens among other things in the past.

The magnet was a photo of Einstein with the quote: "God does not play dice with the universe." In other words there is a pattern to things, a plan. Owen cocked

his head to one side and looked at me with an almost smug look on his furry face.

"'Not only does God play dice but he sometimes confuses us by throwing them where they cannot be seen,'" I said. "Stephen Hawking."

I raised one eyebrow at Owen in my best Mr. Spock–from–*Star Trek* fashion and returned his smug expression. Then two things occurred to me. One, I was being smug over besting a cat. And two, both Einstein and Hawking were talking about quantum mechanics, not murder.

After supper I walked across the backyard to Rebecca's. I found her cutting lettuce from her own small garden with a tiny pair of kitchen shears. She smiled when she caught sight of me. "Kathleen, your timing is perfect," she said. "The lettuce is taking over. Please tell me you'll take some."

"I'll definitely take some. Mine hasn't grown nearly as well as yours." I held up the brown paper bag I was carrying. "I brought tomatoes and radishes."

"Splendid," Rebecca said. "Everett will eat tomatoes at every meal and I have very few radishes. I think the raccoons are having them for a midnight snack."

I watched as she finished filling her colander with lettuce. Then she gestured at the gazebo. "Do you have time to sit in the shade for a bit?" she asked.

"I do," I said.

Rebecca put the lettuce on the small table in the middle of the space and we each took a chair. She folded her hands in her lap. She was tiny with bright

blue eyes and silver-gray hair cropped into a short cut that showed off her cheekbones and long neck.

"Where would you like me to start?" she asked. "You are looking for information about Michael's family, aren't you?"

There was no point in pretending I didn't understand what she was referring to. "How did you know?" I asked.

"You and Harrison are very close. I knew he'd ask you to see what you could find out about Michael's death." She frowned. "I'm not wrong, am I?"

I shook my head. "No, you're not."

"So tell me, what would you like to know?"

"The thing is, I'm not really sure," I said. "Did Mike have any enemies? Was there anyone who would have had any reason to want him dead?"

"Your Marcus asked me the same questions," Rebecca said, "and the answers are no and no. Michael was a good man. He was generous with his time, with his skills and with his money."

"Some of that was Finnamore family money?"

Rebecca nodded. "The Finnamore family started Black Dog Boots more than a hundred years ago and they also made money in the timber industry. And before you think either of those businesses could be the cause of Michael's death, you should know that the Finnamores only own a tiny share of either business now. Michael's mother, Elizabeth Finnamore Bishop, inherited her father's share of both companies and, as an only child, all of his money. There's also a separate trust that provides for Finnamore descendants—it pays for col-

lege. Elizabeth started a charitable foundation with the money she inherited. It supports several educational organizations—education was one of Elizabeth's favorite causes—as well as a number of school food programs all over the state. I know that Michael continued his mother's work and expanded the school food project. He also started a project to provide basic dental care to children who wouldn't otherwise get it. I don't think anyone is going to commit murder over feeding hungry children or fixing their teeth."

Neither did I.

She nudged her glasses up her nose. "I'm guessing all of that will go to Lachlan now."

"Not Eloise or Jonas?" I asked.

"Eloise lives in California. I don't see how she could run the foundation from out there."

"And Jonas isn't a biological Finnamore."

"Yes." She picked a dried rose petal off the front of her shirt. "Jonas is probably the trustee for now, but the Finnamore money always stays in the family." She made a face when she said the word "family." "The older generation—Leitha's generation—cared way too much about the bloodline as far as I'm concerned."

"What about Mike?" I asked. "He was digging into the family tree. Do you think he cared about the bloodline?"

"Goodness no!" Rebecca said, gesturing with one hand. "I once heard him tell Leitha it was all a bunch of foolishness. He said the sainted Finnamores weren't any better than anyone else."

"What about Jonas?" I asked. "Do you think his not being a Finnamore matters to him?"

"I'm not sure. I think in some ways he might be relieved not to be. He inherited some land from his father and some investments from Mary-Margaret and he's done well for himself. He's smart and hard-working. Leitha used that family money like a whip to get people to do what she wanted them to. She couldn't do that with Jonas and he was always pretty good at keeping Lachlan out of that." She smiled. "I can see both of their mothers' influence in Michael and in Jonas."

"You knew both women." I pulled one foot up underneath me.

"I knew Mary-Margaret better," Rebecca said. "I used to cut her hair and she adored both of her boys, Jonas and Colin, Lachlan's father. When Jonas had mumps as a teenager and ran a very high fever, Mary-Margaret wouldn't leave his side at the hospital and Elizabeth had a doctor removed from treating the boy when the doctor tried to send Mary-Margaret home because Jonas wasn't her 'real' son."

"I think I would have liked both of them."

Rebecca smiled again. "You would have. Mary-Margaret was the quieter of the two. Michael is . . . was very much like his mother."

I tried to picture the rough family tree Mike had sketched out as he found new family members. I wasn't sure if any of his family history had anything to do with his murder but it was a place to start, something

to at least eliminate. "So Leitha was Elizabeth and Mary-Margaret's aunt," I said.

Rebecca nodded. "That's right. Leitha and John were brother and sister." She tapped one finger on the table as though she was plotting out the family connections. "Leitha had one child, Eloise. Her brother, John, had two daughters, Elizabeth and Mary-Margaret, which made Leitha great-aunt to Michael—and Jonas as far as I'm concerned. Did you meet Eloise when she was here for her mother's service?"

"I did," I said. "She came into the library to see all the work that had been done."

"She was estranged from her mother, you know."

I shook my head. "I didn't know that, but I'm not really surprised. Leitha had a strong personality." And equally strong opinions I'd learned the first time we'd met. She told me with no beating around the bush that she believed the money spent on renovating the library had been nothing more than "foolish sentimentality." She thought the building should have been torn down and replaced with a new, modern structure.

The Mayville Heights Free Public Library was a Carnegie library and much of the town's history was tied up with it. Not to mention it was an excellent example of the architecture of its time. All of which I had nicely explained to Leitha. None of which had changed her mind.

"The woman had some very old-fashioned ideas," Rebecca said, pursing her lips with disapproval. "Eloise has two daughters. They're both adopted."

"You think that estrangement had something to do with them not being biological Finnamores?"

Rebecca sighed. "I hope not, but knowing Leitha, it wasn't impossible. She was missing out on so much not being in those girls' lives. Look how blessed I am by having Ami."

Ami was Everett's granddaughter. Rebecca had been part of her life since she was a little girl. Even when Everett and Rebecca weren't part of each other's lives, she and Ami had stayed close.

"There's no blood tie between us, but I couldn't love Ami any more if there was. What binds people is love, not strands of DNA." She reached out one hand and gently waved a butterfly away from the lettuce. "You know, some people think the Finnamores are cursed."

I shifted in my chair. The foot I'd been sitting on was going to sleep. "Do you?"

Rebecca shook her head. "No. I don't believe in silly things like that. The rain falls equally on sinner and saint and there were both in that family, just like in any other family, no matter what Leitha would have liked the rest of us to believe."

"Do you know how the family came to start Black Dog Boots?" I asked. I had found very little about the history of the company when I'd been prowling around on their website at lunchtime.

"Leitha's grandfather started Black Dog. He started out as a lumberjack, but he saved every penny and eventually had his own crew of men. Black Dog began because he couldn't find durable work boots. Except for a minor share, the business was sold years ago, so if

you're thinking Michael was killed by a disgruntled employee"—she held up both hands—"I think you're looking in the wrong direction."

"Do you think there could be any connection between Mike's death and the band?" I felt like I was just pulling random ideas out of the air now.

"I don't see how," Rebecca said. "Everyone was thrilled that they had gotten together again. In fact, I wouldn't have been surprised to see them do more shows together. No one thought that was a bad idea, but Harry or Johnny could tell you more about that."

I couldn't think of anything else to ask her, especially since I had already taken more of her time than I'd intended. We talked about our respective vegetable patches for a moment and then I thanked Rebecca for the lettuce and the information and headed home.

Owen had moved from walking around the vegetable bed to sitting on the arm of one of the Adirondack chairs. I joined him. He sniffed the lettuce out of curiosity but made a face. Salad didn't interest him, other than the croutons if there were any, although he had been known to lick the ranch dressing off a bit of cucumber that accidentally landed on the floor.

The cat glanced over toward Rebecca's yard and then gave me a curious look.

"Nothing useful," I said, assuming he wanted to know what I'd learned from Rebecca when maybe he was just wondering if she had any yellow catnip chickens. "I did learn that Mike's great-grandfather was a lumberjack but I don't see how that's going to help me."

Marcus came around the side of the house then. He was carrying one of Burtis's potato baskets.

"Hi," I said.

"Hi, yourself," he said. He held up the basket. "New potatoes for you from Burtis via Brady."

I smiled. Burtis grew some of the best potatoes I'd ever eaten. "Please thank both of them and thank *you* for bringing them over."

"You're very welcome," Marcus said. He leaned down to kiss me, set the basket on the grass and lowered himself into the other chair.

Owen jumped down from his perch on the arm of my chair and walked over to peer at the potatoes. Before I could stop him, he jumped into the basket.

"Get out of there," I said.

He looked at me, not even blinking.

"Get out," I repeated.

His response was to disappear.

I blew out a breath in frustration, lifting my bangs off my face. "I know you're there, Owen," I said.

Marcus laughed.

"Don't laugh," I said. "It just encourages him."

"Did you know that researchers in Montreal have been looking at ways to change a light's frequency to make it pass through an object, which then makes the object seem to be invisible?"

We could both see a potato moving in the basket.

"Clearly those researchers weren't working with any cats," I said.

Marcus stretched out his long legs and raked a hand through his hair. He was frustrated.

"The Bishop case?" I asked.

He nodded. "I have no suspects and almost no evidence. Mike Bishop died of a head injury, but no one in the area heard or saw anything and the man was universally well-liked."

"According to Rebecca, some people think the Finnamore family is cursed." The potato was still moving, pushed I knew by a furry gray-and-white paw.

"You think Rebecca really believes that?" Marcus asked.

I pulled both feet up onto the seat of my chair and wrapped my arms around my legs. "No. And for the record, neither do I. As Rebecca put it, 'The rain falls equally on sinner and saint and there were both in that family.' The quote comes from the Bible, in case you were wondering."

"I don't believe in things like jinxes or curses," he said.

I gave a snort of laughter. "This from the man who wouldn't wash his hockey jersey during the playoffs last year."

He was already shaking his head. "That's different. When I don't wash my jersey, I'm connecting with the collective mindset of hockey fans all over the country. Our shared energy supports the team."

"More like a shared delusion, but who am I to argue?" I said. I rested my chin on one knee.

"Something else I don't believe in?" Marcus said. "Coincidences. The deaths of two people in the same family in just three months doesn't feel right to me."

"It happens," I said.

I'd always felt a little sad about Leitha Anderson's death. She had come to the library for a talk about the history of the area given by Mary. Previous lectures in the series had included two talks by Harrison and one by Everett. Mary and Leitha had had a very loud and very public argument after Mary's talk. On the drive home, Leitha had suffered a heart attack, gone off the road and died before paramedics arrived.

"Mike was murdered. Leitha was old and her death was an accident," I said.

Marcus looked away for a moment; then his eyes met mine again. "What if it wasn't?"

7

I had no words. I just stared at him. "Are you serious?" I finally managed to say. "You really think there's a connection between Mike's death and his great-aunt's? Leitha died in a car accident. Mike was murdered. I don't see it."

"I'm not saying there is a connection," Marcus said. "Right now all I'm doing is speculating, but I do know there is a lot of money in the Finnamore family trust."

"'If money go before, all ways do lie open,'" I said softly.

"Shakespeare."

I nodded. *The Merry Wives of Windsor.* I lifted my chin from my knee and stretched out my legs again. "So who benefited from their deaths?" It was a question Marcus often considered in a murder case.

"As far as I can see, Jonas and Lachlan Quinn."

"You can eliminate Jonas, because he isn't a biological Finnamore, so he didn't benefit from either Mike's

or Leitha's deaths because he can't inherit anything involving the trust. And as for Lachlan, he's seventeen. C'mon, you can't really believe a teenager engineered Leitha's death to look like an accident and did such a good job that up to now no one suspected anything and *then* on top of that he managed to kill Mike. Lachlan seems like a bright kid but I remember myself at that age and I wasn't smart enough to pull that off. Were you?"

Marcus leaned over and kissed the side of my face. "I couldn't figure out how to get girls to notice me when I was seventeen. I wouldn't have been capable of plotting to kill anyone." He laughed; then his expression became serious again. "Just between the two of us, hypothetically, what do you think happened?"

"Hypothetically, I keep coming back to the idea of some random thief who was surprised by Mike and panicked."

"But?" He raised an eyebrow. "There is a but, isn't there?"

I leaned my head against the back of the chair. "Again, hypothetically speaking, if the police, if you, had any evidence that led in that direction—any sign of a break-in, missing valuables, someone suspicious seen around Mike's house or if there had been other break-ins in the neighborhood—you wouldn't be looking for a connection to Leitha's death."

He didn't say anything, which in itself told me I was right.

Hercules came across the lawn from the direction of Rebecca's yard. He eyed the basket of potatoes and

then jumped onto my lap, nuzzling my chin before murping a hello to Marcus.

"This isn't going to be easy," I said as much to myself as to Marcus or the cat.

"No," Marcus agreed, "it isn't."

Harry arrived at the library about midmorning on Tuesday. I was reshelving some reference books and spotted him out the window. I set the last book on the shelf and walked over to the circulation desk. "I'm just going outside to talk to Harry for a minute," I said to Susan, who was working the desk.

She was sorting through a stack of children's picture books, pulling an odd assortment of things that seemed to have been used as bookmarks from between the pages. There were a folded sticky note, a scrap of red yarn, a swizzle stick and three squares of toilet paper piled next to her right arm. She looked up at me, nudging her cat's-eye glasses up her nose with one knuckle. "Take your time." She dipped her head at the heap of would-be bookmarks. "People use the oddest things to mark their place."

"Yes, they do," I agreed, struggling to keep a straight face since Susan herself was anchoring her topknot with a bamboo knife and fork.

I walked across the parking lot and Harry got to his feet when he saw me approaching, brushing the dirt off his hands.

"Good morning," he said. "The old man told me next time I saw you to be sure to tell you that those tomatoes are the best so far."

"I'm glad he liked them. I'll get some more out to him. I have more than I can use." I looked over the flower bed. "The marigolds still look good."

"They should be fine until the first frost." He adjusted the brim of his ball cap. "You didn't come out here to talk about tomatoes and flowers, Kathleen."

"No, I didn't," I said. "I need you to tell me about Mike. The real person. Don't get me wrong. I liked him. But I know that people tend to make a person into a saint when they're dead."

Harry smiled. "Mike definitely wasn't a saint, but he was a good guy. In all the years I've known"—he stopped, took a breath and let it out and then continued—"knew Mike, I think I may have seen him lose his temper five or six times if that. He was just one of those people who could roll with whatever was happening. That was the real Mike."

"How did you all manage to practice for the show without the people around you finding out?"

"I think a few people did guess, but they were just good at keeping the secret," Harry said. "I'm pretty sure the old man figured it out, although he says he didn't. Mike came over to the house every Thursday night for weeks so we could practice together because it was the only time we could make it work. Monday through Wednesday he worked later at the office and Friday night he was checking out new music somewhere in the area. Peggy works late on Thursdays, so dad was always around and you know he doesn't miss a thing."

I smiled. "No, he doesn't." I also knew Harrison was very good at keeping his own counsel, to use one of his own expressions.

"Eventually, we worked things out so the others could join in on Zoom. Mike set everything up. I did ask Larry a couple of computer questions, but I don't think he figured it out." He shrugged. "Then again, for all I know, maybe I'm selling him short. I can tell you that Mike was never late, so I'm guessing someone in his office knew he was doing something even if they didn't know what the something was, because they got him out on time every single Thursday. And we all spent a couple of Saturdays at Paul's camp. It's likely Paul's wife, Sonja, knew or guessed what was going on."

He frowned. "Do you think someone had been watching Mike's comings and goings and broke into the house when they thought he wouldn't show up?"

I played with my watch, twisting it around my arm. I wasn't sure about anything. "I don't know," I said. "Right now anything is possible."

Later that morning Johnny Rock came in to the library. I was standing in the doorway to our smaller meeting room talking to Patricia Queen, head of the quilters group that met each week in the library, when Susan came to find me. Patricia and I were talking about a fall workshop for beginning quilters. We'd already had one quilt show at the library, which had shown me there was lots of interest in the craft.

"Kathleen, I'm sorry for interrupting," Susan said.

"Johnny Rock is here to see you and he says it's important."

"That's all right," Patricia said before I had a chance to speak. "We covered everything I had on my list and I'll e-mail you the notes on our meeting this afternoon." Patricia was nothing if not organized.

"Thank you," I said. "If anything else comes to mind after I've read your notes, I'll be in touch."

Patricia picked up her quilted tote bag, tucked the small notepad and pen she'd been using inside, nodded to both of us and strode purposefully through the stacks.

Susan and I followed behind her, a little less briskly.

"Kathleen, do you think Patricia would come to my house and teach the boys some organization skills?" Susan asked.

Her boys, twins, were incredibly smart, genius-level-IQ smart. They were always coming up with some new project, which always seemed to take the entire house to put together.

"You know, she probably would," I said.

Susan made a face. "Doing that seems kind of mean," she said, "to Patricia."

"You know, if the three of them teamed up, between the boys' creative thinking and Patricia's organizing skills, they could take over the world."

She grimaced. "Did I say getting the three of them together would be mean? Make that scary. Very scary."

Johnny was waiting for me by the circulation desk. He gestured to the carved wooden sun over the front

entrance with the words *Let there be light*. "You know, I'm a bit embarrassed to admit I never noticed those words before," he said.

"You're not the only one, I promise. The same words are over the entrance to the very first Carnegie library in Dunfermline in Scotland."

Johnny looked around the large open space. "I'm glad the building was restored," he said. "It would be a shame to lose such a big part of the town's history."

"I agree," I said.

He turned his attention back to me. "Kathleen, could we talk somewhere a little more private?"

"Of course." I gestured toward the stairs to the second floor. "Come up to my office."

I led the way up and unlocked my office door. "How about a cup of coffee?" I asked.

"Yes, please," he said. "Black with one sugar would be great."

"Have a seat." I indicated the two chairs in front of my desk. "I'll be right back."

I went down to the staff room, got coffee for the two of us and went back to my office.

"What did you need to talk to me about?" I asked after I'd set our mugs on my desk. Instead of sitting across the desk from Johnny, I had taken the other chair next to him.

"You brought the library back to life," he said. "And I don't just mean with the restoration of the actual building. You've made the library a big part of

the community, the way it used to be. The way it should be."

I took a sip of my coffee before I answered. "Thank you," I said. "It took a lot of work from a lot of people to make it all happen. I can't take all the credit. I shouldn't."

"Mike talked a lot about how much help you gave him while he worked on his family history."

I smiled. "He was so caught up in learning more about the family, it was easy to get carried along with his enthusiasm. I enjoyed myself. He brought coffee and muffins for my staff twice. We all liked him."

Johnny handed me an envelope.

"What is this?" I asked.

"Mike wasn't one for showy remembrances, but I wanted . . . I *need* to do something in his memory." He cleared his throat. "Harry said the library is fundraising for new computers." He indicated the envelope. "I hope that will help."

I lifted the flap and was stunned to see the amount of the check inside. It would take us past our fundraising goal. I pressed my lips together and swallowed down the sudden press of tears. "Thank you. This is so incredibly generous. I promise to make sure everyone knows the new computers are in memory of Mike."

Johnny smiled. "Thank you. I think Mike would get a kick out of that. I'll let the guys know and Mike's family as well." He got to his feet and I did the same, still holding tightly to that check. "You know, it's going to be odd on Thursday nights not to be getting

together with the guys online to make music. Those few hours feel as though they've left a gaping hole in my life."

"You gave everyone who was at the concert something we're going to remember for the rest of our lives," I said.

I walked Johnny back downstairs, thanked him again and then stood in the entrance and watched him cross the parking lot to talk to Harry. I went back inside to find Susan stacking books on a cart. She looked up at me.

"Johnny made a donation in memory of Mike, didn't he?" she said.

I nodded. "Enough to put our new-computer fund over the top."

She grinned and did a little fist pump. "Do you remember that Saturday Mike was here and he fixed the computer monitor for that kid who was working on a paper for school? Last minute, of course."

I nodded. Mike had tried so hard not to swear because there were kids around. After the monitor was working again, he'd told me our computers were a bunch of boat anchors with a few colorful adjectives added. I pictured him standing by the circulation desk, just about where Susan was standing now, hands gesturing in the air.

"You're going to figure out who did this, right?" Susan asked.

"That's Marcus's job," I said.

Susan nudged her glasses up her nose and brushed

a stray strand of hair off her face. "I know," she said. "And you're going to figure out who did this, right?"

I could still see Mike, in my mind, standing there telling me that the library needed to have computers from this century. I nodded. "Right," I said.

8

I got home to find Hercules on the back step with a grackle feather under one paw and a triumphant look on his face.

"Don't tell me that you two are at it again?" I said.

He looked down at the feather and then looked at me. "Merow," he said.

The cat and one particular grackle—or maybe it was several different birds for all I knew—had had some kind of war going on for quite some time. Basically neither wanted to share the backyard with the other. They had seemed to reach a détente earlier in the summer, but now it seemed the battle was on again.

I had always had the feeling that the two of them liked their little skirmishes. If one took down the other, the fun would be over. I'd seen the grackle sweep low, just inches over the cat's head, several different times. To me, it looked like the same bird. I'd discovered that the average life span of a grackle was about seventeen years, so it wasn't that unlikely that

Hercules had been warring with the same bird from the beginning. This wasn't the first time he had snagged one of the bird's feathers. Last week the grackle had swiped two sardine crackers from the arm of one of the Adirondack chairs, just inches from Herc's nose. Was this some kind of retaliation or had Hercules found the feather on the lawn and brought it home as a trophy?

I unlocked the porch door. "Leave that out here," I said, indicating the feather.

He wrinkled his nose at me.

"The spoils of battle stay outside," I said firmly.

He looked at the feather, sighed and came inside.

I changed for tai chi class and warmed up a bowl of noodles and veggies for supper. Hercules sulked around the kitchen. I found the little mechanical mouse Marcus had brought back for him after a recent trip. He'd gotten Owen a catnip frog, Ferdinand the Funky Frog, to be precise, sibling, via adoption, to Owen's beloved Fred the Funky Chicken. Since Hercules didn't get the attraction of catnip his gift was the mouse.

I set the mouse going and put it on the floor. Hercules liked to watch it run randomly all over the kitchen and then whack it with a paw. Once he'd smacked the little toy so hard, it skidded across the floor all the way to the living room doorway.

Owen wandered in for a drink, and when the tiny mouse suddenly veered in his direction, brushing against the end of his tail, he started with a loud meow. His paw hit the edge of the dish and flipped it into the air like someone doing a trick with a Frisbee. I sucked

in a breath, picturing water everywhere and a wet, indignant cat, but luckily the bowl was empty and it landed right side up on the floor.

"You're fine," I said. "No water. No harm done."

I spoke too soon.

The mouse was still moving, veering to the right, toward Hercules, who slapped a paw on it and looked at us with triumph in his green eyes.

Owen glared at his brother, taking a step back and unfortunately putting his foot in Herc's water dish. Owen let out a yowl of annoyance, vigorously shaking his back right foot. Hercules made an equally annoyed grumble because he very much did not like Owen putting even a whisker near his dishes. Somehow the mouse got out from under Hercules's foot, spun around in a circle and headed for the back door as though trying to get away from what was shaping up to be a monumental cat argument.

I walked around the table and pointed a finger at Hercules, who was already starting for his brother. "Not another step, mister," I said.

"Merow!" he replied with a fair amount of indignation, pleading his case as it were.

"It was an accident. They happen." They seemed to happen a lot in this house but that wasn't the point.

Owen gave me his best I-have-been-injured look and shook his foot. I bent down and picked him up, using the hem of my shirt to wipe his foot. It was only a little damp. I stroked the top of his head.

"It was just an accident," I repeated. "It's not your brother's fault."

He continued to mutter almost under his breath.

I set Owen down next to the basement door. I looked from one cat to the other. "Don't move."

Owen's front left paw twitched.

"Don't push it," I warned.

The paw stopped moving and Owen contented himself with making a show of *not* looking in his brother's direction, while Hercules darted sideways looks at his sibling.

I gave each cat a cracker. "I'm probably weakening your character by doing this," I told them. That didn't seem to be a concern for either one of them.

I wiped up the tiny bit of water on the floor and rinsed all four bowls. Roma had suggested a fountain for the cats. Maybe it was something I should consider.

I retrieved the mouse from the back door and put it in the cupboard with the cat treats. I realized I just had time to change my T-shirt before tai chi if I wanted to walk down to class.

Owen had eaten his cracker and he followed me upstairs, immediately going to sit in front of the closet door. I thought of him as the feline fashion police. I held up a T-shirt and he wrinkled his whiskers. He didn't like my second choice, either, but he seemed happy with my third pick. I pulled my hair into a ponytail and went back downstairs.

I didn't have time to do my own dishes, so I stacked them in the sink and grabbed my bag with my towel and tai chi shoes. Hercules was in the porch looking out the window.

"Please give Owen some space," I said.

"Mrr," he said.

I hoped that was acquiescence.

It was the perfect night for walking, warm but not overwhelmingly hot. When I got to the studio, I discovered that the stairwell and the area where we hung up our things and changed our shoes had gotten a fresh coat of paint. The clean, bright white walls made the space seem a little larger.

Maggie was inside, standing by the window with a mug of tea. I walked over to join her.

"The entry looks great," I said.

She smiled. "I can't believe what a difference just a coat of paint makes. I didn't realize how dingy the walls looked until the painters started working."

"Who did the work? I know you couldn't have used Oren because he's out of town." Oren Kenyon was a very talented carpenter and a meticulous painter. He was away for a few days supervising the installation of several pieces of his father's artwork in a gallery in Madison.

"It's a company run by a bunch of students just for the summer," Maggie said. "And it was actually Oren who suggested them, so that was enough of a recommendation for me. *And* you'll never guess who one of the painters turned out to be? Zach Redmond."

Zach had been bartending at The Brick, a club up on the highway. He was one of Maggie's yoga students and I'd met him when my brother and his band had visited and we'd gone to the club to listen to a group

Ethan had wanted to check out. Zach wore his thick dark hair in a man bun most of the time. He had dark skin and beautiful blue eyes.

"I thought he'd gone back to school," I said.

She took a sip of her tea. It smelled like marmalade. "He's still working on his degree and he's doing some shifts at The Brick and painting during the day."

Zach was still trying to figure out what he wanted to do with his life. I remembered how Maggie had described him to me: "He's like a big untrained puppy. Sometimes you have to smack him on the nose with a rolled-up newspaper."

Maggie smiled. "You know how Zach has always lacked, well, focus?"

I nodded.

"I overheard him talking to the young woman he was working with, warning her about drinking too much, staying out late and borrowing stuff from her grandmother without asking."

"Sounds like he's maturing," I said.

Roma joined us then. Her dark hair was pulled back in a stubby ponytail and she was wearing a sea green sleeveless T-shirt and cropped gray leggings. "We match," she said, holding out the hem of her shirt. My top was just a slightly darker version of the shade of green she was wearing.

"Truthfully, Owen picked it out," I said.

"Hey, you have a fashion consultant. That's great," she said, grinning and bumping me with her shoulder. "I was going through photos Eddie took at the concert

and there are some good ones of you and Marcus. First chance I get this week, I'll send them and some of the others to you."

"Thank you," I said. "I didn't think about taking pictures and now I wish I had."

"You're welcome. Eddie loves any chance to use that fancy camera. Ruby has been giving him some tips."

Ruby Blackthorne, a very talented artist and photographer, was a member of the local artists' co-op.

"I need to go speak to Rebecca," Roma said. "Eddie got a beautiful shot of her and Everett dancing."

As though saying her name had suddenly conjured her out of thin air, Ruby appeared in the doorway. She crossed the room and joined us.

"I have something to show you," she said, a huge smile lighting up her face.

"Is it the new calendar?" I asked.

Ruby had taken some photos of Owen and Hercules, and that had morphed into a very successful promotional calendar for the town. So successful that now there was a second one, once again featuring the boys at various locations around town.

Ruby nodded and held out the large envelope she was holding. "Take a look."

The calendar's cover photo was Owen and Hercules on the deck of a sailboat. I remembered that shoot. Owen had shown no trepidation about getting on the boat but Hercules had been very reluctant. Given his intense dislike of wet feet, that hadn't surprised me.

Ruby had shamelessly bribed him with a dish of chopped roast beef.

Maggie and I flipped through the calendar pages. "Oh, I like this one!" I exclaimed about the photo that had been taken of the boys in the same spot we were standing. Owen was on his back legs with his front paws on the window ledge. Hercules was sitting on the ledge, one paw in the air almost as though he was working on his tai chi form.

"Look, Owen's doing Cloud Hands," Maggie teased. "He's good, too." Cloud Hands was one of the 108 movements of the form that still gave me grief.

I stuck my tongue out at her and she laughed. Then she bent her head over the calendar again.

"I like the lighting in this one," she said to Ruby. "You've done an incredible job."

I nodded my agreement. "I didn't think it was possible, but this one is even better than the first calendar."

Ruby's cheeks flushed at the compliments. "You can keep that one and take it home for Owen and Hercules to see."

"Thank you," I said, slipping the calendar back inside the envelope.

"I'm going to get a cup of tea," Ruby said. "I'm glad you like the calendar."

Maggie took another sip of her own tea while stretching one arm over her head. "How was your day?" she asked. Maggie was the kind of person who was genuinely interested when she asked a question like that.

"Johnny Rock came in to make a donation in Mike's memory to our computer fund," I said. "It put us over the top."

"I think that's a great memorial for Mike."

"It is. There are a lot of people who depend on us for Internet access and just for the chance to even use a computer. I'm happy that now we have the money to replace all the old ones."

"But you wish it wasn't because Mike's dead." She switched arms, stretching her left one now.

"Exactly," I said. "He called the old ones boat anchors, which isn't far from the truth."

"So he'd be happy you're getting new ones."

I rubbed the back of my neck with one hand. "I think so, yes."

"So you should be happy, too."

"What would I do without you?" I said.

"You'd never master Cloud Hands, you and Marcus would not be a couple and you'd let your cat pick out your clothes all the time," she teased.

I wrapped her in a hug. "Then lucky for me that I came to Mayville Heights."

"Lucky for me, too," Maggie said.

It was almost time to begin. Maggie and I walked over to the tea table.

"Has anyone from Mike Bishop's office called you?" she asked.

I frowned at her. "No. Why would they be calling?"

Maggie ran a hand over her blond curls. "Well, I heard from them because I had an appointment

coming up and Caroline wanted to let me know what my options are."

Caroline was Mike Bishop's office manager. She was someone I should talk to, I realized.

"They're going to call every patient at some point to see what people want to do with their records." She set her cup on the table. "Has Marcus come up with anything yet?"

I sighed softly. "No."

"Have you?"

There wasn't any point in denying that I was asking questions about Mike's death. I shook my head. "No."

"You'll figure it out," Maggie said, giving my arm a squeeze as she moved to the center of the room. She clapped her hands and called, "Circle, everyone."

I darted out to put the calendar in my bag. Then I moved into my usual spot next to Roma and it struck me that I didn't know if Maggie had been referring to both Marcus and me when she'd said, "You'll figure it out," or if she'd just meant me.

When we finished the form at the end of the class, I was surprised to see Marcus waiting by the door. He walked over to me. "Can I lure you out for frozen yogurt at Tubby's?" he asked. "Or do you need to get home?"

I smiled. "I can always find time for Tubby's," I said.

"Good," he said. He turned to Maggie. "Brady showed me your design ideas for the T-shirts for the girls' hockey team. I don't know how we're going to pick just one."

"It was fun working on them," Maggie said. "And

it wasn't just me. Kathleen and Owen both offered their input."

Marcus smiled. "I'll make sure both of them are rewarded."

I changed my shoes and we headed down the stairs.

"Where did you park?" Marcus asked as we stepped outside. "I didn't see the truck anywhere."

"I walked," I said. "It was such a nice evening and I spent a lot of time sitting today. I wanted to stretch my legs."

His SUV was parked just ahead. "That works out perfectly. We can drive over to Tubby's for yogurt and find a place to enjoy it along the Riverwalk. I'll take you home after that."

I recognized his matter-of-fact tone. He was in detective mode.

We got to the car, and before I got inside, I stopped, resting one hand on the roof. "Marcus, I'm always happy to see you and I'm always up for frozen yogurt, but I know you're here for more than that. So please tell me what's up."

He looked at the keys in his hand for a moment; then he looked over the roof of the car at me. "I need you to tell me all about Leitha Anderson's visit to the library on the day she died."

My heart began to thump in my ears. "Did you actually find a connection between her death and Mike's?"

He thought for a moment. "Can we just get in, please?" he said.

We both climbed into the SUV and I turned to face him before I even fastened my seat belt. "What's going on?" I said. "Is Leitha's accident connected to Mike's death?"

He stuck the key in the ignition without saying anything, then looked at me. "At this point I can't be sure, but I have reason to believe Leitha Anderson's death wasn't so accidental after all."

9

I stared at him, wondering if I'd heard him right. "I don't understand," I said. "Leitha had a heart attack. Her car went off the road. Everyone agreed it was an accident."

Marcus did his hand-hair thing. He looked tired. There was dark stubble on his face and lines pulled at his mouth. "I know, but I couldn't let go of the idea that something was off about her death, so I went back through the file on the accident and I noticed that Leitha had been involved in a study on heart disease and longevity."

I nodded. "I know. Mike told me that Leitha was the only person in two generations of their family to live into her nineties."

"It was a long shot, but I contacted one of the doctors who is involved in that study and I sent him a copy of the medical examiner's report. He called me back less than an hour later and he told me that he had concerns over the levels of potassium chloride in blood samples taken at Leitha's autopsy. According to the doctor, she

had used a salt substitute in the past that contained potassium, but not enough to explain the levels found in her blood in his opinion. And as far as he knew, she hadn't been using that substitute anymore."

"If those levels were too high, they could have caused an irregular heart beat and heart failure."

"Exactly," Marcus said.

He fastened his seat belt and started the SUV and we drove over to Tubby's. I got strawberry frozen yogurt. Marcus chose orange cream. We walked along the Riverwalk and sat down on the second bench we saw with our cups of frozen yogurt.

"Tell me what you're thinking," he said.

"I'm thinking that I've always felt bad about Leitha's death," I said.

"Why?" he asked.

"She came to the library for the presentation about the history of Mayville Heights that Mary was giving."

The talks on the history of this part of the state had turned out to be extremely popular. All of them had been well attended.

"And she and Mary ended up having a very loud and very public argument about the early settlement of the town," Marcus said.

I nodded. "Yes." My chest tightened at the memory of their raised voices, particularly the disdain in Leitha's tone. "I had to step in to put a stop to it."

I remembered how Leitha had given Mary her steely gaze and said, "Breeding will tell."

Mary had met the other woman's stare with an equally undaunted look and said, "Yes, it certainly will."

I licked a bit of frozen yogurt off my thumb. "Some people found Leitha to be too blunt and abrasive and they liked seeing Mary stand up to her. I know Mary was sorry for making a scene. She apologized immediately and she came out to the house that night to apologize again."

I had been surprised to see a somber-looking Mary at my door. "May I come in?" she'd asked.

"Of course," I'd said.

"I know I told you this afternoon how sorry I am for getting into an argument with Leitha and making a scene at the library. It was petty and childish of me," she'd said as she stood in the middle of the porch.

"But understandable. Leitha is a challenging person."

"I want you to know that something like that will never happen again. I give you my word. And I'm sorry that I put you in a difficult situation."

"I appreciate that," I'd said. "I don't understand what happened? What made you so angry?"

Mary had looked at the floor for a moment; then her eyes met mine. "Leitha was going on about the Finnamores being among the first settlers in this area. The fact of the matter is it was Ruby's family—the Blackthornes—not the Finnamores who first settled this area. And Keith King's family and Lita's have been here almost as long. I reminded Leitha of that and that the town was actually built where there had been an earlier indigenous settlement." There was a flush of color in her cheeks. This was obviously something she felt strongly about. "You know about Ruby's indigenous ancestry, I'm guessing."

"I do," I'd said.

"In fact Ruby's family was here a couple of generations before the Finnamores, or anyone else for that matter. Leitha was dismissive as though they weren't important because they didn't come over on the *Mayflower*. So I got my knickers in a knot. I should have known it was a waste of time, trying to talk to that woman." Her cheeks got a little pinker and she stuffed her hands in her pockets. "I was wrong for calling Leitha an old bat."

I'd nodded. "It didn't help."

"And I will apologize to her for that," Mary had said.

"Of course she didn't get the chance," I said to Marcus. "She felt bad that maybe their argument had contributed to Leitha's heart attack, which then led to the accident. Leitha was very angry when she left the library. I think Mary still feels a little guilty."

"I can see why she would," he said. "Do you want some of my frozen yogurt?"

"Maybe just a taste," I said.

He held out the cup and I scooped out a spoonful. The orange cream flavor was tart and rich all at the same time. "Oh, that's good," I said. "I'm getting that next time." I offered my own cup. "Would you like to try mine?"

He smiled. "Kathleen, you ate it all," he said.

I tipped up the container to take a look. It was empty. How had that happened?

"Was Mary's talk like the previous ones?" Marcus asked. "Did you offer tea and coffee again?"

"Yes, we did," I said. "Oh, and there were maple cookies from Eric's."

"Did you see Leitha eat a cookie or drink a cup of tea or coffee?"

"You don't think she was poisoned, do you?"

"I didn't say that," he said. "Did you see her eat or drink anything?"

I tried to picture the aftermath of Mary's talk. People had been milling around, getting tea or coffee, talking. More than one person had commented on the cookies.

"Mary offered a cookie to Leitha," I said.

His blue eyes narrowed. "Offered or gave?"

"Mary would not poison Leitha or anyone else. You know Mary. You have to know that."

"I didn't say she did." He waited.

"Offered," I said firmly. "I remember that she was holding the tray." I set my empty yogurt cup on the bench. "You can't possibly think that Mary killed Leitha—that Mary *planned* to kill Leitha—because it's not like she would have had potassium chloride in the pocket of her sweater."

Marcus held up one hand. "I don't believe Mary killed Leitha. I don't believe she would kill anyone—give them a stern talking-to, yes, or in a worst-case scenario maybe drop-kick them across the room, but I don't see her resorting to murder."

I tapped my spoon against my bottom lip. "When would Leitha have to have ingested the potassium chloride for it to have caused her heart attack?"

"The doctor thinks it would have to have been in her

system about an hour before the heart attack that caused her to go off the road."

"So at the library," I said.

"It's possible that Leitha had pills on her and took too many by mistake, but I can't find any reference to any kind of medication in any police reports and she hadn't been prescribed potassium chloride by her doctor."

"I didn't see her take anything."

"But you weren't watching her all the time."

I shook my head. "No. There was a lot going on." I looked out over the water for a moment. "Marcus, do you think it's possible that Leitha committed suicide?" I asked.

Marcus stretched one arm along the top of the bench. "I admit that did occur to me, but it doesn't make sense. She was in good physical health, especially for her age and her mind was sharp. I checked with her doctor *and* the doctor running the study—she had no cognitive issues at all. No one who knew Leitha said anything about her seeming depressed. She had plans made several months ahead. Nothing suggests suicide."

"So what happens now?" I asked.

"The medical examiner is doing more tests and consulting with Dr. Faraday, the doctor in charge of the study."

The breeze lifted my hair and I tucked a stray strand back behind my ear. "What happens if they decide that Leitha was murdered? And how does that all connect to Mike's death? Or does it?"

Marcus shrugged. "That's the part I still don't know."

10

I reached over and laid my hand on Marcus's arm. His skin was warm under my fingers. "So what do you do until you get some answers?" I asked.

"I keep working on the Bishop case. Do you remember? Was Mike at the library for Mary's talk?"

"He was. It was a Friday afternoon and his office was closed, so Mike was there."

Marcus linked his fingers with mine. "Do you know if he had started digging into his ancestry at that point?"

I shook my head. "I don't think so. He told me that Leitha's death was actually what inspired him to learn more about the family, but he seemed very interested in what Mary had to say. I know he talked to her a couple of times about his great-grandfather when he was working on the family tree."

"Do you remember if Mike came to any of the other lectures?" Marcus asked.

"He was at the second one Harrison gave, and I

did see them talking afterward, but they knew each
other well, so it didn't mean they were talking about
Mike's family tree. Why are you asking? Do you think
something Mike uncovered in his family's past has
something to do with his death?"

He shrugged. "Right now I'm not ruling anything
out. Do you remember when he first came into the
library to start researching his family history?"

I straightened the neck of my T-shirt, running my
fingers over the stitching around the neck, as I searched
my memory for the first time Mike had asked for
my help. "I think it was roughly about a month after
Leitha's death. He showed up one Friday morning right
after we opened.

"Mike said he'd been poking around online on one
of those ancestry sites, but he wasn't finding a lot of
what he was looking for, and he wanted to know what
to do next.

"I made some suggestions—there were some old
documents that had been digitized but weren't ac-
cessible through the library's website yet and we had
some other papers he could look at if he took the
proper care, plus old microfilm he could go through.
Mike asked if there was a way to borrow certain other
documents."

"Do you remember which documents?" Marcus
asked.

"A diary, some passenger manifests and some photos. Pretty much all the things he asked about were
too fragile to be in circulation, so I told him if he could
let me know specifically what he wanted, I should be

able to get copies or images of most things for him. And I know he went to Minneapolis to do some research at least once."

Marcus looked thoughtful and I knew he was filing away everything I said, already looking for connections between what he knew and what he was learning.

"Do you remember me telling you about an old map they used on the *Great Northern Baking Showdown*?" I asked.

Eugenie had been very good about working local references into the show whenever she had the chance. When she and Russell had filmed a segment at Wild Rose Bluff, they had used a map from the library in their intro.

Marcus frowned. "It was a map of the area around Wild Rose Bluff?"

I nodded, pushing my hair back off my face again. "Mike looked at that and he was very interested when I told him about an even earlier map showing land claims in the area that had just recently been donated to the library in Red Wing. The librarian there made a copy of it for me."

"Can you think of anything else?"

I shook my head.

"Okay, let's go back to Mary's presentation for a minute. Did Mike sit with Leitha?"

I thought for a moment, trying to picture the meeting room. "Yes," I said. "Leitha was on the end of a row, Mike was beside her and Jonas Quinn was next to him." I motioned with one hand, slotting people in

their seats in my mind. "Harrison was in the row in front of them. And Keith King. Keith has been tracing his family tree ever since Ella got him one of those DNA test kits. And I remember seeing Keith and Mike talking before Mary got started."

Marcus nodded and I knew he was making a mental note to talk to Keith. "Were there people there that you didn't know?" he asked.

"Of course. There always are. There were several tourists and those kinds of presentations always bring out the history buffs—at least based on the other ones we've done. I know there were a few people who came from Minneapolis. During Everett's talk I remember there were several real estate developers in the audience."

"Developers?" Marcus frowned. "Why?"

"Everett told me they showed up for one of two reasons—he was talking about old buildings in Mayville Heights and Red Wing, and developers want to know some of the history of a property they want to restore to exploit those details for financing. Or they want to know a property's past to be sure they won't face too much opposition because they want to tear it down. Do you remember that old bank building in Red Wing that was turned into condos? The plans had to be adapted because of the historical significance of the property."

Marcus rubbed the back of his neck with one hand. "How did Leitha act while she was at the library that day?"

"Like I said before, I wasn't watching the woman all the time."

"Anything you saw might be helpful."

I sighed. "You know how she could be. She had a rather superior attitude."

He nodded.

"Every time I looked in Leitha's direction while Mary was speaking, she had a look of disdain on her face. Now, if Mary noticed and if it bothered her at all, you couldn't tell. And to be fair, Leitha had acted the same way during Everett's talk, so I don't think it was personal."

"Is there anything else you can remember?"

My fingers were still linked with his. I traced my thumb along the side of his hand. "I'm not really sure what you're looking for."

He gave me a wry smile. "That makes two of us. You did say that Leitha had one of Eric's cookies. I know she drank a cup of tea at some point. According to her stomach contents, she'd had tea with milk and sugar. Was that at the library?"

"Yes," I said.

"Did she get the tea herself or did someone else get it for her?"

I knew what he was getting at. If Leitha's death hadn't been an accident, if she had died because of an overdose of potassium chloride—and I was having trouble with the idea—then maybe she had ingested it at the library.

"Someone else got it—Well, sort of."

"Wait a second. What do you mean, someone else got it 'sort of'?"

I exhaled loudly, feeling frustrated. "This is secondhand, so you should really talk to Rebecca. She told me this story the day after Leitha died." I remembered Rebecca saying she didn't like speaking ill of the dead.

"And I will," Marcus said. "Please, just tell me what you know for now."

I picked up the spoon from my frozen yogurt container and turned it over in my fingers. "As far as I know, this happened right before the argument between Leitha and Mary. Leitha did have a cup of tea, but it was actually Jonas's cup that she had taken from his hand, which according to Rebecca was her entitled way of behaving."

"Do you know if he poured the tea himself?" Marcus asked.

I nodded. "Rebecca said that he did and she remembers him drinking from it while the two of them were talking. I don't see how there could have been anything in the tea. Who could have guessed Leitha would take his cup? And anyway, Jonas is fine."

"I know," he said. "I might be completely off base about all of this but I need to be certain."

It was starting to get dark. "Are you ready to go?" Marcus asked, gathering up both of our empty yogurt containers. We started walking back to his SUV.

"When do you expect the medical examiner will have something?" I said.

He shrugged. "I'm not sure. Maybe a week."

Actually it took fewer than three days to get some answers. On Friday, after some investigation by the police and more tests by the medical examiner, the cause of Leitha Finnamore Anderson's death was changed from accident to homicide.

11

I was sitting at the kitchen table with Owen on my lap, eating a toasted bagel topped with tomato slices when Marcus called with the news. "You were right," I said.

"It might have been better if I'd been wrong." I heard the squeak of his desk chair. "Now I have two murder cases and no idea if they're connected or not."

"You'll figure it out," I said. Owen bobbed his head seemingly in agreement. "Owen and I have faith in you."

He laughed. "Well, then, how can I go wrong?"

Midmorning I got a call from Mike Bishop's office. It was the office manager, Caroline. I'd been expecting to hear from her ever since I'd talked to Maggie.

"Hi, Kathleen," she said. "I see from our records that you were coming back for a recheck on the tooth where we did the root canal. I don't mean to push you but I was wondering what you want to do."

"I don't really know," I said, dropping onto the footstool. "What are my options?"

"Well, there are several endodontists in Minneapolis. We could forward your records to one of them and I'm sure they would check the tooth for you. Is it giving you any trouble?"

Owen came down the stairs and over to me, looking quizzically at the phone.

"It's not. I don't have any pain at all now."

"Then you'd probably be okay not having it checked. It was just something Dr. B. liked to do."

"He was very conscientious," I said.

"Yes, he was." Caroline cleared her throat. "So I could just send your records over to your regular dentist. I can tell you that we know of an endodontist who is planning on setting up a practice here in Mayville Heights, probably this winter. If you did have any problems down the road and you didn't want to drive to Minneapolis, that would be an option."

Owen jumped onto my lap and pushed his face close to the receiver. I shifted him sideways and he gave me a sour look.

"I'm not sure what to do," I said. "That tooth gave me so much trouble before the root canal—"

"You're afraid something's going to go wrong again."

"Yes," I said. "I know how silly that sounds."

"It's not silly at all," Caroline said. "I have a suggestion. Why don't you stop by the office sometime? Lorraine is here. You could ask her any questions you have. That might help you make up your mind."

Lorraine was one of the dental assistants in the practice. She was kind and very reassuring.

"I could stop in on my way to the library just before lunch."

"We'll see you then," she said.

Owen looked from the phone to me as I hung up.

"I'm going to stop at Mike's office," I said. "Teeth stuff."

He made a face. Owen hated having his teeth cleaned.

"Maybe I'll learn something useful."

The cat gave a noncommittal murp and followed me out to the kitchen.

"What do you think?" I asked. "Is Marcus right? Is there some kind of connection between Mike's and Leitha's deaths or is it just one weird coincidence?"

He seemed to think about my words for a minute; then he blinked his golden eyes at me. Okay, so he wasn't sure, either.

I poured a cup of coffee, and when I turned around again, Owen was sitting on my chair, eyeing the laptop that was on the table. Roma had sent the photos from the concert and I wanted to take a look at them. Apparently, Owen did as well.

I set my coffee on the table, well away from the computer, scooped up the cat and sat down. He looked over my shoulder at the toaster and then looked at me.

"We don't need toast and peanut butter," I said.

The photos were terrific. There were two of Marcus and me from the side. We were holding hands while

I leaned against his arm. There were three of Roma and me singing along with the band, arms across each other's shoulders. In one of the shots Eddie had taken of Mary and Marcus dancing, he'd caught her in midtwirl.

"I think that's my favorite," I said, pointing at the screen.

Owen's response was to put a paw on the keyboard and suddenly we were looking at an image of Maggie. "Merow!" he said. It was clear which photo was his favorite.

Roma had included several shots of the band. I smiled as I scrolled through the pictures and felt my throat tighten over an image of Mike and Harry grinning at each other as they played.

It wasn't fair. Mike had been one of the good guys. When I got to the library, he should be there flirting with the ladies in the Seniors' Book Club and laughing about some family scandal he'd uncovered with Abigail.

"We have to find the person who did this," I said to Owen.

He nuzzled my chin. He was in.

I decided I'd eat once I got to the library, so I packed my lunch and drove down to Mike Bishop's office. Caroline was at the reception desk.

"Hi, Kathleen," she said. "I'll let Lorraine know you're here."

I took a seat in the waiting room. Lorraine appeared a couple of minutes later. She smiled when she caught

sight of me. She was short and curvy and seemed to smile all the time. She had gorgeous red curls that she generally wore in a high ponytail. Before today I didn't think I'd ever seen her in the office with her hair down.

"How are you?" I asked.

Her mouth twisted to one side. "Still a bit in shock like everyone else." She looked around. "It seems so quiet in here. I'm still having trouble with the idea that the concert was the last time I'm ever going to see Mike."

She swallowed and I reached over and put a hand on her arm for a moment.

"The concert was incredible," I said.

Lorraine's smile returned. "It's funny. That Thursday Mike was just about bouncing all around the office and I chalked it up to him being a bit wired about Johnny Rock performing again. I had no idea we were going to see the band. I can't believe he managed to keep it all secret, because trust me, he was lousy at keeping secrets."

"But we really should have guessed," Caroline said.

Lorraine and I both turned to look at her.

"What makes you say that?" I asked.

Caroline gestured at the computer. "Mike was insistent that he had to leave on time on both Wednesday and Thursday. I had to schedule anything that had the possibility of running late for earlier in the day. More than once he missed lunch to get caught up. I can't believe that it never entered my mind that the band was getting back together."

Lorraine went over my options again and I decided

to have my records sent to my regular dentist for now. "I don't think you're going to have any problems with that tooth," she said, "but if you do, any of the end-odontists in Minneapolis are good."

I thanked her for her help and headed for the library. Mary was at the circulation desk. I hadn't seen her in a couple of days.

"You're early," she said.

I held up the cooler bag. "I had a stop to make, so I thought I'd have lunch here. Maybe out in the gazebo." I pulled out my phone and brought up the photos of her and Marcus. "Eddie took these," I said. "Roma is going to send you copies."

"I look pretty good," Mary said. "And that guy of yours is a real hottie."

I felt my cheeks getting red. "I'm just going to pretend you didn't say that," I said.

Mary laughed; then her expression became serious. "I heard the news about Leitha Anderson's death. And I've already talked to Marcus."

"Was there really anyone who would have wanted Leitha dead? I know she was—"

"Arrogant, rude, condescending?" Mary finished. "A lot of people might have wished she wasn't around, but as far as actually killing her? I don't think so. There's a big difference between wishing someone were dead and actually making it happpen." She picked up a pen and tapped it on the desk. "Leitha just had a way of getting under people's skin. The day she was here, the day she died, she was annoyed at me because I could show the Finnamores had very little to do with settling

the town. And Lordy, she was constantly nitpicking with Mike when he was alive because she wanted him to settle down and make little Finnamore babies."

"Do you think it bothered him?" I asked.

Mary gave a snort of laughter. "Not in the slightest. I remember her complaining that he didn't think about how his choices in his personal life affected her. She was always disappointed because Jonas wasn't a biological Finnamore—or as she put it, a 'real' Finnamore—like anyone cared. Before she died she was even butting in on where Lachlan was going to go to college and what he was going to study."

"It really mattered to her?"

"You'd better believe it did," she said, tapping the pen again for emphasis. "She wanted him to go into medicine or business, which is what the Finnamore men do. The Finnamore name and its legacy were the most important things to Leitha. From what I've heard, it was the same way with Leitha's grandfather, so she got it honestly. The two disappointments in the family were Mike working on people's teeth and Jonas becoming a college professor and PhD. Those were *not* the career paths she had chosen for them."

I shook my head. "It sounds exhausting."

"I think in some ways it was more exhausting for her."

"What happened to Lachlan's parents?" I asked. "I know they were killed in an accident but I don't know any of the details."

Mary shook her head. "That was before you got here. It was heartbreaking. They were on their way

back from Minneapolis and hit a patch of black ice that spun them into the path of a furniture delivery truck. Colin was killed outright. The driver of the truck and Ainsley were badly injured. The truck driver had to have his left leg amputated below the knee, but he did recover. Ainsley spent months in a coma before she died. Lachlan was just eleven. Luckily, he had stayed with Jonas. And I have to give credit where credit is due, for all of Leitha's abrasive ways, she rallied around the child just the way everyone else did."

It was good to hear the woman had had a heart after all. I hadn't really seen that.

I dropped my things in my office and had my lunch outside in the gazebo. Marcus called to say he was on his way to Minneapolis to talk to the doctor heading the cardiac study again.

"I don't know when I'll get back," he said.

"I love you," I said. "Drive safe."

I wasn't that hungry when I got home, so I toasted another bagel, cut a slice of cheddar and poured a glass of lemonade, promising myself I'd eat extra vegetables tomorrow.

The house felt warm and stuffy. I took my food and the laptop and went to sit in the backyard. I was halfway through my bagel, looking at the concert photos again when Hercules came through the porch door. Literally. He walked across the grass, sat at my feet and meowed. I patted my lap. "You can come up."

He meowed again.

"You're perfectly capable of jumping," I said. "It's not that far."

He still didn't move.

"I guess you don't want a bit of cheese, then."

He was on my lap almost before I got the words out, his black-and-white face looming in front of mine. I broke off a tiny bite of cheese and handed it to him. He murped a thank-you and ate it. Then he poked at my legs until he was settled in to look at the computer screen with me.

I scrolled through the photos so the cat could see all of them and I told him about my visit to Mike's office and about what I'd learned from Mary. He tipped his head to one side as though he were thinking about everything I'd said. Then he swiped a paw at the touch pad and a shot of Mike and Harry filled the screen. He turned to look at me as though he expected me to do or say something.

I studied the photo but saw nothing that would help figure out who had killed Mike. "I know you're not trying to suggest that Harry is the killer, so I don't see what you want me to see," I said.

I moved on to one of the images of Roma and me, arms over each other's shoulders. When I took a drink from my lemonade, Hercules managed to go back to the photo of Harry and Mike. I had a cat with computer skills that were better than those some people had.

I narrowed my gaze at him. "Quit it!" I said.

He gave a huff of impatience.

I broke the last little piece of cheese in half and gave

one piece to him. I ate the other one. "Sometimes I wish you could talk," I said.

He made an indignant meow.

"Talk in a language I understand, I mean." I looked at the image on the laptop and thought about how much fun Mike and Harry had been having that night and how magical it had been to be there.

Hercules peered into my lemonade, wrinkled his nose and then began to wash his face, shooting looks at the computer and me from time to time. Whatever I was supposed to see, I didn't. Or maybe the cat wasn't trying to show me anything.

"The guys worked so hard to make it a surprise," I said. "And if anyone did guess, those people kept it to themselves."

"I'm pretty sure the old man figured it out, although he said he didn't," Harry had said when he'd told me about Mike being out at the house every Thursday night for weeks. "Monday through Wednesday he worked later at the office and Friday night he was checking out new music somewhere in the area. . . . Eventually, we worked things out so the others could join in on Zoom."

Johnny had told me how odd it felt not to be getting together online with the others anymore on Thursday nights.

Thursday. Not Wednesday. *Thursday.*

"That's not what Caroline told me," I said slowly.

Hercules paused the face washing with one paw in midair. It almost seemed as though there was a look of anticipation on his face.

"Mike was insistent that he had to leave on time on Wednesday and Thursday. I had to schedule anything that had the possibility of running late for earlier in the day." That's what Caroline said: *Wednesday* and Thursday.

Hercules made a soft "mrr," glanced at the screen and went back to washing his face with a murp. Had I stumbled on what he'd been trying to tell me?

A moth fluttered by only a couple of inches from the cat's face. He leaped into the air, lost his balance and landed awkwardly—albeit upright—on the lawn. He gave himself a shake and looked kind of embarrassed. The moth was fine.

Was it possible that Mike Bishop was doing something on Wednesday nights that he didn't want anyone to know about? I knew I needed to check with Harry and maybe the rest of the band to make sure he hadn't been practicing on Wednesdays, too. Was I onto something? Or was my leap of logic as ungainly as Herc's leap after that moth? Had Mike had a secret of his own?

12

I decided that I would call Harry once the library closed for the day, but when I pulled into the parking lot Saturday morning, his truck was already there and he was unloading the lawn mower.

"I thought I'd get an early start," he said. His mouth worked as though he were trying out what he wanted to say before he actually said the words. "Kathleen, I don't mean to push but I just wondered if you've come up with anything yet."

I knew he meant about Mike's killer.

"I'm sorry," I said. "I haven't. Not yet, but I do have a question. Did you and Mike ever practice on Wednesday?"

He shook his head. "As far as I know, he was at the office getting caught up with paperwork on Wednesday nights. That's what he said."

"Could he have been getting together with someone else to rehearse?"

"Not with Paul. He had something going on with

his kids on Wednesdays. I can check with Ritchie and Johnny if that will help."

"I'll talk to Johnny myself," I said. "But if you could ask Ritchie, that would help."

"What does this have to do with who killed Mike?"

I shrugged. "At this point I don't know."

"Okay," he said. "I'll see what I can find out and I'll talk to you later. I'll be out this afternoon to do the mowing and clipping at your place and I'll take a look at the problem with the downspout."

I thanked him and went inside.

About half an hour later, as I was wrestling with a shelf that seemed to be permanently stuck at a thirty-degree angle, Maggie called to invite me to join her and Roma for a late lunch at Eric's. I was already feeling frustrated and too warm. Lunch that I didn't have to make sounded wonderful. "I'll walk over right after we close," I said.

When the mail arrived on Friday, I had found the copy of the map I'd requested for Mike along with a note from the reference librarian in Grand Rapids. I called Jonas to let him know he could come and get the map along with the copies of the census. I'd also found a zippered folder of notes and papers that Mike had left behind. Everything was in my office sitting on my desk.

I had expected to get Jonas's voice mail but I got him instead.

"I'm free at the moment," he said. "Would it be all right if I came over now?"

"Of course," I said. "I'll see you soon."

Jonas walked in about half an hour later, just as I was pushing an empty book cart back to the front desk. He was wearing jeans and a gray T-shirt and something about the measured way he moved made me think of Lachlan. They didn't really look like they were related. Lachlan had the Finnamore green eyes while Jonas's eyes were dark. Jonas kept his wavy hair short, while Lachlan's hair brushed his shoulders when it wasn't pulled back in a ponytail. Like Mike, Lachlan was very animated when he spoke, but his Quinn DNA showed in the way he moved.

"Everything is in my office," I said. "C'mon up with me."

He followed me up the stairs. I unlocked my office door and picked up the folder and the file of papers from my desk. I handed everything to Jonas.

He stared at the papers for a moment before he took them from me. "Is . . . is this everything?" he asked.

"As far as I know. I think the last time Mike was here, he was in a bit of a rush. It was the day of the concert. That's probably why that folder got left behind, but if I find anything else, I'll set it aside and call you."

"I appreciate that," he said. "Mike and Lachlan were close and I like to think all this information about his family may be important to Lachlan someday."

"I hope it will," I said. "Mike shared a few of the stories with me. The Finnamores are a very colorful family."

He gave me a gentle smile. "That's a very diplomatic way to put things, Kathleen."

"I'm serious. For example, it turns out there's more than one musician in the family tree. An eighteenth-century bagpiper among others."

"I always said Mike had music in his blood. I guess he did. That night at the Last Bash he was so happy."

"Did you have any hint that the band was getting back together?" I asked.

His gaze softened. "I didn't. I was oblivious. There were a couple of times that Lachlan invited Mike for supper and he couldn't come, but he just said he was working late and I didn't think twice about it. That wasn't unusual. Mike was either working, out somewhere listening to live music or lately working on the family tree."

"How's Lachlan doing?"

He took off his glasses and rubbed the bridge of his nose. "Losing Mike was horrible and now learning that Leitha's death wasn't an accident . . . it's a lot for anyone to deal with. I'm not saying she wasn't a difficult person, but we have so little family left that any loss is painful. I don't mean to put you on the spot, but do you know if Detective Gordon has any suspects, or are you even allowed to answer that?"

I wanted to give Jonas some kind of hope that the person or people who had devastated his family would be brought to justice, but I didn't know what I could say that would do that. "At this point the police are still gathering information and asking questions. I know it's probably not much comfort, but they need to be slow and meticulous so they don't miss anything that might be important."

He nodded. "Leitha was a prickly person who said what she thought, whether or not it was thoughtful or kind or helpful. She made her share of enemies over the years, but she pretty much outlived them all. You saw her argument with Mary Lowe?"

"I did."

"At the time she was annoyed at Mike over something. I don't even remember what now. I was on her good side. In a few days Mike would have gotten back on the A-list and I would likely have been on the naughty list, so to speak, once again. It was just the way Leitha was in her personal life as well as in business. I don't think she cared what people thought of her."

"She was a woman in the business world when it wasn't that common," I said, treading carefully because I didn't want to offend Jonas. "She must have developed a thick skin."

"Like a rhinoceros hide." He smiled to take the sting out of his words. "As a young woman, Leitha worked with her grandfather at Black Dog and over time she built up a small portfolio of properties that she was still very hands-on with right up until she died. In fact, she had a potential deal with Everett Henderson that had fallen apart just before her death—I don't know any of the details—and I'm not trying to suggest that Everett had anything to do with her death."

He paused, almost as though he was weighing what he wanted to say next. "Kathleen, I hope I'm not being, well, rude, but I know you have some experience in this kind of thing. Do you think it's possible that Leitha's death and Mike's death are somehow

connected? I thought that Mike had walked in on someone in the middle of breaking in to his house."

I shifted uneasily from one foot to the other. The conversation made me uncomfortable. I understood that Jonas wanted answers but I wasn't the person who could give them to him. "I think it's way too soon to know at this point."

"I admit I'm still having trouble with the idea that Leitha's death wasn't an accident. I keep thinking that maybe she took the potassium chloride by accident or even by design, not realizing it could hurt her. She did seem to be getting a bit fatigued on occasion, but she was in her nineties. She was very private about her health along with everything else. It was her generation. Now I wish that I'd pushed."

I gave him what I hoped was a reassuring smile. "From what I knew of Leitha, I don't think pushing would have worked with her."

Jonas nodded. "Her response to being pushed was to push back even harder."

"Give the police time, Jonas," I said. "They're good at what they do."

"You're right," he said. "Thank you for listening and for all of this." He held up the papers.

"If I find anything else, I'll be in touch," I said.

Jonas left and I sat down at my desk and looked at the phone. I didn't think for a moment that Everett had had anything to do with Leitha's death, but I was curious about their failed deal. I decided to call Henderson Holdings and leave a message for Lita. To my surprise she answered the phone.

"Hi. I didn't expect to actually get you," I said when she picked up.

She laughed. "That begs the question: Then why did you call?"

"I was going to leave a message."

"You can still do that if you want to," she teased. "I just came in to clean up a few things from yesterday that had to be put aside because the power went out. I only picked up because I recognized the number and guessed it was you. What do you need?"

"Information," I said. There was no need to beat around the bush with Lita.

"That I have. Whether or not it's the information you're looking for, I can't say."

"Tell me about the deal between Everett and Leitha Anderson."

She didn't ask why I wanted to know. "Leitha owned a property in Red Wing that Everett was interested in turning into condos or apartments."

"It's something he's done before."

"Oh yes, restoring an old building instead of tearing it down." Like Mary and Harrison, Everett cared about the history of the state, and as he'd said at his presentation, not every old structure could be saved or should be, but they shouldn't all be torn down, either. "You know how Everett—and Rebecca—feel about not losing our ties to the past."

"'A people without the knowledge of their past history, origin and culture is like a tree without roots,'" I said. "Marcus Garvey."

"Mr. Garvey was a very wise man," Lita said.

I propped an elbow on my desk and leaned the side of my head against my hand. "So what made the project fall apart?"

"Leitha's pigheadedness. John Stone came to see Everett. He wanted to buy that building himself. John believed it had been the home of the first music school in the state, predating the MacPhail School by about two years. He wanted to turn the property back into a school. Everett agreed and tried to convince Leitha to sell to John instead."

"I take it that didn't go well."

"No, it did not," she said emphatically. "Leitha didn't like John. I don't think she ever liked the idea of Mike being in the band. She found that kind of thing unseemly for a Finnamore man. So she didn't want to be accommodating. And she saw John's desire to save the building as nothing more than just foolish sentimentality. Those were her exact words, 'foolish sentimentality.'"

The same expression she'd used with me about renovating the library.

"She decided to sell to someone else who was going to tear down the building and turn it into a parking lot. John was furious and Everett wasn't too happy, either."

"There was nothing either of them could do?" I asked.

"No. Leitha and Everett had no agreement in place on the property. And it was impossible to reason with her. It was weeks before John got over his anger. Fi-

nally, he just seemed to accept there was nothing he could do. He even told Everett to let it go."

"That's not exactly something Everett is good at."

Lita laughed. "No, it isn't." There was silence for a moment. "Kathleen, I heard that the police think Leitha's death wasn't an accident after all. Does any of this have anything to do with that building?"

I shook my head even though she wasn't there to see me. "I honestly don't know."

"Well, if you think any of this will help Marcus, go ahead and tell him. He knows where to find us if he has any questions."

"I will. Thank you," I said.

After we hung up, I got to my feet and went to stand by the window. I looked out over the water. It occurred to me that to solve one murder, I might just have to solve two.

13

I spent the rest of the morning shelving books and helping several people find something new to read. The latter was one of my favorite parts of the job. It always made my day when I suggested a book to someone and they came back to tell me that they had enjoyed it.

I discovered that someone had put gum on three different shelves in the reference section. Grape-flavored bubble gum, it seemed.

I rubbed the space between my eyebrows. "Some days I think gum should be a controlled substance," I muttered to Levi, who had been helping me get the reference section back to rights. Several students who were taking a summer school history class had just spent the last hour looking for references in "real" books for a class assignment.

"Did you know that the ancient Greeks chewed gum?" Levi asked.

"I did not," I said. "And I hope none of those ancient

Greeks ever stuck their gum on one of the wings on the statue of Nike or on Venus de Milo's shoulder."

He laughed. Then he gestured at the shelf. "I can take care of that," he said.

"Are you sure?" I asked. Getting gum off anything was a tedious job. I thought about Mariah doing the same thing out at the diner.

"It's no problem," Levi said.

"You'll need a scraper. That stuff sticks like super-glue. It took forever to get it out of the book drop."

"I used to be a room service waiter, remember? Everywhere someone can put gum, I've probably seen. Including some that, trust me, you don't want to know about."

He headed upstairs to get the scraper and I thought once again how glad I was that I'd hired Levi. The senior ladies loved his manners and were always bringing cookies to try to fatten him up. He had very wide tastes in reading material, which meant he could help pretty much any reader find something they'd like, and he knew more about graphic novels than I did.

I went back to the front desk to get the last cart of books to put on the shelves.

"You don't want Levi to finish this?" Abigail asked.

"He's scraping gum off one of the shelves."

She shook her head. "I swear some people behave like they were raised by wolves."

"I don't think wolves chew gum," I said.

"Then they clearly have better manners than some of our patrons."

I smiled. "No argument here."

Abigail had been on tour for her most recent children's book in June. She had a contract to write three more books in the series and I wondered sometimes if we'd lose her to a full-time career as a writer. She was very talented. I suspected her main character—a daring little girl with five bossy older brothers—was modeled after the little girl Abigail herself once was. She, too, had five older brothers. She'd even created a secret code so she could write things in what she called her logbook and they wouldn't be able to read it.

The first day she was back at work—which happened to be a Friday—Mike had come in with coffee and muffins for the whole staff, but I'd always had the feeling the gesture was really aimed at Abigail. I'd harbored a secret hope that the two of them might get together. Now that was never going to happen.

Maggie and Roma were already at a table when I got to Eric's Place. "Have you been waiting very long?" I asked as I slid onto my chair.

"I just got here," Roma said.

"And I barely got here before she got here," Maggie added.

Claire came over to take our orders. We all decided on the chopped salad and breadsticks. "And how about the blackberry iced tea?" Claire suggested. She smiled at me. "I know it's not coffee, Kathleen, but I think you'll like it."

"I'll try it," Maggie said.

Roma nodded. "Me too."

They all looked at me.

"So will I," I said.

"Seriously?" Roma said. She looked . . . surprised.

"I do drink more than coffee." Even I could hear that I sounded a little defensive.

"Not very often," Maggie teased.

Claire gathered our menus. "If you don't like it, I'll bring you coffee, I promise," she whispered as she collected mine.

"I heard about the medical examiner reclassifying Leitha Anderson's death," Roma said, picking up her napkin.

"Marcus doesn't think her death is connected to Mike's, does he?" Maggie asked.

I wasn't sure how to answer. I didn't want to say that he did and I was beginning think he might be right. "As far as I know they're two separate cases." I was saved from having to say anything more because Claire came back with the iced tea, which was as good as she had said it would be.

"How's hockey school going?" I asked once Claire had headed to another table. I was genuinely interested and I didn't want to talk about Mike or Leitha right now.

"It's going very well," Roma said. "Eddie is a natural teacher and he's already getting phone calls from high school and college hockey teams looking to work with him."

Despite all the obstacles he'd encountered in getting the school up and running, and despite people telling him he should set up in Minneapolis, Eddie

had never wavered from running his hockey school in his new hometown.

"Maybe I should get him to give me skating lessons," I said, reaching for my glass. I had never learned to skate as a kid. Both Maggie and Marcus had tried to teach me. All I'd managed to learn was how to fall so I didn't break anything.

"He would, you know," Roma said. "I should have thought of that a long time ago."

"You're good at standing up," Maggie offered. She always managed to find something positive to say.

"I'm fantastic at standing up," I said. "It's just moving that stymies me."

"Talk to Eddie," Roma said. "I'm serious. He'll teach you."

"I will," I said. I took another sip of my iced tea.

Roma put both of her hands flat on the table. "Before Claire comes back, I have to confess. I had an ulterior motive for suggesting we have lunch. I need both of your opinions on something."

"We are full of opinions," I said solemnly, squaring my shoulders and laying one hand on my chest.

Maggie nodded in agreement, looking equally serious.

Roma gave her head a little shake. "The two of you are full of something."

Mags smiled at her. "How can we help?"

"Do you remember the burlesque show at The Brick that raised money for the no-kill shelter?"

Maggie's eyes met mine and she grinned.

"Vividly," I said. "Mary put on a push to get me to take part in it."

Maggie was still grinning. "You should have said yes. It looked like a lot of fun."

I squinted across the table at her. "I don't remember seeing you on that stage."

"Mary didn't ask me, but I would have if I'd had the chance."

"You might want to be careful about saying that in front of witnesses," Roma said.

"Why?" I asked, unfolding my napkin and putting it in my lap.

"Because there may be another show."

Maggie eyed her, the remnants of a grin still on her face. "You're serious," she said.

Roma nodded. "Very."

At that moment Claire returned with our food. Once we all had our salads and fat, chewy breadsticks, I turned to Roma. "Another show? Explain please."

"I thought the original show was supposed to strictly be a onetime thing. Basically a last-minute idea to help raise enough money to fix the roof at the no-kill shelter," Maggie added.

"It was," Roma said. "I don't know if you remember, but we were desperate. The roof was leaking in about a dozen places and none of the other fund-raising efforts were bringing in the kind of money we needed. Mary suggested a burlesque-style show—nothing that involved nudity or anything obscene, just a little slightly naughty fun. She convinced The

Brick to give us the stage for a night and to kick in a percentage of the drink totals."

Mary might look like someone's kindly cookie-baking grandmother, but she was also an example of the old saying that looks could be deceiving. She was the state kickboxing champion in her age group and she danced regularly at amateur night at The Brick. Like the burlesque show, there was no nudity, just fishnets, feathers and flirtation.

In the weeks before the first show, I'd learned a lot about burlesque from Mary. She'd explained that shows usually featured a master of ceremonies whose job it was to keep the show moving forward. The MC not only introduced each act; he or she also interacted with the audience. Most acts ran five minutes or less. The performers included dancers, singers, magicians, comedians and, yes, striptease artists.

"But not in this show, I promise," Mary had said when my eyebrows went up, "although . . ." She'd winked and given me a sly smile.

Mary had used all of her persuasive skills to try to get me to take part in the fund-raiser. "First of all, I don't dance," I had told her. "And second, I'm not the kind of person to put on fishnets and feathers."

"Everyone can dance," she'd retorted, "and fishnets and feathers are flattering to every body type."

In burlesque everything was big: lots of makeup, lots of hair, especially wigs, and costumes that were detailed and elaborate. There were rhinestones and sequins on everything. Burlesque, I discovered, was

intended to make the audience laugh. It poked fun and skewered people and ideas alike.

We had sold tickets at the library in advance and they were available at the door as well. People were also encouraged to sponsor a cat. There were posters all over the bar on the day of the show. Ticket sales had been decent but donations to sponsor cats were slow despite the fact that the audience was clearly having a lot of fun.

Then Zorro came out. The lights went down and the theme song from the 1950s show began to play; then the music changed to a dance mix.

No one knew who the man was, but he put on the performance of a lifetime. He was bare chested under a satiny cape with black leggings and what looked to me to be black Docs. A silky bandanna with eyeholes covered the top of his face and his hair. He also wore a black hat. And he'd gotten a genuine fencing foil from somewhere. What he lacked in skill, he more than made up for with his enthusiasm.

Most of the time it's not acceptable to call out to a performer while they're in the middle of their act or to whistle at them from the back. With burlesque, it's expected. The audience doesn't have to wait to politely clap at the end. They're expected to show how they feel during the performance with comments, whistles, claps and screams of laughter. That audience loved Zorro. People laughed but because they were having fun, not at his expense. As he left the stage, the crowd erupted in even louder applause, hooting and stomping their feet.

Mary came out and promised another dance from the masked man when they reached a certain dollar value in sponsorships. It worked. The masked man danced again at the end of the evening and the event surpassed its goal. Since then Mary had refused to give even a hint as to the man's identity. I knew I had a better chance of finding out the secret ingredient in her cinnamon rolls.

I pulled my attention back to the current conversation.

Roma speared a chunk of cucumber with her fork. "You know the shelter never really has enough money, not for long-term things like work on the building."

Maggie and I both nodded.

"Well, about a month ago, Sandra mentioned in passing that we should do another show—maybe make it an annual thing—to raise money for the shelter."

Sandra Godfrey was a mail carrier. She was *my* mail carrier. She was also a member of the library board, which was how she'd gotten to be friends with Mary.

"I've been thinking about the idea on and off since she mentioned it," Roma continued. "And it strikes me that maybe it's not such a bad idea. What do you two think?"

"I think you should do it," Maggie said, gesturing with her fork. "I'm not sure if The Brick is the best venue, though. You might get a larger audience if you held the show somewhere else."

"I thought about that," Roma said. "There are other possibilities." She looked at me.

"I'm sorry, not the library," I said.

She and Maggie laughed. "No, not the library, but what do you think about the idea?"

"I think it could work. Could you get enough performers?"

Roma grinned. "Well, apparently Maggie is in."

Maggie looked up from her salad. "I am."

"Sandra has really taken to the dancing since Mary got her started. She's done more than one workshop herself and she's been teaching a few women the art of erotic dancing over the past few months. I don't think there would be a problem getting enough participants."

"What, no would-be Zorros?" Maggie asked.

"Maggie's right," I said. "If you could get Zorro again, whoever he was, that would be a big draw."

"I think it was Burtis," Maggie said.

"Did Brady say something to you?" I asked.

She shook her head and her blond curls bounced. "No, but Burtis does love animals and the body type was right."

I held up one hand. "No, no, no. I don't want to think about Burtis in a cape. Now that's going to be in my head all day."

"What about Thorsten?" Roma asked.

Maggie wrinkled her nose. "Too tall."

"Maybe Everett?"

Even I had to laugh at that suggestion. I couldn't imagine Everett dancing in a mask and a cape. "I'm not going there," I said. "I have to work with the man and I don't want to be in a meeting and suddenly find myself wondering if that was him in that cape and

mask. Besides, I don't believe Rebecca would have been able to keep the secret from everyone."

Maggie and Roma continued to speculate as I spotted Eric and got up to talk to him. "I'll be right back," I said.

Eric smiled when he caught sight of me walking toward him. "How are you?" he said. "I haven't seen you since the funeral."

"I'm well, thank you. I wanted to thank you for sending the extra cookies from the service over for the Reading Club kids. They were a big hit."

Eric smiled. "Hey, no problem. There were two plates that didn't even have the tops removed and I didn't want to see them go to waste. And you know Mike was a softie when it came to kids. I figured he'd be happy that they got the leftovers." He looked away for a moment and then his gaze came back to me. "It's funny, you know. He was in here a lot in the weeks before he died. I keep expecting to see him come through the door, telling me he needs the largest cup of coffee I have."

"I know what you mean," I said. "Mike was at the library working on his family tree. I keep expecting to come around a corner and see him at a table with a stack of reference books."

"He told me about that. He'd come in after work every Wednesday for takeout, and if it wasn't busy, we'd talk for a few minutes. I didn't think of it at the time, but it's clear in retrospect that he was going to practice with the rest of the band." He shook his head. "Marcus is going to catch whoever did this, right?"

"He's doing his best," I said. "Hold a good thought."

We talked for a minute or two longer and then I went back to the table. So Mike had been getting take-out every Wednesday night. Eric's words matched what Caroline had told me. Mike had been doing something on Wednesday nights. I had no idea what it was but he'd definitely had a secret. Had it gotten him killed?

14

I went back to the table to find that Maggie and Roma had given up trying to figure out who Zorro was and were now trying to pick a piece of music for Maggie to dance to if there was in fact another show.

"And I think you should give Sandra a call," Roma was saying as I sat down again. "You could have a couple of lessons so you'd feel more comfortable onstage."

After lunch we parted company on the sidewalk in front of the café. Maggie had a shift at the artists' co-op store and Roma was on her way over to take lunch to Eddie. I hugged them both.

"You know, Sandra does take students for one-on-one lessons," Roma teased. "I mean, if you happen to be interested."

"You're as persistent as Owen," I said.

"Since I know the little furball, I'm going to take that as a compliment," she said with a grin.

"I don't dance. I'll hang posters. I'll sell tickets. I'll help make costumes. *I'm not dancing.*"

"Put her down as a maybe," Maggie said. She grabbed Roma by the arm and pulled her down the sidewalk. I could hear them both laughing.

I was meeting Marcus at the bookstore in a little while. Mary had told him about a book on forgotten landmarks in the state that he wanted to get for his father. Since I knew Marcus should be there in less than half an hour, I decided to take a walk along the Riverwalk. It was too nice a day to go back to my office and do paperwork.

I hadn't gone very far when I saw Johnny coming toward me. He smiled when he saw me. "I thought I was the only person who didn't find it too warm to be out walking," he said as we got closer to each other.

"The Riverwalk is one of my favorite places," I said. "I did a lot of walking here when I first came to town. I'd go all the way to Wild Rose Bluff and back sometimes."

"I've been walking down by the marina. Mike and I were working on a song and I keep going back there, hoping inspiration will hit so I can finish it."

"I'm sure it will," I said.

"I'm glad I saw you," Johnny said. "I'm looking for some information on a former music academy in Red Wing. I'm hoping you might know of a reference book that could help."

"You mean the property you tried to buy from Leitha."

"Yes." He looked a little surprised that I knew.

"Kathleen, I'm angry about Mike's death. So angry some days I could punch someone, which wouldn't do me or anyone else any good. But I'm not sorry Leitha is dead and I won't be a hypocrite and pretend I am now that it seems her death wasn't an accident."

"Leitha brought out strong feelings in a lot of people," I said, matching his quiet tone.

"Very diplomatic," he said.

"It doesn't make the words any less true."

"She was managing to estrange her whole family. Her daughter had very little to do with her. In fact she moved to the other side of the country. Lachlan avoided Leitha as much as he could and she and Mike were on the outs when she died but Mike didn't even know what over. It's hard to feel grief-stricken over someone who alienated so many people. Mike on the other hand, that wasn't fair."

I shook my head. "No, it wasn't."

I could hear my mother's voice in my head saying, *Life is not always fair, Katydid. Sometimes bad people win. Sometimes good people lose.*

"She tried to sabotage your project." We started walking back the way I'd just come.

"She went out of her way to try to make sure it didn't happen. I offered her a good price for the property—ten percent over Everett's offer and his was more than fair. But that wasn't the only reason I didn't like her," he said. "I didn't like the way she was always trying to interfere in Lachlan's life. He's a good kid."

It was impossible not to hear the intensity in his voice and see the angry lines pulling at his mouth.

"I know she had some pretty rigid ideas about what he should do with his life."

"In her mind there was a very limited list of careers for Finnamore men and anything related to music was out. I think Lachlan could have said he wanted to play for the Chicago Symphony Orchestra or the Berlin Philharmonic, and that wouldn't have satisfied her. Jonas put up with way too much of her meddling and threats to hold back money for Lachlan's college education. I like the guy, but he's always been too much of a soft touch. I think he should have stood up to her. He always said he wanted to make sure that Leitha wouldn't be able to interfere with Lachlan getting his money for college. I told him more than once that he should have told her to stuff her Finnamore money. Lachlan is really talented. Even if the old crab had somehow managed to hold back the trust money, Lachlan could get a scholarship."

I'd had no idea Johnny had so much animosity for Leitha. In a moment of anger, could he have done something stupid? I didn't want to believe it.

"You know I was at the library for the presentation the day of Leitha's accident," Johnny said. "I guess I shouldn't say 'accident' anymore."

"I remember seeing you." I wanted to ask him what he was getting at, but I'd learned that if I just let people talk, sometimes I found out more than if I asked a lot of questions. It took patience I didn't always have.

"Mary wasn't the only person who had words with Leitha." He exhaled loudly. "I did as well. It was the same old conversation about not letting me buy that

building. She took great pleasure in telling me that she had sold the property to another developer."

"You must have been angry," I said.

He shrugged. "Some days you eat the bear. Some days the bear eats you. And so far the building is still standing, so you never know what might happen."

The intensity that had been in his voice earlier was gone and the lines in his face had smoothed out. Why was he so calm now about something that had left him so angry when Leitha was alive? Leitha meddling in her great-great-nephew's life had gotten more of a re-action from Johnny than that deal that had fallen through.

Johnny suddenly smiled. "We got tattoos, you know," he said, "about a week before Leitha died."

"You and Mike?" I didn't see Harry going to get a tattoo. On the other hand, I'd been learning that Harry had layers I didn't know about.

"Yeah," he said. "Nothing wild. Just the sign lan-guage symbol for rock and roll." He touched his left hip. "I have no idea how but Leitha found out. You can imagine how she reacted. Mike didn't give a sh—Mike didn't care. She blamed me. Mike told her it was his idea. She wouldn't hear it."

"But it was your idea, wasn't it?"

He grinned. "Oh yeah!"

We stopped by a bench at the spot where I'd first crossed the street to reach the Riverwalk trail. I gave Johnny the name of the reference librarian in Red Wing. "They have an excellent collection of old pho-tographs. I think it's the first place you should start to

try to document the building's history. I'll call her on Monday and tell her to expect to hear from you."

"Thanks, Kathleen," Johnny said. "I appreciate this."

"This is probably going to sound a little odd, but do you know what Mike was doing on Wednesday night for the last few months?" I asked.

"As far as I know, working late, having supper and this time of year watching the Twins play on TV." His eyes narrowed. "Why?"

"He'd been leaving the office on time on Wednesday and Thursday but he was only practicing on Thursday."

He shrugged. "So? Maybe he was seeing someone or maybe he just wanted to watch the ball game with a beer."

Something over my shoulder caught Johnny's eye and his face darkened. "You can't honestly think it had anything to do with Mike's death. Mike wasn't the kind of person to have secrets." He raised his voice. "And if the police were working harder instead of manufacturing cases, maybe they'd have his killer by now."

Marcus joined us, putting a hand on my back. "We are working hard on Mike's case," he said, his face devoid of emotion.

"Well, from my perspective, you seem to be spending all your efforts on Leitha Anderson's death, which no one even knew was a crime. You're wasting your time going down that road."

"Leitha deserves justice just as much as Mike does," Marcus said. "And I'm going to keep working so that they both get it."

"Mike Bishop didn't have an enemy in the world." Johnny's voice was getting angrier. "Mike made friends everywhere he went, unlike Leitha. He was ten times the person she was." He stood with his feet apart, hands jammed in his pockets. "There were some break-ins and some vandalism to cars in the area of Mike's house. Are you trying to find those people? Why aren't you checking out people who got out of prison recently? Or known drug addicts?"

I lifted a hand to touch Johnny's arm and then thought better of it. "Marcus knows how to do his job," I said gently.

He didn't look at me. "Then do it," he said, his gaze locked on Marcus's face.

"I am," Marcus said. "I'm not going to insult you by telling you to trust me, but I am looking into all of those things. And more. I give you my word."

Johnny couldn't have known how serious a promise that was, but I did.

Johnny swiped a hand over his face. The anger seemed to drain out of him. "All I care about is bringing Mike's killer to justice."

Marcus nodded. "I get that. I want the same thing. But I have to put just as much effort in for everyone. Otherwise the whole system falls apart."

They stared at each other for a long moment; then Johnny turned to me. "Thank you for the information," he said. He turned and headed across the grass.

"'Justice cannot be for one side alone, but must be for both,'" I said in a quiet voice. I knew Marcus would agree with Eleanor Roosevelt's words.

I watched Johnny cross the street and head into Eric's. I turned back to Marcus. "Did it look as though Mike had walked in on a robbery, just between us?"

He shook his head. "It did look to me as though someone might have gone through his desk. Or maybe he was just someone who had a messy desk. What bothers me is, why was he killed? If Mike had walked in on someone, why not run? None of the break-ins and vandalism out there have been anything other than stupid kids showing off, not someone who would try to rob someone's house and then kill the owner when he surprised them. And Mike was an average middle-aged person, not some big muscular guy or a martial arts expert. Killing him seems like an over-reaction when it would have been so much easier to run."

"Maybe the person couldn't get away," I said.

"If Mike had come in the front door to the house, the thief could have gone out through the kitchen or through the French doors to the deck. Someone who was looking for a few dollars or something to sell would have panicked and gotten the hell out. It doesn't make sense."

That was the problem. Everywhere I turned, nothing about this case made sense.

15

There's something I need to tell you," I said. "I'm not sure if it's important or not."

"Okay. What is it?"

"Wednesday nights, Mike was making sure to leave work on time."

"Because he was going out to Harry's to practice."

I shook my head. "No, he wasn't. They practiced on Thursday. I checked with Harry."

"So he was probably just going home."

We headed for the street.

"I don't think so," I said. "He stopped at Eric's for takeout on those Wednesday nights. I don't think he was going home."

Marcus frowned. "So you think he was doing what? Leading some kind of secret life?"

"No. Maybe." It sounded silly when he said the words out loud.

"I don't think so," Marcus said. "I'm not saying

your instincts aren't good, but so far from what I've learned, Mike Bishop's life was an open book."

"I hope you're right," I said.

We walked over to the bookstore and got the book for Elliot and then headed to Marcus's house. The plan was to do some yard work and figure out a permanent spot for the bench he'd bought.

I changed my clothes and started weeding the vegetable garden. Micah perched on one corner of the raised bed, watching me, while Marcus tried to decide on the best location for the bench.

"I thought you were going to paint it first," I said.

"I am," he said as he stood in the middle of the yard, looking around. "I just want to know where it's going to go when I'm finished."

I didn't follow the logic. "Okay." I looked at Micah, who seemed to shrug.

"What do you think?"

"On the deck," I said.

Micah meowed her agreement.

Marcus looked around the yard again. "I think by the rosebushes," he said, muscling the bench over the grass into place.

"Bees," I said.

He thought for a moment, then moved the bench to the other side of the bed I was working in. Micah and I exchanged another look, which this time he saw.

"What?"

I hesitated.

"You don't think this is a good spot? Why?"

"It's not a big deal. It's just that the ground is kind of uneven right there."

He pushed at one end of the seat. "There. I've found a level spot."

"Good," I said without looking up. I knew there were no level spots on that part of the lawn.

Marcus dropped onto the bench. It immediately canted sideways, almost knocking him to the ground. Micah walked around the edge of the vegetable bed, peered at Marcus and gave a concerned meow.

"I'm fine," he muttered.

"Why don't you try it on the deck?" I suggested.

He moved the bench under the maple tree instead and stood back with a look of satisfaction on his face.

Micah looked skyward, then glanced at me and meowed once more.

Marcus shook his head. "What's wrong with right here? There's shade. There are no bees. The ground is level. It's perfect."

Before I could answer, a bird flew overhead and made a direct hit on the center of the bench seat.

Micah ducked her head. I bit my lip to keep from laughing and watched Marcus from the corner of my eye.

He stood silently for a long moment. Finally, he said, "You know, I think the bench would look great on the deck."

I nodded. "Good idea."

* * *

Later, once the weeding was done and the grass had been clipped around the flower beds, we sat on the deck steps with glasses of lemonade and lots of ice. Marcus seemed lost in thought.

"You weren't wrong to take a second look at Leitha's death," I said, "no matter what Johnny says, no matter what anyone says."

He put his free hand on my knee and gave it a squeeze. "Thanks. I know, but it has complicated the investigation into Mike Bishop's death."

"I'm not second-guessing you, but is there any chance his death is connected somehow to those car break-ins?"

He shook his head. "It's not." He ran a hand through his hair. "They're just kids—you know that, teenagers—and more important, they have alibis for the night Mike was killed. I'm glad that Mariah Taylor isn't hanging around with that bunch, though."

"She's a bright kid," I said, reaching for my glass, which was two steps below me between my feet.

"There are three kids involved as far as I can tell—a girl and two boys—and I feel confident that the girl is the ring leader. She's smart and articulate and she's got a bit of a chip on her shoulder. She's being raised by a single dad, and from what I could see, money is tight. We have them on the whipped cream incident and a couple of other car break-ins, but that's as far as it goes. They didn't have anything to do with Mike's death."

"Why didn't you tell that to Johnny? He thinks you're not working on the case."

He leaned sideways, kissed my neck and straightened up again. "Because it just happened and the lawyers and the prosecuting attorney are still talking, hopefully working out some kind of a deal that involves restitution and community service. Cleaning garbage out of ditches sounds pretty good this time of year. And I think right now nothing I could say is going to make a difference to Johnny."

"It would be such an easy solution if you found out that Mike had been killed just by some random thief."

"I don't think this case is going to be that easy," he said.

I leaned my head against his shoulder. Neither did I.

Marcus kissed the top of my head. "Could you make a list of everyone you remember being at the library for Mary's talk? I should have asked for that sooner."

"I can do that, but there's no way I'll remember everyone."

"I know," he said. "But it's a place to start."

We sat there for a little while longer, talking about the backyard and whether or not it needed another raised bed. Finally Marcus stretched and got to his feet. "Do you want to try those veggie burgers Maggie recommended?"

I looked at Micah, who wrinkled her nose. "No," I said.

"Let me rephrase." He gave me an over-the-top smile that made me think of SpongeBob SquarePants for some reason. "Hey! Let's try those veggie burgers Maggie recommended!"

"Merow!" Micah said. Rephrasing had not changed her opinion.

I laughed. "I'm willing to try them, but if they taste terrible, you have to promise we can order pizza."

"Deal," he said. "And Maggie said they're good."

I stood up and kissed the side of his mouth. "Maggie thinks herbal tea is better than coffee. I love her, but she's not a reliable source of information on this kind of thing."

The veggie burgers were actually good. Even Micah tried a tiny bite and seemed to like them. After supper I pulled up some paint swatches on my phone and we tried to decide what color to paint the bench with Micah weighing in with her opinion from time to time. Later on, we drove out to The Brick to listen to a new band. We didn't talk about Mike or Leitha and I tried not to think about them, either.

Marcus and I went out to feed the cats at Wisteria Hill the next morning.

"Do you know if Leitha shopped online?" I asked as we drove up the hill. I was thinking out loud as much as I was talking to him.

He shot me a quick glance. "Where did that come from?"

"I'm just trying to work out a couple of things. Did she shop online?"

He kept his eyes on the road but gave his head a little shake. "Lots of people in their nineties have embraced technology, but Leitha Anderson was not one of them. No computer. No tablet. No smartphone. What is it exactly that you're trying to work out?"

"How she ended up with potassium chloride in her system. What if she took too much by mistake?" I held up a hand before he could say anything. "Just hear me out. Leitha was stubborn and opinionated. Maybe she thought it would benefit her somehow. Potassium does help the heart and the kidneys work properly, among other things, although as far as I know, most people get enough from what they eat."

"I don't disagree with your reasoning," Marcus said. "But we're still left with the same question. How did she get it? She didn't order anything online. She didn't buy it in town. There was no potassium chloride in her house. No charges for it on her credit card. And before you suggest she bought it in Minneapolis, when she went there, Jonas Quinn always drove her. She'd have had no opportunity to buy anything he wouldn't have seen."

"Maybe she stole it," I said.

"You mean, from the hospital?"

I nodded.

He shook his head. "I had the same thought. Again, no opportunity."

I sighed softly.

"Kathleen, your own timeline puts Leitha at the library for close to two hours. The medical examiner says the potassium chloride had to have been ingested

there. There's not a lot of wiggle room in that. All she had in her stomach was the partly digested cookie and tea with milk and sugar."

"Did she take any pills?" I knew I was reaching.

"She took a multivitamin every day. It was a large yellow pill, not a capsule, which could have been tampered with a lot more easily. I don't see how it could have been the source of the potassium chloride."

I rubbed the back of my head with one hand. This whole thing gave me a headache. "What about blood pressure medication or something to manage her blood sugar or thyroid?"

Marcus shook his head. "There was nothing like that. The woman was as healthy as a horse. That's why she was part of that study."

"I remember that when the accident happened you didn't find any evidence that Leitha's car had been tampered with," I said. "That hasn't changed?"

He turned his head to look at me for a moment. "No, it hasn't. Leitha's death was not an accident, Kathleen. I wish it was. But it wasn't. Why are you having such a hard time with that?"

There was a knot in my stomach. "Because if someone deliberately killed Leitha, then maybe that same person also killed Mike. Maybe . . . maybe it wasn't some random burglar who panicked." I straightened up, linked my fingers together and rested my hands on the top of my head. "I know this is more emotion than logic talking. It's just how I feel right now."

"The car was checked from top to bottom. There

were no mechanical issues. In fact, Lachlan had taken
the car in for service the day before Leitha died."

"Harry's looking for answers. So is Johnny. So is
pretty much the entire town."

"And you're afraid they're not going to like those
answers."

I sighed, dropped my arms and adjusted my seat
belt. "I'm afraid they're not going to get any answers,"
I said.

"I'm not going to give up," Marcus said. "Are you?"

I studied his profile. I knew what that determined
jut of his chin meant. I shook my head. "No."

"Then everyone will get their answers eventually."

The cats all looked healthy and they seemed to still be
happy in the new home Eddie had built for them. The
girls' hockey team had a training session and Marcus
needed to stop in at the station, so I drove home right
before lunch.

Hercules was waiting in the porch. I brought him
up-to-date on what I'd learned from Marcus while I
made coffee. Since I hadn't had any at lunch, I decided
it was okay to have a cup of coffee now. I was very
good at rationalizing my coffee drinking.

I sat at the kitchen table with my cup, a banana
muffin and two sliced tomatoes. Hercules climbed
onto my lap and helped me make the list that Marcus
had asked me for. When I couldn't come up with any
more names, I e-mailed it to him, but I didn't shut
down my laptop.

"What do we know about Leitha's daughter, Eloise?" I asked the cat.

He blinked his green eyes and gave me a blank look.

"Exactly," I said. "Really, we know nothing."

I didn't actually believe Eloise had snuck back into town twice, once to kill her mother and a second time to get rid of her cousin, but maybe there was something in her life or her background that might help me. I was grasping at straws, but right now I didn't really have anything else to hold on to.

As usual, Hercules was happy to help me see what we could find online, making occasional comments about what was on the screen and swiping at the touch pad when he wanted to check out something else.

Eloise Finnamore Anderson-Hill was a fascinating person, I learned, very different from her mother. She had two daughters adopted from Korea, Nari and Min, and ran a children's clothing company that focused on sustainable practices and provided shoes and clothing to kids in need. And she had established a scholarship in her father's name—Markham Anderson. There was only one mention of the Finnamore name in a newspaper article about the scholarship.

"I know I can't change the world," Eloise had said in an interview. "But I can work on making my small corner of it better."

Hercules and I looked at Eloise's social media and her company's website. Most people called her Ellie, I learned. She was divorced. She was a vegan. She liked to hike and camp.

"How could Leitha not have been wildly proud of her daughter?" I said to Hercules. I thought about my own mother. She was my, Sarah's and Ethan's biggest cheerleader.

He blinked his green eyes at me again. It didn't make any sense to him, either.

An errant paw took me to a photo of Eloise at her mother's funeral, which had been private. She wore a navy coat over a gray dress. Mike's hand was on her shoulder, and even at a distance, she looked profoundly sad. Other than that one time, I couldn't recall ever seeing the woman in town.

There was a knock at the door.

Hercules looked expectantly at me. "Are you going to get that or should I?" I asked.

His tail flicked through the air and he made a huffy sound, his way of telling me I wasn't as funny as I thought I was.

Keith King was standing at my back door. He was about average height, strong and wiry with dark hair and dark eyes behind a pair of black stainless steel–framed glasses.

"Hi, Keith," I said. I was surprised to see him.

He smiled. "Hi, Kathleen. I'm sorry to bother you at home, but I'm going out of town for a couple of days and I didn't just want to leave this." He was holding a green file folder and he offered it to me.

"What is this?" I asked. Keith was on the library board. Was there a meeting I'd forgotten about?

"I found some papers in a book that I borrowed from the library. They look like they belong to someone

tracing their family tree. You know I'm doing some of that myself. I didn't get a chance to look at the book before now, so that's why I didn't find them sooner."

"Thanks for dropping them off," I said. "Maybe I can figure out who they belong to."

"That's what I was hoping," Keith said. "There are several pages of notes in there, which means a lot of research someone will have to do again." He smiled. "We're going to see Taylor."

Keith's daughter had a summer job in St. Paul.

"Tell her we miss her at tai chi."

"I will," he said. "She's going to be home for a few days at the end of the month. I know she'll want to see you."

"We all want to see her, too."

I thanked Keith again and he left.

I took the file of papers into the kitchen. Hercules was sitting on my chair, washing his face. I pushed the laptop aside and laid the folder on the table. Hercules abandoned his beauty routine and stood up on his back legs, one white-tipped paw on the edge of the table, craning his neck for a look.

I picked up the top sheet of paper and right away I knew who had made the notes. I recognized Mike's cramped, angular handwriting. I'd seen it many times. I flipped through the pages. Some were just copies of documents with notes in the margins. Others were paragraphs of information and one page was covered with what looked like several Punnett squares. It looked as though Mike had been trying to figure out someone's eye color. Maybe he'd been trying to

eliminate someone from the family tree. I remembered him telling me that back in the 1800s, the Finnamores had been a randy lot.

"I should get these to Jonas," I said to Hercules.

He yawned and jumped down to the floor. It seemed the eye color of errant Finnamores didn't interest him.

I looked up Jonas's address. There was a flea market close to where he lived that would be wrapping up in about an hour. I was searching for some old maps for a display I had planned at the library, but so far I hadn't found anything that would work. I could swing by the flea market and then drop Mike's notes off to Jonas if he was around.

I called Jonas, crossing my fingers that he was home. He was. I explained about Keith finding the papers and bringing them to me. "I'm heading to the flea market. I can drop them off afterward. I won't be that long."

"I appreciate that," Jonas said. "Do you know how to find me?"

"I do," I said.

"Then I'll see you soon."

I grabbed my bag and the folder and stepped into my canvas shoes. "I'm leaving," I called.

There was silence and then an answering meow from upstairs. I locked the back door, walked around the house to the truck and climbed inside, setting Mike's notes on the seat beside me. Out of nowhere Owen appeared on the hood of the truck. "Merow," he said, cocking his head to one side.

I knew what he wanted. Owen loved going out in the truck, but there was no way taking him with me was a good idea. I knew what would happen. Owen would do his disappearing act and then go on a self-directed tour of Jonas's house as I tried to nonchalantly swing my arms around and make contact with him while at the same time making casual conversation with Jonas.

I shook my head. "Not this time."

He got a sulky look on his face and disappeared.

I jumped out of the truck, leaving the driver's door open, felt around on the hood and somehow managed to grab him. He reappeared, looking even more disgruntled than he had before.

"Not this time," I repeated.

I set him on the path. He refused to look at me, starting around the house in a snit. He flicked his tail in my direction just as he turned the corner and then once again he disappeared.

I got back in the truck, wondering what it was like to have normal cats.

The flea market was winding down, so there weren't many people around. I didn't unearth any maps, but I did come across a poster of a large tree covered with dollar bills that would be good for Money Week in the fall.

I found Jonas's house without any difficulty. It was a beautiful Victorian, larger than I had expected, painted a creamy white with dark gray accents. It was set back from the road and the grounds looked like a park with a well-trimmed lawn, beautiful flower beds

and what might have been an English-style cottage garden at the back.

Lachlan was sitting on the front steps, bent over his phone, as I pulled up. He was dressed all in black: jeans, T-shirt, high-tops. When I got out of the truck, he got to his feet and came over to me.

"Could I talk to you for a minute first before you go inside?" he asked.

"Of course," I said.

"Uncle Mike said you were really good at research and I was wondering if you could teach me how to find some information about . . . something?" He shifted awkwardly from one foot to the other.

I pushed my sunglasses up onto the top of my head. "I could try. Can you give me an idea of what the something is?"

He looked over his shoulder at the house. Whatever it was, he didn't want Jonas to know. "There's this building in Red Wing that my family owns. My Aunt Leitha was selling it to someone but I want to cancel the deal and sell it to someone else instead. She was wrong and I need to correct her mistake."

"You mean, the building that may have been the first music school in the state?" I said. "You want to sell it to Johnny?"

He looked surprised but he nodded. "He told me to just let it be, but I can't do that. If I can find proof that it was the first music school, then maybe I can stop it from being turned into a parking lot."

"You're welcome to come to the library anytime and any of us would be happy to help you, but I

happen to know there are other people researching that same building, so you might want to wait a bit."

"It's Johnny, isn't it?" he said.

"I'm just going to go with 'no comment' for now," I said.

He nodded. "Okay, I can wait for a while but not forever. I can't let that building be torn down."

"How about if I happen to come across anything that might help you, I put it aside and let you know?"

He smiled. "Thank you."

Jonas came around the side of the house then. "Kathleen, hello. You found us without any difficulty?" he said.

"I did. I've driven by several times but I never realized this beautiful house was here."

"This is the Quinn family homestead. Colin—Lachlan's dad—and I grew up here. So did our father."

Lachlan pointed to a large elm tree on the other side of the driveway. "Don't get him started on all the members of the Quinn family who have fallen out of that tree," he said. "I think it's some kind of weird family tradition by now." He darted a look at Jonas and I saw the same mischievous gleam in his eye that I'd seen more than once in Mike's.

"Don't you have a couple of books left on your summer reading list that you should be pretending to read?" Jonas asked.

"Yeah, probably," Lachlan said. He looked at me. "I might come in some time and try to finish the family tree Uncle Mike was working on."

"Anytime," I said. "You might get lucky and Mary might have cookies."

He headed for the house. As he passed his uncle, Jonas put a hand on the boy's shoulder for a brief moment.

I held out the folder of papers. Jonas took them but didn't bother looking inside. "Thank you," he said. He raised an eyebrow. "Do you have time for a cup of coffee?"

"I'd like that," I said.

We walked around the side of the house, and the backyard stopped me in my tracks. "Oh, this is beautiful," I said.

The thick green lawn was bordered by curving flower beds that were bursting with color. I recognized wild roses, black-eyed Susans and lilies with colors running the gamut from pale yellow to a purple so dark, it was almost black. There were daisies, astilbes and other plants I didn't know the names of.

Jonas smiled. "Thank you. My mother, Mary-Margaret, designed the garden. When Ainsley, Lachlan's mother, was alive, they lived in this house and she took care of it. Since then I've mostly been just trying to keep all the plants alive. Thankfully, I've had a lot of help from Harry Taylor."

He gestured to a small wrought iron table sitting on a flagstone patio at the back of the house. "Please have a seat." There were three wicker chairs spaced around the table with fat flowered seat cushions, and on top sat a round wooden tray with an insulated

carafe, a heavy white stoneware mug, spoons, sugar and cream. Another mug sat in front of one of the chairs.

Jonas set the file of papers on the seat of the empty chair and then poured a cup of coffee for me. I added cream and sugar to mine and took a sip.

"This is good," I said. The coffee was strong and rich, just the way I liked it.

He took a sip from his own cup and smiled. "I confess I'd choose a cup of coffee over tea or pretty much anything else. I generally only have tea if it's late in the day. I had a feeling we might be kindred souls on that front."

I smiled back at him. "Guilty," I said.

"I know I'm going to sound like an overprotective parental figure, but Lachlan asked you to help him try to document the history of that building in Red Wing that Leitha was in the process of selling, didn't he?"

I hesitated. "Yes," I finally said. "Is that a problem?"

He shook his head. "Not for me. It's something for him to focus on and right now I think it's good for him."

"I'll do a little digging on Monday and see what I can find."

"I appreciate that," Jonas said. "He's a tough kid, but he's had more loss than most adults ever have to face. We're lucky to have people like Johnny and Harry around us. They've become family."

"'Families are like pieces of art,'" I said. "'You can make them from almost anything.' Mitch Albom."

Jonas nodded. "Smart man."

Out of the corner of my eye, I saw movement. I

glanced sideways as the file folder on the chair between us opened. There was no breeze but I was pretty
sure there *was* a small gray tabby cat sitting on the
chair. Owen had gotten in the truck after all. Somehow
he had darted back and jumped inside, probably because I'd left the driver's door open when I'd gotten out
to lift him off the hood. He was faster than I'd realized
and for once he hadn't given himself away on the drive
out or at the flea market. The little furball was getting
sneakier. Had he gotten out of the truck at the flea market? I didn't want to think about that.

What I needed to do was distract Jonas so he didn't
see the piece of paper that was now seemingly levitat-
ing above the flowered seat all by itself.

I set my mug on the table. "Would you mind if I
took a closer look at the flower beds?" I asked.

"Of course not," Jonas said. He set his cup next to
mine and got to his feet. I stood up as well and we
walked over to the closest bed.

Looking at the paint box of colors, I wished I had
more of a green thumb. I pointed at the plant closest
to me. "I would say that's a black-eyed Susan with
purple petals but I'm thinking I'd be wrong."

He smiled. "Those are *Echinacea purpurea*, purple
coneflowers. They attract bees and butterflies and
they're easy to grow."

I smiled. "My kind of plant." Behind us the piece of
paper was moving, seemingly of its own volition,
across the grass. I fervently hoped it and Owen were
headed in the direction of my truck.

Jonas and I spent about ten minutes walking

around, looking at the various plants. "You're welcome to come out again for another look anytime you'd like," he said. "And if you describe pretty much any of these plants to Harry, he'll know what they are."

"Thank you for the tour of the garden," I said as we walked back to the truck. I had no idea where Owen was or what he'd done with that piece of paper. "When I get to the library on Monday, I'm going to be looking for some gardening books."

"Thank you for bringing out those papers," Jonas said. "And thanks for offering to help Lachlan."

I opened the driver's door, hoping Owen was close by and would hop in. I felt something move across my foot and looked down to see my shoelace was untied. I set my bag by my feet and bent down to fasten it and just under the edge of the truck spotted the piece of paper Owen had swiped.

I didn't want to leave it there covered in cat drool and I didn't want Jonas to see me pick it up. Luckily he was checking out the truck and I managed to pick up my bag and the paper and set them on the front seat in one more or less smooth motion.

"Kathleen, where did you get this truck?" he asked. There was something in his expression I couldn't quite read, an almost wistfulness.

"Harrison Taylor gave it to me. It's old, but it'll push through a fair amount of snow and pretty much anything else that gets in its way."

"Colin, my brother, had one just like it. It brings back a lot of good memories." He laid his hand on the front

fender for a moment and I thought how Lachlan wasn't the only one who had lost way more than was fair.

I drove away with my fingers crossed that I had a furry—and invisible—stowaway. Once I was down the road beyond the Quinn driveway, I pulled over to the side of the road.

"Show yourself, Owen," I said.

Nothing.

"Right now. I'm not kidding."

Still nothing.

Was I wrong? Was he still out prowling around Jonas's yard? How on earth would I explain that I had left my cat behind?

And then I felt the tiniest brush of something against my right arm. It felt like a piece of dandelion fluff grazing my skin. Or a cat's tail. I stretched both arms over my head and then shifted sideways and brought my right hand down onto the seat. I had timed it perfectly. I had a handful of invisible cat.

Owen winked into sight and there was something cocky about the look he gave me.

"You're in so much trouble," I said, glaring at him. "Jonas almost saw you and you stole one of those pieces of paper."

He peered at the seat, spotted the piece of paper in question and set one paw on it, looking at me as though he was expecting some kind of praise. As usual, he wasn't sorry. I reached over and picked the paper up, wondering what it was that had attracted the cat's attention.

The paper was half of a page from a lined yellow notepad. I'd seen Mike making notes on a similar pad at the library and it was his writing filling the lines.

There were two Punnett squares drawn on the page. Like the notes I'd glanced at earlier, it seemed as though Mike had been trying to work out eye-color probabilities. His handwriting was hard to read. "Leitha" with a question mark was written just above the tear line. What had Mike been trying to figure out and why was Leitha's name written on the page? I had no idea.

Once again, none of this made sense.

16

Owen sat next to me all the way home, eyes fixed on the road.

"You're in trouble," I said.

"Mrr," he said.

We both knew I was wasting my breath. First of all, how did you punish a cat with klepto tendencies and the ability to disappear whenever he felt like it? It's not as though I could put him in a time-out or take away his cell phone. I couldn't even take away his supply of catnip chickens because they were stashed all over the house in hiding places I hadn't discovered yet.

I glanced over at him again. He definitely looked cocky.

I spent a good chunk of the evening trying to figure out the Punnett squares that Mike had drawn. It had been a long time since I'd had a biology class, but I remembered more than I'd expected about genetics

and I found a couple of texts in the library's online catalogue.

"'A Punnett square is used to predict which traits offspring will have based on the traits of the parent,'" I read to Owen. "'It's a visual representation of the principle—put forth by Gregor Mendel by the way—that certain traits are dominant over others. It's not infallible because there can be other factors at work, but the results are a lot better than just making a wild guess.'"

Working out eye color wasn't as simple as we'd once thought it was. At one time geneticists had believed it was controlled by a single gene, which meant, for instance, that blue-eyed parents could never have a brown-eyed child.

"Except they can," I told the cat. "It's rare, but it does happen. The idea of just one gene controlling eye color was too simplistic." I remembered my professor explaining that eye color is an example of a polygenic trait. In other words, it's controlled by several different genes.

Owen wasn't the slightest bit interested in genetics. "Did you know that cats with white in their fur are believed to have a mutant gene?" I asked him as he washed his face.

Hercules had just walked into the kitchen and Owen immediately turned to look at him with an inquiring murp.

"Yes, like your brother. And you."

Hercules gave me a blank look as though he was wondering what he'd just missed. Or not.

Owen disappeared and a moment later the basement door opened a little wider.

I turned back to the computer. Maybe if I could find out what color Leitha's eyes were, I could sort out what Mike had been doing.

All of a sudden I had a lap of cat.

"Hello," I said to Hercules. "Would you like to help?"

"Mrr," he said, shifting around on my legs. Finally he was settled, eyes fixed on the screen, one paw next to the touch pad. I sometimes got the weird feeling that when I wasn't home Hercules was on the computer watching Netflix. He pretty much had the skills for it.

It took some digging, but I finally managed to find two photos of Leitha that were close enough for me to see her eyes.

"They were green," I said. I was remembering correctly.

Hercules murped his agreement. It took more poking around but I managed to learn that Leitha's mother had blue eyes. I couldn't find any photos or any references to the color of John Finnamore Senior's eyes.

I looked at the tables Mike had drawn. There were a couple of reference sources I could check at the library in the morning.

I shut off the laptop. What had he been trying to work out? And did it even have any connection to his and Leitha's deaths? Maybe this was just a waste of time. I slumped in my chair and stared up at the ceiling. There weren't any answers up there, either.

* * *

It was busy at the library in the morning. A couple of
teachers came in to look around our reference section
and get a jump on planning for fall assignments. Two
boxes of new books were delivered, and Patricia
Queen sent me a detailed plan for the proposed quilt-
ing workshops. I pulled one genetics reference, hoping I'd have a chance to look at it during my lunch
break. Then I moved over to the local-history section.
I was hoping to find an article about some event that
John Finnamore Senior had attended. Many of them
were written with a lot of extraneous detail, like the
style of shoe a man had been wearing, the cut of his
suit or the color of his eyes.

"Looking for something?" Susan asked as she came
around the shelving unit. I was twisted sideways,
reading the call numbers on the spines of the books.

I straightened up. My left shoulder had kinked and
I rubbed it with my other hand. "We have a book
about the so-called upper echelon of Mayville Heights'
society in the late 1800s. I can't find it."

"I think I saw it on one of the carts," she said. Today
there was one thin knitting needle and one black lac-
quered chopstick stuck in her hair. "Do you want me
to set it aside for you?"

"Please," I said.

"Are you finishing Mike's research for his family?"

"Just trying to tie up a couple of loose ends." That
was true as far as it went.

"It's quiet right now," Susan said, pushing a collection of bracelets up her arm. "I could look something up if that would help."

I hesitated. "All right. I'm looking for some reference to John Finnamore Senior's eye color. I remember Mike saying he usually went by Jack."

I waited for her to ask me why I wanted that information. She just smiled and said, "No problem. I'll let you know if I find anything."

"And will you keep an eye out for any notes Mike might have left behind. Keith King found some papers that belonged to Mike in a book Keith had borrowed. I just want to make sure we haven't missed anything else."

"Will do," Susan said.

Roma came by midmorning with four large zucchini. She handed them to me. "This is partly a thank-you for feeding the cats and partly a 'please take these' because I have so many."

"You're welcome," I said. "I'm thinking chocolate zucchini bread sounds good."

She smiled. "I'm thinking I need to bring you more zucchini."

"Rebecca would probably take some. She makes a wonderful vegetarian lasagna."

"I'll call her," Roma said. "Or maybe I'll just leave a bag on the front step, ring the doorbell and run."

I laughed. "It can't be that bad."

"Oh, but it is. They're taking over my garden. I get

up in the morning and I swear there are twice as many of the things as there were the night before." She looked around. "Is Mary here?" she asked.

"She is," I said. "She's putting out new magazines. Do you have zucchini for her as well?"

Roma smoothed a hand over her dark hair, tucking it behind one ear. "No. I need to talk to her. After I had lunch with you and Maggie, I called Sandra to talk more about doing another burlesque show. It looks like the shelter is going to need a new heating system."

I made a face. "That's not good."

"The reality is that they need a new building, which means a major fund-raising push. I asked Sandra if she would talk to whoever Zorro was and see if he'd do another show as a way of launching a fund-raiser for a new home for the shelter. She refused."

"Did she say why?" I asked. Working with Sandra on the library board, I'd found her to be a very reasonable, easy-to-get-along-with person.

Roma shook her head. "That's the thing. All she said was no and that Zorro's performance was a one-time thing. There's no point in putting on the show without him, not if we want to generate a lot of attention for the fund-raising campaign, but Sandra won't budge. I want to try to appeal to the person myself if Mary will tell me who he is. Sandra wouldn't. It's not just the heating system. When they were working on the roof, they uncovered some structural problems with the building. The shelter can probably get through this winter but beyond that they need a new home. As

it is they're going to have to close one room, which means they're going to have to turn animals away."

"C'mon," I said. "I'll walk you over to her."

Mary listened to what Roma had to say but she wouldn't budge.

"I'm sorry," she said. "I'll help you in any way I can, but as far as Zorro is concerned, that was something that isn't going to be repeated."

"If I could just talk to him," Roma said.

Mary just shook her head. "I'm sorry."

I walked Roma back to the front entrance. "I really thought she'd tell me who he is," she said. "I don't understand why they're both being so secretive."

"I can't promise anything," I said, "but give me some time. I'll talk to Mary again."

Roma hugged me. "Thanks, Kath," she said.

I stood outside on the steps, trying to figure out who had played Zorro and why, after dancing onstage bare chested in a cape and tights, he did not want anyone to know who he was. I tried to think of who would bring out such unequivocal loyalty from both Sandra and Mary. The two most likely candidates were Everett and Burtis, and from what I'd seen of Zorro's performance, it wasn't either of them.

When I went back inside, Susan waved me over to the desk. "Blue," she said with a smile.

"I thought we settled on gray," I said. It had taken a month for us to come to a consensus on a paint color for the walls of the staff room, and now she was changing her vote?

She frowned at me for a moment and then the frown cleared. "I'm not talking about the staff room. I'm talking about John Finnamore. His eyes were blue. Light blue by all accounts. I read three of them."

"Thank you," I said.

She smiled again. "You're welcome. I hope it helps."

I nodded. "So do I."

I went up to my office. There was a slim chance that Leitha's blue-eyed parents could have had a green-eyed child. So what had Mike been trying to work out? Once again it seemed I was left with nothing but a handful of straw.

When I went back downstairs about an hour later, I spotted Mary shelving in the children's department. I walked over to her.

"I know what you want and you're wasting your time," she said without preamble as she straightened a row of picture books. "If it were possible to help Roma, believe me, I would, but it's not."

"Could you at least ask Zorro if he'd talk to Roma?" I said.

She looked at me. "Do you think I like the idea of cats being put down because there's no shelter for them to go to?"

"I know you don't," I said.

Mary might have been able to take someone down with just one well-placed kick, but she was very much a mushball inside.

"Then take me at my word when I tell you that there is no way Zorro will ride again and you just need to accept it."

* * *

Lachlan showed up around two o'clock. He was dressed all in black again. "If it's okay, I thought maybe I would see what I can find about the old music school in Red Wing after all. I mean, I wasn't doing anything else."

"Of course it's okay," I said. "I'm thinking the best place to start would be with the newspaper. The only problem is, the older issues haven't been digitized, so you'll have to use the microfilm reader."

"Okay," he said with a shrug.

I got him set up at the machine and showed him how to scroll through the pages. "Try looking for references to the school in articles and photographs but keep an eye out for any ads for classes or recitals."

He nodded. "I can do that."

"If you have any problems, I'm around and Susan is at the desk."

I left him to it, thinking how much he reminded me of Mike, who had also spent some time going through back issues of newspapers. It wasn't that they looked alike, but Lachlan seemed to be capable of the same level of concentration and the ability to tune out everything else that Mike had had. Right now Lachlan was leaning forward, watching the screen, just the way Mike had, his eyebrows drawn together in a frown in exactly the same fashion.

I was in the staff room about half an hour later getting a cup of coffee before I started to work on the staff schedule when Harry appeared in the doorway.

"Hi," he said. "Susan said you were up here."

"I'm getting fortified for some paperwork," I said, holding up the pot. "Would you like a cup?"

He shook his head. "No, thanks. I just wanted to let you know that I talked to Ritchie and he wasn't spending Wednesday nights with Mike."

"Thanks," I said. "It was a bit of a long shot."

"Do you really think it's important?" Harry asked. "Maybe Mike was seeing someone and just wanted to keep it to himself."

I leaned back against the counter and folded my hands around my cup. "You're probably right."

"I have faith in you, Kathleen," Harry said. "I know you can figure out what happened." He gestured toward the back of the building. "I'll be out at the gazebo if you need me."

Instead of going back to my office, I stayed where I was, leaning against the counter. Harry had faith in me but I wasn't so sure that I had faith in myself.

Mike had probably just been seeing someone that he wasn't ready to introduce to his family and friends. And he'd likely been killed by some random prowler. It happened, even in a place as small and safe as Mayville Heights. My problem was the fact that I couldn't shake the feeling that that *wasn't* what had happened. I didn't know why I felt that way. I just had some feeling, some instinct that there was more to Mike Bishop's death than it seemed on the surface. I thought about what Harrison had said to me, "Just rely on your instincts and everything will be just fine."

I was probably tilting at windmills à la Don Quixote but I wasn't going to give up on figuring out where Mike had been on Wednesday nights for the past couple of months.

I did some work on the schedule and then went downstairs to give Susan a break at the front desk.

"It's been quiet so far," she said. "Did Harry find you?"

"He did," I said. "Thanks for sending him up."

"Lachlan Quinn is still on the microfilm reader and the monitor on the second computer is acting up again. I did your 'whack it on the side' thing and it seems to be okay for now."

"The board meeting's this week. After that, I should be able to order the new computers." I held up my crossed fingers.

"I can't wait," Susan said. "I may make a bonfire out of the old ones and dance naked around it in the moonlight."

"I'm pretty sure you can't burn computers," I said. "They release toxic chemicals into the air."

"Okay, so naked dancing in the moonlight it is." She grinned.

"Or we could just have cake."

She thought about it for a moment. "Yeah, or we could just have cake." She stretched and yawned. "Please tell me there's coffee."

I smiled. "I made a new pot."

Susan smiled back at me. "I knew there was a reason I like you."

There were three books sitting on the counter. She put a hand on top of them and her smile faded. "Mike requested those," she said.

It wasn't the first time books had come in for someone who had died. That little bit of unfinished business always left me feeling sad, even if I hadn't known the person beyond what they had liked to read.

The top book on the stack was about the *Mayflower*, the second one was about life in England in the early 1600s and the last was *The Genetics of Eye Color*.

"I'll send them back," I said. "Go take your break."

She headed for the stairs and I picked up the books. I had suggested the one about the *Mayflower* and another source had mentioned the book about life in seventeenth-century England. The genetics text had to have something to do with those Punnett squares.

Holding the book in my hands, I had a crazy thought that maybe Mike had gotten the idea that Leitha wasn't a Finnamore because of something he had learned during his research. I thought about the picture he had shown me of Leitha with her parents. Leitha didn't look a lot like them but that might have been her stern appearance in the photograph. Was it possible? And if bizarrely it was true, then did that have anything to do with either of their deaths?

17

I spent the rest of the afternoon with questions about what Mike had been trying to work out turning over in my head. If she'd been faced with proof that she wasn't a Finnamore, what would Leitha have done? It had been such a huge part of her identity. If—and that was a very big if—Mike had found some reason to suspect she hadn't been part of the Finnamore legacy, I didn't see her just accepting that. She would have needed more solid proof than just his suspicions. And the color of her eyes proved nothing with respect to whether or not she was biologically part of that family.

Mike was smart enough not to just rely on eye color to prove something like that. Maybe I needed to look at another Finnamore family trait that was more genetically straightforward. I was probably tilting at windmills again. I rubbed both temples. I had a headache again.

Lachlan had found some information about the music school in the newspaper. "I'm on the right track,"

he said to me. "I know it. Thanks for suggesting the newspaper and showing me how to look at it. I'll be back to see what else I can find."

I was happy to see him smile.

"Do you know where Levi is?" I said to Susan. "I need some help carrying in some boxes."

"He's scraping gum off the bottom of one of the tables in the children's section," she said. "What is it with people and gum in the library? Don't they know what garbage cans are for?"

"I don't know," I said.

Gum stuck all sorts of odd places in the building was a chronic problem for us.

"Would it be okay if I made some signs?" Susan asked. "Just something that says, 'Please put your gum in the garbage can,' or something like that?"

"It's fine with me." I wasn't sure signs would make a difference but it wouldn't hurt to try.

Levi was on his hands and knees under one of the big round tables in the children's department, scraping at the underside with the plastic scraper. His mind was clearly somewhere else because, when I called his name, he started and banged his head on the table.

"I'm sorry," I said as he backed out from underneath. "I didn't mean to scare you. I just need some help carrying some boxes up to the workroom."

"It's not your fault," he said. "That's the second time I've done that in the last ten minutes. My brain can't seem to remember there's a table just four inches above my head." He held one hand just above his hair and moved it through the air.

Levi looked tired. He'd missed a patch on his left jawline when he'd shaved and he wasn't quite looking me in the eye.

"What's wrong?" I asked.

"I'm okay," he replied just a little too quickly.

I could easily think of half a dozen things that could have been wrong in the life of someone his age. I hoped it was one of the minor ones.

"I didn't ask if you were okay. I asked what's wrong." I waited.

He didn't seem to quite know what to do with his hands. He ran them back through his hair, then tugged at the front of his shirt.

"I don't want to get anyone in trouble."

"Are you trying to convince someone to break the law or hurt themselves or another person?"

"No," he said. "I would never do anything like that."

"Then you're not going to get anyone in trouble. They might get themselves in trouble but that's on them, not on you." My mother had used that logic on me many times. Some of them it had actually worked.

"Mrs. Anderson, the woman who died in that car accident a few months ago—is it true what I heard? That it wasn't an accident."

I nodded. "It looks that way." My stomach suddenly felt like I was on a roller coaster.

"She was going home from here," Levi continued, "after Mary's talk, right?"

"That's right." I wanted to push him to get to the point, but I was afraid if I did, he'd stop talking altogether.

He rubbed his hands on his black jeans. "That day, I heard Mrs. Anderson arguing with someone. She was really angry."

"Do you know who she was arguing with?"

He nodded. "Yeah. And the thing is, I just know that . . . that he wouldn't have killed her."

"So then you can't get that person in trouble."

He looked doubtful.

"Levi, who was it?" I asked. I had a feeling I knew the answer.

He looked down at his feet. "Johnny Rock."

That was what I had expected him to say. "I know they argued. Johnny told me."

Levi still looked troubled. "Did he tell you what he said to her?"

"He told me they'd had words over a business deal."

He couldn't seem to keep his hands still. He ran a hand over his head. He pulled at a loose thread on his shirt. "He wouldn't have killed an old lady. I don't want him to be in trouble because of what I heard."

"Levi, is this something the police need to hear?" I asked.

He looked down at his feet. "I don't know. Maybe. It's just that Johnny said something they might take the wrong way."

I slowly let out a breath. "I don't think Johnny could kill anyone, either—old or not. So what did he say? 'I wish you were dead'?" I smiled. "I'll tell you a little secret. When I was not much younger than you are, I said that to my mother more than once when I was

fighting with her. But I didn't mean it and no one really thought I did."

Levi almost smiled. "I can't picture you as a teenager," he said.

"Sometime, I'll show you some slightly embarrassing photos from back then," I said.

He scuffed one foot on the floor. "Okay. Johnny didn't exactly say he wished she was dead but it was pretty close. He said, 'When you're dead, I will dance on your grave, old woman, and it can't come soon enough for me.'"

Given how angry I knew Johnny had been at the time, the words didn't surprise me. It also didn't surprise me that he hadn't volunteered that he'd said them.

"So do I need to talk to the police?" Levi asked.

"How about I tell Detective Gordon what you just told me, and if he needs to talk to you, he'll let you know."

His shoulders sagged with relief. "Thanks, Kathleen," he said. "I'll go get those boxes for you."

Once the cartons of books were upstairs, I called Marcus and explained what Levi had told me. "I don't think it's a big deal," I said. "But I thought I should let you know."

"Thanks," he said. "Johnny's feelings about Leitha are pretty clear. I don't need to talk to Levi."

"For the record, I don't think Johnny killed Leitha no matter what he said to her, and I'm certain he didn't kill Mike."

I pictured Marcus probably shaking his head at the

phone. "For the record, right now I'm just going to say, 'no comment.'"

Marcus showed up just after we'd closed the library. I was about to get in the truck and Harry was sweeping the back end of the parking lot. The Reading Club kids had taken some vegetables home, and there were dirt and the odd radish all over the pavement.

I waited by the truck as Marcus walked over to me. He raised one hand in hello to Harry. "Kathleen, did you by any chance talk to Johnny this afternoon?" he asked.

"If you mean, did I call and warn him that Levi had heard him telling Leitha how happy he'd be when she was dead? No."

He had the good sense to look a little embarrassed. "I'm sorry," he said. "I didn't mean to accuse you of anything. I just wondered if he might have come in or called for any reason. You did say he made a big donation to the computer fund."

"I haven't talked to Johnny at all today. Why?"

"I need to talk to Harry," he said.

That didn't answer my question, so I followed him across the lot. He asked Harry the same question: Had he talked to Johnny this afternoon?

Harry shook his head. "I haven't talked to Johnny for a couple of days." He pulled off his hat, ran a hand over his bald head and put it back on again. "More than any of the rest of us, Johnny is struggling with Mike's death. They were close and I think Mike would have ended up going on the road with Johnny for at

least part of the time, even if the rest of us didn't." He stopped and took a couple of deep breaths. "Mike was the reason we ended up getting together for the Last Bash. It was his idea and he nagged the rest of us until we were all in. The two of them had plans and I think Johnny's having a hard time letting go of them." He focused on Marcus. "No offense, but we need answers and the sooner the better."

"I know," Marcus said. "I'm trying to get you those answers. There are a couple of things I need to talk to Johnny about, but I haven't been able to find him."

"If I hear from him, I'll tell him to call you," Harry said.

Marcus nodded. "Thanks."

I said good night to Harry and walked back to the truck with Marcus. "You can't actually think Johnny killed either one of them?" I said. "He had no reason."

"My job is to gather the evidence."

I gave him a look.

He sighed. "The problem is, no one had a reason to want Mike dead as far as I can see. No one had a motive to kill Leitha, either. She was difficult, no question, but she was an annoyance, like a mosquito buzzing around your head, not a threat to anyone. I'm going to check Eric's. I'll call you later."

I watched him drive away and then I unlocked the truck, set my messenger bag on the seat and climbed inside. When I turned to head toward Mountain Road and home, I looked out over the water and the Riverwalk and it occurred to me that I might know where Johnny was. I headed in that direction instead.

As I drove, I thought about the argument Levi had overheard between Leitha and Johnny. Those words "When you're dead, I will dance on your grave, old woman, and it can't come soon enough for me" didn't sound like a threat to me. It almost sounded like Johnny had been gloating.

I thought about Lachlan, working so hard to find some justification to stop the deal for that property in Red Wing. Lachlan had said Johnny didn't want the teen to waste his time researching the old building. That gave me an idea.

I parked in the lot where the concert stage had been set up. That night felt like such a long time ago. A man was standing by the edge of the embankment, looking out over the water, hands stuffed in his pockets.

I walked across the grass toward him. "Hey, Johnny," I said when I got close.

He turned and gave me what passed for a smile from him these days. "Hey, Kathleen. What are you doing here?"

"Looking for you."

The water was dark and angry and the clouds were low and heavy. It was going to rain soon.

"You were the new buyer for the building in Red Wing, weren't you?" I asked. "The buyer who was going to turn the property into a parking lot. You scammed Leitha. That's why you weren't worried. That's why you told Lachlan to let go of his plan to stop the sale. You didn't want to stop the sale."

He was nodding before I finished speaking. "Yeah.

I bested her. You have no idea how hard it was not to rub her face in that, to keep it secret."

"I can imagine."

"It wasn't just about the building. It was the way she treated Mike and Jonas. Part of it was because I hated how she kept pressuring Lachlan about college and threatening not to let him have the Finnamore money for his education, as though studying music was somehow not good enough. I wanted her out of the kid's life but I didn't make it happen. Mike cared about the old bat, you know. And that tells you everything you need to know about him right there."

I nodded because I couldn't get any words past the lump in my throat.

"So why were you looking for me?" Johnny asked.

I cleared my throat. "Marcus needs to talk to you. I think you should tell him what you just told me."

Johnny pulled out his phone. "What's his number?"

18

I waited with Johnny until Marcus arrived.

"I would never tell you how to grieve," I said when I caught sight of Marcus pulling in next to my truck in the parking lot, "because something like that is so intensely personal, plus it annoys the crap out of me when people do that."

Johnny gave me a small smile, the first genuine one I'd seen from him in a while.

"But I am going to remind you that if Mike were standing here instead of me, he would tell you to grab life by the—" I pictured Mike onstage explaining his definition of a good friend. I smiled. "By the athletic supporter and live every second you've got because none of us knows how long that's going to be."

I put a hand on his shoulder for a moment and then headed over to meet Marcus.

"Thank you for getting Johnny to call me," he said. "I thought you were going home."

I knew that meant *Why didn't you just tell me where*

you thought Johnny was? Since he hadn't asked me that directly, all I said was "I'm going home now."

I started for the truck. Marcus didn't say, *I'll call you later*, and neither did I.

After supper, once again I sat at the table with my laptop. I checked my e-mail. Susan had scanned the documents she'd found that referred to John Finnamore's eye color and e-mailed them to me. I also had an e-mail from Roma with a fairly large attachment. The subject line was THE BURLESQUE SHOW.

I opened Susan's e-mail first. Two different society-page articles mentioned John Finnamore's blue eyes and dark hair. I had the feeling I'd gotten way off on a tangent. I hadn't learned anything that put me closer to figuring out who had killed Mike.

"Does any of this really matter?" I asked Hercules, who was sitting at my feet, carefully washing his chest.

He looked up and meowed loudly and enthusiastically. He seemed to think it did. I wasn't so sure anymore.

I heard the washer shut off. I went down to the basement and discovered Owen sitting in the empty laundry basket on top of the dryer, both paws up on the end of the basket.

When Ethan and Sarah were very small, I would take the two of them sledding in a park close to where we lived. I'd stick them in our laundry basket—leaving behind a pile of dirty clothes on the floor—tie the basket to an old metal toboggan we had and then I'd jump on

the back and we'd go like stink down the steepest hills there.

Ethan was always in the front of the basket, two little mittened hands holding on to the end, a huge grin on his face, with Sarah behind him with an equally big smile on her face. Dad insisted that that was the reason they both had lead feet.

The cat reminded me of Ethan. For all I knew, maybe Owen was imagining himself hurtling down a snowy hill.

I moved the wet towels into the dryer. Owen leaned his head over the side of the laundry basket and watched. "You know, if you could just learn how to set the timer, I could get you to do this and save me a trip up and down the stairs."

He looked at me and yawned. Cat for *Not happening*.

When I got back upstairs, I found Hercules standing up on my chair, looking at something on the laptop. Somehow, he'd managed to open Roma's e-mail and get into the photos from the burlesque show.

"How did you do that?" I said.

He ducked his head as though modestly trying to say, *Oh, it was nothing*.

A photo of Zorro strutting his stuff on the middle of the stage out at The Brick filled the screen. I smiled, then leaned over and closed the image. I thought of Roma's frustration with trying to organize another show. I wished there was a way to convince Mary to at least plead Roma's case to whoever Zorro was.

I scooped up Hercules, sat down and settled him

on my lap. He immediately reached a paw toward the computer and Zorro filled the computer screen again.

"I don't have time for this right now," I said.

He gave an insistent meow that I knew meant he wanted me to look at the photo.

I yawned and stretched. "You're so stubborn," I said.

His whiskers twitched. A pair of green eyes was locked on my face. I glared back at him, which was a waste of time because he never lost a staring contest. Neither did Owen. "Fine," I said. "I will look at the picture."

I pulled the laptop a bit closer, centered the photo of Zorro and studied it. His fencing foil was thrust forward, his cape swirled behind him and he was giving the crowd a wicked grin as he swiveled his hips from side to side. I couldn't see what Hercules thought was so important about the image. Maybe he'd just been poking at the touch pad because it was fun. Maybe the photograph didn't matter at all.

And then I noticed something on Zorro's left hip. I used the magnifying feature to get a close look. The image was blurry but I could just make out the tops of two tiny fingers, spaced apart like they were part of some hand gesture tattooed on the man's hip.

I zoomed out again and looked at the man carefully: his body type, his smile. And suddenly I got it. I slumped against the chair back. "Mike Bishop was Zorro," I said aloud.

Hercules had already jumped down to the floor

and was washing his face. He meowed his agreement without looking up from his ablutions.

Mike was Zorro. Suddenly it all made sense. That was why both Mary and Sandra had refused to put Roma in touch with the mystery dancer. They couldn't. "Take me at my word when I tell you that there is no way Zorro will ride again," Mary had said to me. I looked at the photo one more time. It seemed so obvious now. Why hadn't it occurred to me before? Mike had the soul of a performer and a huge, kind heart. Getting up on that stage to help the no-kill shelter was exactly the kind of thing he would have done.

Hercules had stopped washing his face and was looking up at me as though he wanted something.

"Thank you for pointing out the photo," I said. "I'm sorry I didn't take you seriously at first."

And then, in case he hadn't been looking for a little vindication, I got him a couple of sardine crackers.

It was raining when I got to the library the next morning. I was unlocking the main doors and juggling my messenger bag, my coffee mug and my umbrella when Mary came up the steps and grabbed my cup just before I dropped it. I didn't have a good record with coffee mugs.

"Thank you," I said as we stepped inside.

I shut off the alarm and unlocked the second set of doors. Mary handed me my coffee. Then she flipped on the lights and pushed down the hood of her yellow slicker.

"It's not fit for man nor beast," she said, patting her hair.

I looked at her, thinking it must have been hard to keep her emotions in check when Roma and I were pressuring her to tell us Zorro's real name. She'd known Mike forever.

"I'm sorry," I said.

Mary was patting the pockets of her raincoat, looking for her keys or her phone probably. "I don't think you're responsible for this weather, Kathleen," she said without looking up.

"I didn't mean that. I mean, I'm sorry Roma and I pushed you so hard yesterday."

She did look up then. Something she saw in my expression made her shake her head. "Sometimes I think you can look right into people's heads," she said. "You figured it out, didn't you?"

"That Mike was Zorro? Yeah, I did."

"How the hell did you do that?"

I explained about the tattoos he and Johnny had gotten. "Roma sent me some photos from the show. It was really just chance that I spotted it." Chance and a small tuxedo cat, to be specific.

She laughed. "Shows how much attention I paid. I didn't even notice he had a tattoo."

We headed for the stairs. "It really was a last-minute thing, Mike getting up there as Zorro?" I said.

"Very last minute," Mary said. "We needed to get people's attention and I knew Mike was comfortable onstage."

"How did you come up with the costume?"

She laughed. "A little ingenuity and a lot of luck. The pants were his bike pants. His gym bag was in the backseat of his car. We made the mask out of one of my scarves."

I unlocked my office door and dropped my things on my desk chair, stopping to hang up my damp jacket. Mary waited in the doorway.

"What about the cape?" I asked.

"Remember I said it took a lot of luck? The cape was one of those lucky things. Sandra made it for a vampire routine and then decided the rest of the costume probably crossed a line. The hat was something we had in our costume stash and the fencing foil was another piece of luck. It came from the high school. It was used in a play they put on last year. One of the history teachers drove down and grabbed it for me. She's a cat person."

"How did you manage to keep Mike's identity a secret?"

We went down to the staff room and I started the coffee while Mary hung up her things.

"We were using the office as a dressing room, but there was a small bathroom back there as well for staff. I basically waited until no one was looking and pushed Mike inside." She made a shoving motion with one hand.

"I thought if we could keep Zorro's identity a secret that would keep people talking and keep the fundraiser on people's minds. Mike was game." Mary pressed her lips together for a moment. "I don't think I've ever laughed so hard in my life as when I was

trying to get all of his hair under that scarf. I knew if people saw those curls, the jig would be up." She looked at me. "The reason we kept the secret for so long was that Mike wanted to bring back Zorro for another fund-raiser—ironically just the thing Roma wants to do. In fact, he'd been getting together with Sandra on Wednesday nights to work on a new routine."

Wednesday nights. Now I knew what Mike had been doing. Now I understood why he'd kept it a secret. I also knew that secret had had nothing to do with his death.

I glanced at Mary, who seemed lost in thought. "I don't think he'd mind you telling Roma," I said as I got the cream out of the small refrigerator.

Mary nodded. "It was such a good night. To tell the truth, I was looking forward to doing it all over again."

She swallowed a couple of times and I had to blink away the unexpected sting of tears.

"I will call Roma," Mary said, her voice suddenly hoarse. "Make sure you tell that man of yours that someone needs to be held accountable."

Despite the rain—or maybe because of it—it was a very busy day at the library. It was close to two o'clock before I got to have lunch and I got only half my sandwich eaten before Abigail came up to tell me that the door to the loading dock was leaking. I called Harry, who was able to do a temporary fix that stopped the water coming in.

"It might—*might*—be possible to order a new seal for that door," he said. "Otherwise you're going to need a new door. Water's coming in now. It's going to be a lot worse this winter." He made a face. "Let's hope this is the last bit of substandard work from Will Redfern."

Will Redfern was the original contractor for the library renovations. He and his crew had done some quality work and some that was outright shoddy. Harry and Oren Kenyon—with some help from Harry's brother, Larry, who was an electrician—had fixed most of the problems. Luckily there had been nothing major until now. A new loading dock door wasn't in the budget.

"Let me see if I can track down a door seal," Harry said. "We might get lucky."

"Fingers crossed," I said.

When I got home, I found both cats in the living room. Owen was on the chair by the phone and Hercules sat on the footstool next to the calendar Ruby had given me. It had somehow been flipped open to April and it almost seemed like they had been admiring themselves.

"Get down," I said.

Hercules looked at Owen. Owen looked at me. Neither one of them moved. I didn't have time to argue with them. I started for the stairs.

"I could have gotten some nice, well-behaved goldfish," I said. "Or a cute little hamster." We'd had this one-sided conversation before.

I looked back at them in time to see Owen exchange a look with his brother. I'm pretty sure he was rolling his eyes.

Since I'd had just part of a sandwich for lunch, I was hungry. The refrigerator and cupboards weren't quite in the realm of Old Mother Hubbard, but they were close. I found an onion, a rubbery carrot and two suspiciously soft tomatoes. I cut them all up and added half of one of the zucchini Roma had given me. I stir-fried the veggies with hot sauce and added a fried egg on top. It was filling and healthy, but I needed to get groceries soon.

It was still raining, so I drove down to tai chi and was lucky to snag a parking spot not too far away. I opened my umbrella and ran through the puddles to the studio door, where I shook the umbrella before I darted inside.

Ruby was sitting on the bench at the top of the stairs, changing her shoes.

"The calendar definitely gets two paws of approval," I said. I told her how I'd found Owen and Hercules when I got home. "I think fame is going to their heads."

Ruby smiled. "'In ancient times cats were worshipped as gods; they have not forgotten this.'"

I smiled. "Terry Pratchett."

Maggie worked us hard and I was sticky and warm by the time we finished the whole form at the end of the class. And I was hungry again. I drove over to Eric's for something to eat, promising myself I'd make a grocery list in the morning.

I ordered a turkey sandwich to go, which I knew

Eric would make with Swiss cheese, tomato, sun-
flower sprouts and cranberry mayo. Because it was
raining, I also got a cup of coffee.

"It should be only about five minutes," Claire said.

I sat on a stool at the counter. My cell phone buzzed
in my jacket pocket. I pulled it out and checked the
screen. It was Roma.

"I need a favor," she said.

"Name it," I said.

"Could you and Marcus feed the Wisteria Hill cats
in the morning?"

I wasn't sure about Marcus but I could. "Of course."

"I'm sorry it's such short notice. I have to go to Red
Wing to assist on an emergency surgery on a police
dog. Eddie's gone to Minneapolis. His plan was to
drive back early in the morning and go right to the
rink."

"It's not a problem," I said. "I love any chance I get
to see Lucy and the other cats."

I heard her exhale with relief. "Thanks," she said.
"You're a lifesaver."

I wished her good luck with the surgery, we said
good-bye and I put my phone back in my pocket.

The diner was quiet. Maybe because it was raining.
There was a man standing in front of me at the counter
in a dark blue slicker. It was Jonas Quinn, I realized. I
touched his shoulder and he turned, smiling when he
saw it was me.

"Kathleen, how are you?" he said.

"A little damp. Otherwise I'm fine. How are you?"

"I'm on my way to what I expect will be a very

boring meeting. Otherwise *I'm* fine. And by the way, thanks for the help you gave Lachlan the other day."

"It was no trouble," I said. "He's a great kid."

Jonas's smile got wider. "Yes, he is."

His fingers were tapping out a rhythm on the edge of the counter and it struck me that he seemed to have the same musical bent as his nephew. Claire came out then with four take-out cups in a cardboard tray plus a paper take-out bag. She ran down the contents— three were coffees, each with a different permutation of cream and sugar, and the fourth container was tea.

"Would you like milk and sugar for the tea?" Claire asked.

"Just some milk, please," Jonas said. "The tea is mine and I don't like my drinks sweet."

She smiled. "My grandfather says the same thing. He says, 'I'm sweet enough already.'" She leaned sideways and looked at me. "Your food will be ready in just a minute, Kathleen," she said.

Jonas picked up the tray of drinks and the take-out bag. "It was good to see you, Kathleen," he said.

"You too," I said. "I hope your meeting is short and interesting."

He raised both eyebrows and smiled. "Me too."

I was restless when I got home. Marcus hadn't called, probably because he was working on one or both cases. I thought about what he'd said: "The problem is, no one had a reason to want Mike dead. . . . No one had a motive to kill Leitha, either. She was difficult,

no question, but she was an annoyance . . . not a threat to anyone."

I kept coming back to those Punnett squares Mike had drawn. Even though I'd told Hercules they didn't matter, I couldn't seem to let go of the idea that somehow they did. I thought about all the times I'd seen Mike working at the library, all the times he'd waved me over. I couldn't think of a single time when he'd been drawing one of those squares.

I looked at the half sheet of yellow paper again. Something about it seemed wrong. I could think of only one occasion when I'd seen Mike with his head bent over a sheet of yellow paper. He'd mostly used wide-ruled white paper. I closed my eyes and tried to remember what I'd seen. Jonas and Lachlan had come in to take Mike to lunch. I had taken them upstairs because Mike was in our workroom. As he looked up, I remembered him jamming several pages into a book and closing the cover. Several yellow sheets of paper. I'd thought he had been marking his place but now it struck me that maybe he had been hiding them instead. But from whom? From me? From Jonas and Lachlan? I didn't know. Was I seeing something that hadn't really happened?

I found a marker and pulled a flattened cardboard box out of the recycling bin. I spread the cardboard out on the table and drew out the Finnamore family tree starting with John Finnamore Senior. Below Finnamore Senior I added his two children, Leitha and John Junior. The next generation, Eloise Anderson-Hill, Elizabeth

Bishop and Mary-Margaret Quinn followed. Underneath, I wrote in Mike, Jonas and his brother, Colin, along with Eloise's daughters, Min and Nari. Lachlan had the last row to himself. I added spouses where I knew their names.

The diagram looked a little lopsided. Because there had been so many years between Leitha and her brother, Eloise was actually closer in age to Mike, Jonas and Colin—than she was to their mothers, her first cousins.

Plotting everyone's eye color was just too complicated, so I decided to try doing hair texture instead. It was simpler.

Leitha Finnamore Anderson had had curly hair. I wrote *CC* beside her name. I remembered that Susan had included a photo of Leitha and her parents when she'd sent me the information about John Senior's eye color. I got my laptop and looked at it again. Leitha's father had had curly hair. *CC* went next to his name as well.

I studied the photo carefully. Leitha's mother had had wavy hair I realized, not curly. It was a distinction some people had trouble making. That meant she had one curly-hair gene and one straight-hair gene. I put *Cs* by her name. So Leitha could easily have been their child. Eloise had the same hair as her mother. Min and Nari were adopted, so they had no Finnamore DNA.

It wasn't hard to find photos of Mike's parents. They had the same curls their son did. I kept going mostly out of curiosity. Mary-Margaret Finnamore Quinn had wavy hair, not curly. Her son, Colin, had a head full of

those Finnamore curls. And Jonas, who wasn't a Finnamore, had wavy hair like their father. Ainsley Quinn, Colin's wife, also had a gorgeous head full of blond curls.

I stared at my handiwork. I thought about Lachlan's unruly hair. I pictured him with his head leaning in close to the microfilm reader. "A tangle of curls," Mary had called his hair. But it wasn't really curly, I realized.

Lachlan's hair was wavy, which wasn't possible.

I got the piece of paper that Owen had swiped and looked at it again. What if Mike had been trying to work out Lachlan's eye color, not Leitha's? I thought about Jonas coming into the library that day with Lachlan. It had been just a few days before the concert. What if I was right about why Mike had stuffed those pages in the book and closed it? I looked at Owen. "What if he *was* hiding them?" I said.

I had wondered why none of the staff had checked the pages of the book in which Keith had discovered Mike's notes before Keith borrowed it. Mike had been around the library enough to know how things worked. He could have easily put the book with other ones Keith had requested. Whoever had checked Keith out could have missed those sheets of paper stuck inside the book, especially if it had been busy.

I took a sip of my coffee. There were only a couple of mouthfuls left now, and they were cold and a bit too sweet for me since some of the sugar had settled to the bottom of the cup even though Claire had stirred it well before she handed it to me.

I tapped the marker on the table. "Leitha was

adamant about the importance of the family line," I said, "and she thought telling the truth was more important than discretion or hurt feelings." I remembered hearing her tell Mary the day that they had argued, with a great deal of pride in her voice, that the Finnamores could trace their family tree, unsullied, back to the *Mayflower*. Jonas had said that family was more than biology. Leitha had snorted and said of course *he* would say that.

I thought about my own family and the similarities between Ethan, Sarah and me, how Ethan made me think of Mom in so many ways. They were both born performers.

I thought about Lachlan's wavy hair, his green eyes and his gentle manner so different from the more outgoing Finnamores, so much like soft-spoken Jonas.

"Lachlan is Jonas Quinn's son," I said. It was the only explanation that made sense.

Behind me a voice said, "Yes, he is."

19

I turned around slowly. Jonas was standing in the kitchen doorway, pointing a gun at me.

"You're very smart. I knew you'd figure it all out," he said. "I wish you hadn't, though."

I swallowed against the sour taste in the back of my throat and tried not to panic. Owen leaned around the side of the chair and stared with curiosity at Jonas.

"Mike figured it out, too," I said.

"Not at first." Except for the gun, Jonas seemed just like the man who had come into the library, who had shown me around his garden, who had laughed with us all at Eric's.

"Leitha figured it out first."

He nodded. "She never let me forget that my mother was really my stepmother and I wasn't a real Finnamore."

"And she was going to tell Lachlan," I said.

Jonas loved his nephew—his son. You had to spend only a few minutes with them to see that. It was the

only reason I could think of that could explain why he had killed Leitha, because I was suddenly sure he had.

"Lachlan adored his mother and father and they felt the same way about him. If there were any fairness in the world, any justice, they would be alive and Leitha would have died years ago." He took a deep breath and slowly let it out. "It's her fault they're dead, you know," he said.

The lines around his mouth tightened. It was the only sign of what he was feeling. I suspected Jonas had learned to keep his emotions to himself a long time ago.

"Leitha kept pushing Colin to get more involved in the family business," he continued. "She still had shares in Black Dog and she convinced him to go and vote her proxy. The accident happened on the way home. She would have ruined every memory Lachlan had of them. I couldn't let her do that. And I couldn't let her cut him off from the trust money for his education."

My phone was on the table. There was no way I could reach it before he shot me. The only thing I could do was keep him talking. I was Miss Marple in the drawing room of an English country manor, I told myself. I was Hercule Poirot on the *Orient Express*.

"You laced your tea with potassium chloride and put sugar in it so Leitha wouldn't notice the taste."

"Potassium chloride tastes a little salty and slightly metallic, but the sugar hid that quite well," Jonas said. The shoulders of his jacket were damp. It must still be raining, I realized.

I put one hand on the back of the chair next to me, gripping it tightly so Jonas wouldn't see my hand shaking. "How did she figure it out?" I asked. I genuinely wanted to know the answer.

Jonas rubbed his face with his free hand. "It was that study she was part of. They were looking into the genetics of heart disease, looking to see if there was a connection to common physical traits like eye and hair color, and how cilantro tastes to someone. Leitha outlived her brother and lived longer than her parents and her grandparents. She had the Finnamore green eyes. They had become less common over the years."

I nodded. "I remember Mike saying that."

"She didn't want the Finnamore line to die out. It drove her crazy that Eloise had adopted instead of having biological children. I can't remember when she wasn't at Mike to get married and have babies. He'd just laugh and say one of him was enough for the world."

I almost smiled. I could imagine Mike saying that.

"And she was always pestering Colin and Ainsley to have more children. She didn't know that they had been trying for years to have a brother or sister for Lachlan. It just never happened."

I could see the pain in his eyes. "It was only one time with Ainsley, a momentary lapse on both our parts. Colin was the only man for her."

"And she was the only one for you," I said. It was a guess but a good one.

He nodded.

Jonas had slept with his brother's wife—a huge

betrayal. The fact that he had been in love with her forever probably would have made things worse if the truth had come out. But Lachlan was the result. How could Leitha even have considered telling him? It seemed too cruel even for her. As Jonas's child, Lachlan wasn't entitled to any money from the family trust because he was not a biological Finnamore. Did money really matter more to her?

"Did you know Lachlan was your child from the beginning?" I asked.

"Not at first. But when they couldn't seem to have more children, I got suspicious. I finally confronted Ainsley and she admitted that I was Lachlan's father. She didn't want him or Colin to know and neither did I. I didn't want to break up that family. Colin was Lachlan's father. The only father he knew. The only father that mattered. I didn't want to do that to my . . . to Lachlan and I never wanted Colin to know that I had betrayed him. I wanted to be the big brother he believed in."

"Leitha wasn't going to let Lachlan have the money for college from the trust."

Jonas shook his head. "The DNA shouldn't have mattered. Lachlan was Colin's child in all the ways that were important, but Leitha was the trustee and her belief was that only blood Finnamores were entitled to the money. Eloise's daughters should have gotten the money for their education as well. If Leitha wouldn't release the funds for her own grandchildren, she wasn't going to give it to Lachlan and she was determined to tell him why."

"So you decided to kill her," I said. How was I going to get out of this? What would Jonas do when he got to the end of his explanation?

"Yes," he said. "I won't insult you by saying I had no other choice. There were other options. I just didn't like any of them. I knew potassium chloride could bring on a heart attack. I started college as a chemistry major."

"Leitha gave you an ultimatum, didn't she?" I took a step closer to the chair and dropped my hand onto Owen's back. He meowed softly.

"She had given me forty-eight hours to tell Lachlan the truth or she said she would. On the day of Mary's presentation at the library, I had just a few hours left. She was a miserable old woman and the world isn't any worse off with her dead. It was easy to get the potassium chloride at the university. I faked drinking the tea when I was talking to Rebecca. It was that simple."

"And then Marcus got suspicious about two deaths so close together in one family."

"I really wish he hadn't done that," Jonas said. He looked like he felt bad, but the gun he was pointing at me didn't waver.

"When we were at Eric's, I knew the minute the words were out of my mouth that I'd made a mistake with that comment about not liking sweet things. I knew you'd pick up on that. Marcus had told me about the contents of Leitha's stomach. I knew he would have told you as well. And you don't miss details like that."

"So what happens now?" I said. I was surprised how steady my voice sounded since both of my hands were shaking and my chest felt as though an elephant had just sat on it.

"We're going for a ride," he said.

"Where?"

"Out to Wisteria Hill."

My heart sank. He'd heard my conversation with Roma when we'd been at Eric's.

He nodded his head as though he'd read my mind. "Yes, I heard enough of your conversation to know that Dr. Davidson and her husband won't be there. And I know that you're looking after the cats that live out there. For some reason you wanted to check on them tonight. It's been raining hard and you were just worried about them. You're a very kind person." His eyes hardened. He gestured with the gun. "Let's go."

"I need my keys."

"And bring your phone," Jonas said.

"All right," I said. I felt a frisson of hope. If I had my phone, there was a chance I could get help. I leaned down and kissed Owen on the top of his head. "It'll be okay," I whispered. I wasn't sure if the words were for his benefit or mine. At the edge of my vision, I could see Hercules peeking around the living room doorway. At least they were both safe.

We walked out to the truck. "You drive please," Jonas said. He had such nice manners. How could someone who remembered to say "please" and "thank you" kill another person?

"I could put the car in the ditch," I said through clenched teeth as I fastened my seat belt. Anger was beginning to replace my fear.

"And I could shoot you," he said. "I think that puts us on even ground."

"If you're not going to shoot me, what are you going to do?" At least out at Wisteria Hill I had a chance. I knew the woods around Roma and Eddie's house well. Out there Jonas and I were no longer "on even ground." Out there I had an advantage.

"I told you, you're going to drive out to Wisteria Hill to check on the cats. You'll discover one of them is missing and you'll go looking for it in the dark and have a nasty and deadly fall into the brook."

"No, I won't," I said, forgetting for a moment that he was holding a gun on me.

His dark eyes narrowed. "If it comes down to choosing between Lachlan and you, between Lachlan and anyone, it's an easy decision."

I needed him to think about what he was doing. I needed him to think about what he had already done. That meant asking him the question I didn't want to hear the answer to. I tried to take a deep breath but I couldn't. My chest was tight with anger. Still I managed to get the words out. "Why did you kill Mike?"

He didn't say anything.

I glanced in his direction. The pain was raw on his face. Part of me felt compassion for the man and part of me wanted to hit him. I started the truck.

"I kind of understand about Leitha. I'm not saying

what you did was right, but she threatened your child, so that part I get. But Mike would never have hurt Lachlan. Never."

"He didn't see that what he wanted to do would hurt Lachlan." His voice was flat, empty of emotion.

"Maybe Lachlan would be happy to find out he still had one parent," I said as I pulled out of the driveway.

"No. Lachlan adored Colin. He would be devastated to find out Colin wasn't his father." For a moment Jonas didn't speak but I could feel his gaze on me. "Mike was one of those people who saw the best in everyone and he had this idea that the rest of the world did the same thing. You're like that, too."

"He just wanted to tell the truth."

I saw Jonas nod his head out of the corner of my eye. "It was an accident," he said. "It wasn't like Leitha. Mike and I were arguing. He shoved me a couple of times and then I hit him back. He lost his balance and went backward. When I close my eyes, I can still see his head hit the mantel above the fireplace."

"I don't understand," I said. "Why didn't you call nine-one-one? It was an accident."

"He was dead."

I was gripping the steering wheel so tightly, I felt it might snap in half. "You're not a nurse or a doctor. You don't know that." Anger gave my voice a raspy harshness.

"I know how to check someone's pulse. He was dead. And I panicked. I wish I hadn't."

I glanced over at him again. The hand that was pointing the gun at me was shaking.

"I wish I hadn't punched him. I wish I hadn't gone over there. I wish I hadn't . . ." He didn't finish the sentence and I wondered if he'd been about to say he wished he hadn't slept with his sister-in-law.

We drove in silence for a few minutes. I needed to get Jonas talking again. I needed him to see me as a person and not an obstacle to be dealt with.

"Did Mike think Leitha might not have been a Finnamore?" I asked.

Jonas nodded. "You saw his notes. Yes. For a while he did. He found something in a diary of a midwife. Leitha was a surprise baby, coming years after her brother. She was supposed to have been born premature, but she was a robust eight pounds plus at birth according to the midwife."

"Her mother had an affair."

"Maybe. Celeste married John Finnamore on the rebound after a broken engagement. It seems she carried a torch for her former fiancé for the rest of her life."

"Mike tried to work out whether or not Leitha was a Finnamore by looking at eye color." We were almost at Wisteria Hill. All I could think was *Keep him talking*.

"The Finnamore green eyes," Jonas said. "It's ironic that Lachlan probably got his green eyes from me and I'm not a real Finnamore."

He was still holding on to my phone. He looked at it and then set it on the floor by his feet. "Eye color was just too complicated. Too many factors involved. Then Mike looked at the type of everyone's hair, which told him that Leitha *was* a Finnamore—her mother's previous beau had straight hair."

"Which meant Leitha would have had wavy hair, not curly," I said.

He nodded. "But the old eye-color thing had him intrigued. He was trying to work out when green eyes first showed up in the family tree. He wouldn't let it go. He wanted us all to take those DNA tests so we'd know more about our genetic makeup. I couldn't dissuade him."

"You were afraid the truth would come out if Lachlan did the test."

"I gave him every logical reason not to that I could. You know what Mike was like. He told me I was too much of a worrier and everything would be fine."

"He got suspicious because you were so adamant."

"No," Jonas said.

I saw him shake his head out of the corner of my eye. I didn't believe him. I'd seen what Mike was like when he sank his teeth into something, the way he had been with researching his family tree. He wouldn't let go until every question he had was answered.

"He went back to his Punnett squares," I said, "while he was trying to change your mind. And at some point he started looking at everyone's hair again."

"People have always commented on Lachlan's curly hair. It's been like that since he was a baby."

"But his hair isn't curly. It's actually wavy. Curly hair is spiral and wavy is S-shaped. The interesting thing is that hair type is an example of what's called incomplete dominance. It means that if you have one of each version of the gene, you end up with a mix of the two: not straight, not curly, but wavy hair."

"I see why Mike liked you," Jonas said.

"What do you mean?"

"You're a lot alike. You notice things other people don't. And you have a strong sense of right and wrong."

He was right. Were our similarities going to get me killed, too?

"I couldn't let the truth come out. I wanted Lachlan to at least be able to get an education."

"Why didn't you just pay for college yourself?" I looked over at him again.

"I can't. Without the trust there is no money for Lachlan's education. There isn't even enough money to hang on to the house much longer."

"I don't understand."

"It took every cent Colin and Ainsley had to pay for her care after the accident. It took every cent I had and everything I could beg or borrow. Lachlan is as entitled to that trust money as anyone."

"So you finally just told Mike the truth." My eyes were on the road but I could watch him in my peripheral vision. The gun was still pointed at me.

"The night he . . . That night . . . Yes. He didn't think it was such a big deal. He told me we'd figure out college. Lachlan could take out a loan or better yet we could challenge the terms of the trust. He didn't understand that it would blow up Lachlan's life. I swear to God, I didn't mean for him to get hurt."

We were almost at Wisteria Hill. There wasn't anything left to talk about. I felt something brush against my leg then, as light as the sweep of a feather. I froze, my entire body rigid.

Owen. It had to be.

Owen was with us in the truck.

Jonas suddenly leaned forward. I forced myself to keep my eyes on the road. There was no way he could know that Owen was here. Even if the cat accidentally touched him. I could feel my pulse pounding in the hollow at the base of my throat and I made myself take deep breaths and slow down my breathing. Panicking wasn't going to do me any good.

"Detective Gordon sent you a text," Jonas said.

Marcus rarely sent texts. Had he figured out something was wrong? "What does it say?"

"He wants to know where you are."

I swallowed to ease my suddenly dry mouth. "Are you going to answer him?" I asked.

"No," he said.

We drove in silence for maybe a minute; then Jonas spoke again. "I'm sorry I have to do this."

"Then don't do it."

"And what? You'll give me your word that you'll keep all my secrets? You won't. As I said, you're just like Mike." There was an edge of anger to his voice now.

"No, I won't keep your secrets, but I will help you in any other way that I can."

He laughed. "You're honest. I'll give you that. But I would sacrifice my life for Lachlan. And yours as well. Detective Gordon is a good man. I'm sorry he's going to be hurt."

Not if I can help it, I said silently.

20

We were at Wisteria Hill. I drove slowly up the driveway, hoping that somehow Roma had been late leaving or that her plans had changed, but the farmhouse was in darkness. I parked as close to the old carriage house as I could.

"Give me the keys, please," Jonas said.

I handed them to him and laid one hand on the dashboard for a moment. Harrison had given me the truck because Owen and I had found some papers about his daughter, Elizabeth's, adoption. And we'd almost gotten blown up in the process. We had barely gotten clear of the cabin where we'd been trapped when the propane tank exploded. I remembered having no sense of where my body was as the impact propelled me into the brush. I had landed flat on my back in a pile of snow, cold, wet, bruised and bloody.

But alive.

And then I'd caught sight of Owen coming toward me, snow and bits of tree bark stuck to his fur, spitting angry, meowing loudly all the way.

But alive.

We'd gotten out of that and we were going to get out of this as well.

Jonas gestured with the gun and I climbed out of the truck. Could I sprint to the carriage house if I had the chance? I hoped so. From there the woods were dense enough that I could find lots of places to hide.

I stood next to the truck while Jonas stuffed the keys and my phone into his pocket. He'd said that I noticed things that other people didn't. He was right, which meant I'd paid attention when Harry had explained how he'd hot-wired a truck almost identical to this one when he was a lovestruck teenager. I didn't need those keys to get out of here.

"If I had any other option to protect Lachlan, I would take it," Jonas said. "Everything I have ever done has been for Lachlan."

"So tell the truth for Lachlan. Tell him who he really is."

"He's Colin and Ainsley's son. He's a Finnamore."

I wasn't going to get through to him. In a different circumstance, I would have respected his loyalty to his child. But I was in this circumstance.

"I admire you and people who are like you," he said. "I admire the fact that you truly do seem to see and expect the best from people, but I'm not like that. Maybe I was once, but not now. As I said before, I am sorry." Once more he gestured with the gun.

I thought about Marcus and Mom and Dad and Ethan and Sarah and Harrison and Roma and Maggie and the furballs. I thought about what Mary had

taught me about kickboxing and the structure of the human knee.

"I'm sorry, too," I said.

And then I kicked the side of his knee as hard as I could. He yelled and went down, the hand holding the gun flying up in the air. I didn't waste any time trying to look for the gun. I ran and hoped Owen was with me.

I bolted around the side of the old carriage house and sprinted for the trees. I had a bit of a head start, but I knew it wasn't enough to let me double back to the truck. Jonas was taller and faster and stronger. I just hoped I'd connected hard enough that his knee would cause him enough trouble to give me an edge.

I tried to picture the road that ran in front of Wisteria Hill. If I turned left once I got up the graded embankment behind the carriage house, I could make another left turn and then head down toward the road. It made more sense than continuing to cut through the woods in the direction of the back access road. The main road would have more traffic.

It was dark and the air was heavy with moisture but it had stopped raining. Everything was dripping. The ground was saturated with water. I was breathing heavily. My feet in my canvas shoes were already soaking wet. I could hear the sound of rushing water. There was a stream off to the left behind the carriage house, skirting the rise where the trees began. When I got that far, I would need to turn left a second time. I reminded myself that it didn't matter that it was dark. I could hear the water. I knew which way to go. I had an advantage Jonas didn't have.

Owen still hadn't appeared. I was afraid to even whisper the cat's name in case Jonas heard me. I had to keep moving forward, hoping that Owen was here somewhere in the darkness beside me.

I made my way through the dripping trees, trying not to lose my footing on the mud and leaves and pine needles underfoot. Climbing up the embankment was a challenge. My feet kept sliding out from under me. The water sounded louder, closer. I tried to picture the last time I'd been here earlier in the summer. I couldn't be that far from the stream. I could follow it to the road. I just had to keep moving.

I went from one tree to the next, hugging their trunks, trying to stay small and quiet. I had to assume Jonas was behind me. And then suddenly I pitched forward. A tree branch snapped against my forehead and I landed facedown on the ground. I rolled over onto my back, trying to get my breath. After a few moments, I sat up, running one hand down my right leg. The calf, right above my ankle, was bleeding. I flexed my foot and grimaced. It hurt but I didn't think anything was broken. I felt around on the ground. I had tripped over a sharp-edged rock a bit bigger than my hand.

I could feel blood running down my leg. I needed a bandage. I pulled off my shirt, grateful that I had a tank top underneath. I managed to tear the fabric at a side seam. I tore off the whole right-front section and fashioned a makeshift tourniquet, knotting it as tightly as I could around my leg. I had just tied a second knot when Owen appeared beside me. He nuzzled my hand and I had to swallow a couple of times so I wouldn't

cry. I buried my face in his neck. He was muddy and wet and none too happy.

The rock I'd tripped over was still next to my foot. I ran my fingers over it and thought maybe I could use it. I looked around. Even though it was dark, I could see that I was at the upper edge of the embankment. I listened, focusing on tuning out the water rushing over the rocks. I heard a foot slip on the wet ground. Or was it just a raccoon or a skunk? No. They would have been more sure-footed. It had to be Jonas. He was quiet but not quiet enough.

I kissed the top of Owen's head, hoping he'd understand what I wanted him to do. I pointed at a nearby tree and then held up the rock. I pantomimed throwing it. He cocked his head to one side. Then I pointed to him and mimicked throwing back my head and yowling. My face was close to his and I saw his golden eyes narrow. Did he get it? I needed him to draw Jonas over to us. He probably would come this way but I needed to be sure and I needed to be ready.

My heart was pounding. My plan to get away from a man who wanted to kill me depended on a cat playing his part. But Owen wasn't just any cat. I climbed the tree, grateful that it was wet and made my progress quieter. I slid out along a branch about eight feet up, holding the rock tightly with one hand. I pushed my damp hair out of my face and gestured in Owen's direction. His response was to take a couple of swipes at his face with his paw. For a moment I thought he hadn't understood me and then he meowed loudly. He leaned forward and he meowed again and then again.

I was counting on the fact that even though he had killed two people, there was still some part of Jonas Quinn that was a good, kind person. My heart was thumping so hard, I was afraid it would shake me off the branch. The gash on my leg throbbed and the edge of the rock dug into my hand. Then Jonas came through the trees. I didn't see any sign of the gun. Either he hadn't found it after I'd kicked him, or he hadn't bothered looking. Owen meowed once more and to my surprise held up one paw. Was he . . . acting?

Jonas looked around; then he sighed. "What are you doing way out here? You belong down with the other cats."

He thought Owen was part of the feral colony. Owen continued to hold up his paw, his meows becoming more pitiful.

Jonas took a step closer. "I'll come back for you," he said.

It was now or never. I calculated the angle, hoped my math was right and then pushed myself partway up with my free arm and threw the rock with everything I had.

The rock struck Jonas on the side of his head, just above his right temple. His legs buckled and he collapsed. I waited for a moment to see if he'd move. When he didn't, I made my way down out of the tree, slipping on the wet bark and almost landing on the ground next to Jonas. I had scraped the skin on one arm but I was all right. I could see his chest moving, so I knew Jonas was breathing.

I grabbed Owen. "We're okay," I said. "We're okay."

My makeshift bandage was soaked through with blood and my leg hurt but I knew I could retrace my steps back to the truck. I'd crawl if I had to.

I took two steps and Jonas's arm snaked out and grabbed my ankle, pulling me down. I fell hard, knocking the wind out of me. Owen had jumped from my arms and stood by my head hissing as I struggled to catch my breath.

I kicked, gasping for air, and tried to roll over and sit up but Jonas was already on his feet. He grabbed my other leg and began dragging me across the ground. I yelled for help. I tried to grab onto anything, a tree root, a rock, a bush, but he was bigger and stronger.

He was headed for the stream. He was going to push me over the edge onto the rocks and into the water. Panic swirled in my chest. I used the burst of adrenaline to twist and kick even harder. It didn't work. Jonas's hands were clamped around my ankles like a set of handcuffs. I couldn't see Owen anymore, but I could hear him. I wasn't sure if he'd disappeared or was just out of my line of sight.

My face banged against the ground and I got a mouthful of dirt. I spit and choked. I couldn't get away. I could try to pull Jonas over with me or I could do everything I could to survive the fall. I stopped kicking and flailing. I went limp, hoping Jonas might loosen his grip even a little. I couldn't seem to stop shaking, but I promised myself that when he pushed me, I'd curl into a ball and cover my head with my arms. I'd probably break some bones, but as long as I stayed conscious, I'd be all right. I was a good swimmer and the

water was high, but it wouldn't be cold. I would get out of this.

We were at the edge of the gully. Jonas let go of one of my ankles. I tried to kick him but he dodged my foot.

"Get up," he said.

I still had dirt in my mouth, my arms were scraped and I could feel blood running down my leg. I knew physically I was no match for Jonas but I wasn't getting to my feet. I wasn't helping him throw me over.

"No," I said.

He bent down and grabbed my arm, pulling me halfway off the ground. Pain sliced through my left side but I forced myself to go limp again, and as my body slumped forward, I bit his hand.

He let go and I scrambled backward. Owen appeared claws out and hissing. When Jonas came toward me, I used my good leg to kick him in the stomach. I fell to my knees. Jonas doubled over for a moment and I thought he was going to go down again. He swayed but stayed on his feet and pulled the gun out of his pocket. So he had found it. I was out of options.

Jonas pointed the gun at me. I lifted my chin and stared up at him and behind me Marcus shouted, "Drop the gun!"

For a long moment Jonas didn't move.

"Drop the gun," Marcus called out again. "It's over. Just put it down."

Finally, Jonas nodded. He lowered his arm and leaned forward, setting the gun on the ground. I got to my feet, never taking my eyes off of his face. I felt

Marcus's strong arms go around me, pulling me against his chest.

"Are you all right?" he said.

I nodded because I didn't trust my voice to work. Jonas took a step backward.

"Stay where you are," Marcus said.

Jonas took another step backward.

"It's over."

Jonas nodded. "I know." He looked at me. "Kathleen, tell Lachlan he was the great joy of my life. Tell him that Ainsley and Colin loved him."

I realized what he was going to do but it was too late. He jumped.

The next few hours were a blur. Marcus called for backup and wrapped his jacket around my shoulders. He climbed down to the water but Jonas was dead.

We drove to the hospital and Marcus flashed his badge to get me seen right away. The gash on my leg and a cut on my forehead needed stitches. Dirt had to be cleaned out of all my scraped skin. The doctor said my ribs weren't broken. Bruises were already darkening on my left side. But I *was* alive.

Marcus left Owen in the car with the window cracked and a chicken salad sandwich he'd gotten from the vending machine in the waiting room.

"How did you know where I was?" I asked while we waited for the nurse to come back with a prescription and instructions on how to take care of the cut on my leg.

It turned out that Owen had managed to respond

to Marcus's text with a string of nonsense letters and symbols. "I knew you had to be in trouble," he said.

"What made you come out to Wisteria Hill?"

"Hercules. He was pacing back and forth in the kitchen. You know that photo you have on the refrigerator of Roma and Eddie the day they got married?"

I nodded. "He knocked it to the ground. Then he picked it up and brought it to me. I was looking for any clue in the house and he brought me the picture three times. Quinn's car was parked up the street. I ran the plates. It was just too much of a coincidence and then I realized what Hercules was trying to tell me."

I stretched out my arm and caught his hand.

"He killed Leitha," Marcus said. "He was the only person I couldn't eliminate. I figured it had to have been the tea."

"It was," I said. "He just pretended to drink it. Lachlan was his child, not his brother, Colin's. Leitha figured it out."

Marcus shook his head.

I swallowed a couple of times. "He killed Mike, too."

He stared at me. His mouth worked but no words came out at first. "No," he finally managed to say.

"I'm sorry," I said. I told him everything Jonas had told me. "I don't think it was just about the Finnamore money. I think he genuinely thought he would lose Lachlan if the truth came out."

Marcus pulled one hand down over the back of his neck. "This is worse."

"I know," I said softly.

21

One of the nurses found a set of scrubs for me. They were a bit big, but they were clean and I didn't have to leave in one of those gowns that flapped open in the back. Owen was stretched out on the middle of the backseat of Marcus's SUV, asleep with one paw over his nose.

"I can't believe he texted you," I said.

Marcus shrugged. "He can disappear whenever he feels like it. Texting doesn't seem like that big of a stretch."

"Why did you text me in the first place? You always call."

"I did call," he said as he unlocked the passenger door and helped me get settled on the seat. "It went to voice mail. I'm guessing Quinn turned off the ringer as well."

Owen lifted his head, murped hello and came from the backseat to the front, settling himself on my lap. He nuzzled my chin and I stroked his fur.

"You were very brave," I told him, "and very smart."

Marcus leaned down and kissed the top of my head. "So were you," he said.

When we pulled into the driveway, Hercules came around the side of the house as though he'd been listening for the sound of the SUV. I opened the car door and Owen jumped from my lap to the ground. Marcus came and helped me to my feet. I leaned down over his protests and picked up Hercules. He studied my face, green eyes narrowed.

"I'm fine," I said, kissing his furry head. "You saved us. Thank you for telling Marcus where we were."

"Mrr," he said, his nose touching mine.

"I love you, too," I whispered.

We made our way around the house to the back door with Owen leading the way. Marcus unlocked the door and I had the feeling he would have carried me into the kitchen if I'd let him.

"I'm all right," I said, reaching up to put my hand to his cheek. "I knew you'd find me."

He pressed his lips together before he spoke. "I thought he was going to throw you over the side of the gully," he said, a rough edge to his voice.

"He was. But I had a plan."

He looked at me for a long moment. Then he started to laugh, wrapping both arms tightly around me. "I love you," he said.

I felt my throat get tight at the thought that I might never have heard those words again. "I love you, too," I whispered.

Marcus had to head back to Wisteria Hill and he had

no intention of leaving me alone even though I pro-
tested that I had Owen and Hercules. Turned out, he'd
already called Rebecca. She arrived at the door with
one of her poultices for the tub, some poached salmon
for the boys and a basket of still warm blueberry
muffins.

Marcus kissed me twice, told Rebecca to call if I
needed anything and instructed Owen and Hercules
to watch me. Then he left.

"Oh, sweet girl, I am so glad you're all right," Rebecca said, and I saw the gleam of unshed tears in her
eyes. She took my hands in hers and turned them over
to examine the scraped-raw skin. I saw her wince. She
eyed my forehead. "Does that hurt?" she asked.

I shook my head. "Not very much. They gave me
some pills at the hospital."

She reached up and brushed my hair back off of
my face. Something about that simple gesture made
me start to tremble.

"Jonas killed Leitha," I said in a voice that trembled,
too. "He killed Mike. Mike."

"But he didn't kill you," she said.

I started to cry and she folded me into her arms and
I cried for everyone who was lost and everyone who
was still here.

I woke up looking worse than I felt. I discovered Marcus in the kitchen making coffee with two furry helpers
with suspiciously fishy breath. All three of them were
insistent that I needed to stay home.

I didn't put up much of an argument. Marcus went

out to feed the cats at my insistence. Maggie arrived with a cream for my bruises—Rebecca had been teaching Maggie the things Rebecca herself had learned from her own mother for quite some time now. Owen was overjoyed to see her. She praised both cats for their resourcefulness and bravery.

"I think you're part cat yourself," she said, hugging me as though she thought I might break. "You've used up at least three or four of your nine lives."

I couldn't stop thinking about Lachlan. Marcus had told me that he was with Johnny and Ritchie and Elena Gonzalez. The band had closed ranks around him. Eloise had defied her doctor's orders about flying and would be arriving in the late afternoon. After supper Marcus and I were going to share the details of the story that weren't public knowledge with them all, including the truth about Lachlan's parentage. I was trying not to think about how painful that conversation was going to be, but secrets were why all of this had happened. Secrets were why Mike and Leitha—and Jonas—were dead.

I was sitting in the backyard in the sunshine just before lunch, with my leg propped up on an overturned laundry basket, while Maggie and Owen picked tomatoes, when Harrison and Harry came around the side of the house.

I started to get up but the old man raised a hand. "Don't even think about moving," he said.

I smiled up at him. "What are you doing here?" I asked.

"I wanted to see for myself that you're all right."

"I'm fine, I promise."

For a long moment Harrison didn't say anything. He took in the bandage on my leg, the stitches on my forehead and the various scrapes and bruises that were visible. Then he shook his head. "I'm so damn sorry for getting you involved in all of this," he said.

I was shaking my head before he had all the words out. "No, no, no. Nothing that happened is your fault. Mike was my friend, too." I put one hand on my chest. I thought about Jonas dragging me toward the edge of the gully. Those could have been the last moments of my life. They had been the last moments of Jonas's life. I took a breath. "What I did was my choice. What Jonas did was his."

One month and three days later, I was backstage at the Stratton Theatre, which was sold out for the Stars and Garters burlesque revival.

"They sound like a rowdy bunch," Maggie said as we peeked out at the crowd. She grinned. "This is going to be fun."

True to her promise to Roma, she was taking part in the show. She wore fishnets, high heels and a very short, barely there frilly white dress, and she was carrying a shepherd's hook.

"Every guy out there is going to lose their mind over you," I said. "The Little Bo-Peep in my book of Mother Goose stories did not look like this."

Mary was acting as mistress of ceremonies. She passed us all in black satin, carrying a huge feathered headdress like they'd wear in a show in Vegas. "It's

not too late to be onstage, Kathleen," she said over her shoulder.

"I already did my part," I called after her.

Roma peeked out at the crowd, then grabbed my arm. "Are you sure this is a good idea?" she asked. We were about fifteen minutes from the curtain going up.

I laughed. "As my mother likes to say, 'If you have to dance with a bear, put on your high heels and tango.'"

"I take it that means yes?" Roma said.

I hugged her. "Times three!"

There were hoots and good-natured catcalls and waves of applause for each act. It was clear the show was a hit. I headed down to the dressing room to check on what Mary called our showstopper.

I'd taken two steps into the room when Brady grabbed my arm. "My shirt is missing half the buttons," he said.

"Your shirt is fine," I said. "Just put it on."

I clapped my hands. "You have five minutes, everyone."

"Kathleen, I can't go out in public in this outfit," Harry said in a low voice. His shirt was just like the one Brady had been complaining about and like Brady he didn't have it on.

"Of course you can." I pulled at the sleeve of his white T-shirt. "And you need to take this shirt off."

He pointed at himself with one finger. "Nobody wants to see this without a shirt on."

"People paid good money to see that. All of that," I said. "Don't make me take that T-shirt off of you,

Harry Taylor." I gave him my best stern-librarian look. "Mary taught me a few moves. I can do it."

He took a step backward.

I held up four fingers. "Four minutes," I said.

A hand touched my shoulder. I turned around to see Marcus standing there. At least he had his shirt on.

"You so owe me for this," he said.

Silver lamé and sequins had never looked so good. "I can live with that," I told him. And then I winked.

To me, Zorro belonged to Mike and Mike alone. The show needed something that would celebrate the spirit of the man, but not be a pale imitation of his act. And then I remembered what Mike had called out to the crowd at the concert—*C'mon, people, you should be dancin'!*—and I knew what to do.

Ella King had made the guys' outfits with help from Rebecca, and the two of them had used every sequin within a five-mile radius of Mayville Heights. Rebecca had jokingly asked Ella if she could make an extra outfit for Everett—at least I was telling myself she was joking.

Finally Mary walked onstage to introduce the last act. "At our first show our star act was the dashing Zorro and we all miss him very much." She unveiled a large photo of Mike dancing in his costume. "Mike Bishop's absence has left a huge hole in this show and in our lives. Anyone who spent even five minutes with the man knew how much he loved music. So we honor his memory and celebrate his life with Mike's own words: 'You should be dancin'!'"

The throbbing disco percussion of the Bee Gees' hit began to pound in the background.

The guys came out in their silver disco outfits: tight flared pants, boots with heels, chunky silver neck chains and sequinned shirts open to the navel because there weren't any buttons above that. Sandra Godfrey had spent two hours with them working on a routine. She'd walked into the library afterward, laid her head on the circulation desk and said, "They're all hopeless. They have no rhythm, no sense of timing. You know that saying 'You've gotta dance like nobody's watching'? Well, the whole town will be watching and they can't dance!"

She was right, but it didn't matter. All five of them were stiff and awkward at first, but Johnny was the consummate performer. He started to swivel his hips Elvis style, and before I knew it, he was doing a hip bump with Eddie.

Marcus, Brady and Harry were doing their version of disco; at least I thought that was what it was. One hand was on their hips as their other arm pointed sideways à la John Travolta in *Saturday Night Fever*. That was followed by an arm roll and a repeat on the other side. They were even more or less in sync.

I realized that Brady was repeating something over and over. Maybe Sandra had taught them more than she'd thought. I watched his lips. Maybe she hadn't. Brady was a football fan like his dad. He was saying, "False start, defense, false start, offense." The movements all lined up. And it didn't matter that they were more NFL referees than disco stars because the audience loved them.

Sandra moaned and leaned against me. "Someone is going to put this on the Internet and John Travolta is going to sue me," she said.

I would have answered her but I was laughing too hard. And if a couple of tears got mixed in, that was okay, too. Mike would have loved this, I was certain. Once again, I was watching a show where the crowd went wild and I fervently hoped that wherever or whatever Mike Bishop was in the universe, he, too, was dancing.

Acknowledgments

It takes a multitude of people working diligently behind the scenes at the publisher to make my books the best they can be and then help readers find them. Thank you, everyone. Special thanks to my talented editor, Jessica Wade, who always finds all the holes I've left in the story. Her skills make every book better. Thank you as well to assistant editor, Miranda Hill, who keeps us all on track.

My agent, Kim Lionetti, is everything a writer could want—advocate, cheerleader and wisewoman. Thanks, Kim!

A big thank-you goes to the real Dr. Michael Bishop, endodontist extraordinaire, and his staff who have always taken excellent care of this very anxious patient. Dr. B. never played the stand-up bass in a church band, wore his hair in a mullet or danced in a burlesque show—at least as far as I know. He is, however, a very good sport.

And last but never least, thank you to Patrick and Lauren, who always have my back and my heart.

If you love Sofie Kelly's
Magical Cats Mysteries, read on for an
excerpt of the first book in Sofie Ryan's
New York Times bestselling
Second Chance Cat Mysteries . . .

THE WHOLE CAT AND CABOODLE

Available wherever books are sold.

E lvis was sitting in the middle of my desk when I opened the door to my office. The cat, not the King of Rock and Roll, although the cat had an air of entitlement about him sometimes, as though he thought he was royalty. He had one jet-black paw on top of a small cardboard box—my new business cards, I was hoping.

"How did you get in here?" I asked.

His ears twitched but he didn't look at me. His green eyes were fixed on the vintage Wonder Woman lunch box in my hand. I was having an early lunch, and Elvis seemed to want one as well.

"No," I said firmly. I dropped onto the retro red womb chair I'd brought up from the shop downstairs, kicked off my sneakers, and propped my feet on the matching footstool. The chair was so comfortable. To me, the round shape was like being cupped in a soft, warm giant hand. I knew the chair had to go back down to the shop, but I was still trying to figure out a way to keep it for myself.

Before I could get my sandwich out of the yellow vinyl lunch box, the big black cat landed on my lap. He wiggled his back end, curled his tail around his feet and looked from the bag to me.

"No," I said again. Like that was going to stop him.

He tipped his head to one side and gave me a pitiful look made all the sadder because he had a fairly awesome scar cutting across the bridge of his nose.

I took my sandwich out of the lunch can. It was roast beef on a hard roll with mustard, tomatoes and dill pickles. The cat's whiskers quivered. "One bite," I said sternly. "Cats eat cat food. People eat people food. Do you want to end up looking like the real Elvis in his chunky days?"

He shook his head, as if to say, "Don't be ridiculous."

I pulled a tiny bit of meat out of the roll and held it out. Elvis ate it from my hand, licked two of my fingers and then made a rumbly noise in his throat that sounded a lot like a sigh of satisfaction. He jumped over to the footstool, settled himself next to my feet and began to wash his face. After a couple of passes over his fur with one paw he paused and looked at me, eyes narrowed—his way of saying, "Are you going to eat that or what?"

I ate.

By the time I'd finished my sandwich Elvis had finished his meticulous grooming of his face, paws and chest. I patted my legs. "C'mon over," I said.

He swiped a paw at my jeans. There was no way he was going to hop onto my lap if he thought he might

get a crumb on his inky black fur. I made an elaborate show of brushing off both legs. "Better?" I asked.

Elvis meowed his approval and walked his way up my legs, poking my thighs with his front paws—no claws, thankfully—and wiggling his back end until he was comfortable.

I reached for the box on my desk, keeping one hand on the cat. I'd guessed correctly. My new business cards were inside. I pulled one out and Elvis leaned sideways for a look. The cards were thick brown recycled card stock, with SECOND CHANCE, THE REPURPOSE SHOP, angled across the top in heavy red letters, and SARAH GRAYSON and my contact information, all in black, in the bottom right corner.

Second Chance was a cross between an antiques store and a thrift shop. We sold furniture and housewares—many things repurposed from their original use, like the tub chair that in its previous life had actually been a tub. As for the name, the business was sort of a second chance—for the cat and for me. We'd been open only a few months and I was amazed at how busy we already were.

The shop was in a redbrick building from the late 1800s on Mill Street, in downtown North Harbor, Maine, just where the street curved and began to climb uphill. We were about a twenty-minute walk from the harbor front and easily accessed from the highway—the best of both worlds. My grandmother held the mortgage on the property and I wanted to pay her back as quickly as I could.

"What do you think?" I said, scratching behind

Elvis's right ear. He made a murping sound, cat-speak for "good," and lifted his chin. I switched to stroking the fur on his chest.

He started to purr, eyes closed. It sounded a lot like there was a gas-powered generator running in the room.

"Mac and I went to look at the Harrington house," I said to him. "I have to put together an offer, but there are some pieces I want to buy, and you're definitely going with me next time." Eighty-year-old Mabel Harrington was on a cruise with her new beau, a ninety-one-year-old retired doctor with a bad toupee and lots of money. They were moving to Florida when the cruise was over.

One green eye winked open and fixed on my face. Elvis's unofficial job at Second Chance was rodent wrangler.

"Given all the squeaks and scrambling sounds I heard when I poked my head through the trapdoor to the attic, I'm pretty sure the place is the hotel for some kind of mouse convention."

Elvis straightened up, opened his other eye, and licked his lips. Chasing mice, birds, bats and the occasional bug was his idea of a very good time.

I'd had Elvis for about four months. As far as I could find out, the cat had spent several weeks on his own, scrounging around downtown North Harbor.

The town sits on the midcoast of Maine. "Where the hills touch the sea" is the way it's been described for the past 250 years. North Harbor stretches from the Swift Hills in the north to the Atlantic Ocean in the

south. It was settled by Alexander Swift in the late 1760s. It's full of beautiful historic buildings, award-winning restaurants and quirky little shops. Where else could you buy a blueberry muffin, a rare book and fishing gear all on the same street?

The town's population is about thirteen thousand, but that more than triples in the summer with tourists and summer residents. It grew by one black cat one evening in late May. Elvis just appeared at The Black Bear. Sam, who owns the pub, and his pickup band, The Hairy Bananas—long story on the name—were doing their Elvis Presley medley when Sam noticed a black cat sitting just inside the front door. He swore the cat stayed put through the entire set and left only when they launched into their version of the Stones' "Satisfaction."

The cat was back the next morning, in the narrow alley beside the shop, watching Sam as he took a pile of cardboard boxes to the recycling bin. "Hey, Elvis. Want some breakfast?" Sam had asked after tossing the last flattened box in the bin. To his surprise, the cat walked up to him and meowed a loud yes.

He showed up at the pub about every third day for the next couple of weeks. The cat clearly wasn't wild—he didn't run from people—but no one seemed to know whom Elvis (the name had stuck) belonged to. The scar on his nose wasn't new; neither were a couple of others on his back, hidden by his fur. Then someone remembered a guy in a van who had stayed two nights at the campgrounds up on Mount Batten. He'd had a cat with him. It was black. Or black and white. Or

possibly gray. But it definitely had had a scar on its nose. Or it had been missing an ear. Or maybe part of its tail.

Elvis was still perched on my lap, staring off into space, thinking about stalking rodents out at the old Harrington house, I was guessing.

I glanced over at the carton sitting on the walnut sideboard that I used for storage in the office. The fact that it was still there meant that Arthur Fenety hadn't come in while Mac and I had been gone. I was glad. I was hoping I'd be at the shop when Fenety came back for the silver tea service that was packed in the box.

A couple of days prior he had brought the tea set into my shop. Fenety had a charming story about the ornate pieces that he said had belonged to his mother. A bit too charming for my taste, like the man himself. Arthur Fenety was somewhere in his seventies, tall with a full head of white hair, a matching mustache and an engaging smile to go with his polished de-meanor. He could have gotten a lot more for the tea set at an antiques store or an auction. Something about the whole transaction felt off.

Elvis had been sitting on the counter by the cash register and Fenety had reached over to stroke his fur. The cat didn't so much as twitch a whisker, but his ears had flattened and he'd looked at the older man with his green eyes half-lidded, pupils narrowed. He was the picture of skepticism.

The day after he'd brought the pieces in, Fenety had called to ask if he could buy them back. The more I thought about it, the more suspicious the whole thing

felt. The tea set hadn't been on the list of stolen items from the most recent police update, but I still had a niggling feeling about it and Arthur Fenety.

"Time to do some work," I said to Elvis. "Let's go downstairs and see what's happening in the store."

The cat jumped down to the floor and shook himself, and then he had to pause and pass a paw over his face. Elvis knew *store* meant "people," especially tourists, and *tourists* meant "new people who would generally take one look at the scar on his face and be overcome with the urge to stroke his fur and tell him what a sweet kitty he was."

I put on some lipstick and gave my head a shake. I'd gotten my thick, dark brown hair from my father and my dark eyes from my mom. I'd just cut my hair in long layers to my shoulders a couple of weeks previous. If we were moving furniture or I was going for a run I could still pull it back in a ponytail. Otherwise I could pretty much shake my head and my hair looked okay.

One of my part-time staff members, Avery, was by the cash register downstairs, nestling three mismatched soup bowls that had gotten a second life as herb planters into a box half-filled with shredded paper. Her hair was the color of cranberry sauce, and she'd shown up that morning with elaborate henna tattoos covering the backs of both hands. They were beautiful. (She claimed the look was all part of her "rebellious teenager" phase.) Avery worked afternoons in the store—her progressive private school had only morning classes—and full days when there was no school, like today.

I'd had a few rebellious moments myself as a teenager, so Avery's style didn't bother me. She was smart and hardworking, and even though one of the main reasons I'd hired her was because she was the granddaughter of one of my gram's closest friends, I kept her because she did a good job. And my customers seemed to like her.

Mac, the store's resident jack-of-all-trades, was showing a customer a tall metal postman's desk that we'd reclaimed from the basement of a house near the harbor. We'd had to cut the desk apart to get it up the narrow, cramped steps and through the door to the kitchen. Mac had banged out all the dents, put everything back together and then painted the piece a deep sky blue, even though I'd voted for basic black. I watched him hand the customer a tape measure, then give me a knowing smile across the room.

I could see the muscles in his arms move under his long-sleeved gray T-shirt. He was tall and fit with close-cropped black hair and light brown skin. Avery had given Mac the nickname Wall Street. He'd been a financial planner but had ditched his high-powered life to come to Maine and sail. In his free time he crewed for pretty much anyone who asked. There were eight windjammer schooners based in North Harbor, along with dozens of other sailing vessels. Mac was looking for space where he could build his own boat. He worked for me because he said he liked fixing things.

Second Chance had been open for a little less than four months. The main floor was one big open area, with some storage behind the staircase to the second

floor. My office was under the eaves on the second floor. There was also a minuscule staff room and one other large space that was being used for storage.

Some things we offered in the shop were vintage kitsch, like my yellow vinyl Wonder Woman lunch box—with matching thermos. Some things were like Elvis—working on a new incarnation, like the electric blue shelving unit that used to be a floor-model TV console. Everything in the store was on its second or sometimes third life.

Our stock came from lots of different places: flea markets, yard sales, people looking to downsize. Mac had even trash-picked a metal bed frame that we'd sold for a very nice profit. A couple of Dumpster divers had been stopping by fairly regularly and in the last month I'd bought items from the estates of three different people. So far, rummaging around in boxes and closets I'd found half a dozen wills, a diamond ring, a set of false teeth, a stuffed armadillo and a box of ashes that thankfully were the remains of someone's long-ago love letters and not, well, the remains of someone.

We sold some items in the store on consignment. Others, like the post office desk, we'd buy outright and refurbish. Mac could repair just about anything, and I was pretty good at coming up with new ways to use old things. And if I ran out of ideas, I could just call my mom, who was a master at giving new life to other people's discards.

Elvis had headed for a couple that was browsing near the guitars on the back wall. The young woman

crouched down, stroking his fur and making sympathetic noises about his nose. The young man moved a couple of steps sideways to take a closer look at a Washburn mandolin from the '70s, with a spruce top and ebony fingerboard.

Avery had finished with the customer at the counter. She walked over and lifted the mandolin down from its place on the wall and handed it to the young man. "Why don't you give it a try?" she said. I knew as soon as he had it in his hands he'd be sold.

Avery glanced down at Elvis. He tipped his furry head to one side, leaning into the hand of the young woman who was scratching the top of his head, commanding all her attention, and it almost looked as though he winked at Avery.

A musical instrument was the reason I'd ended up with Elvis—that and his slightly devious nature. I'd taken a guitar down to Sam for a second opinion on what it was worth. Sam Newman and my dad had grown up together. I could play, and I knew a little about some of the older models, but Sam knew more about guitars than anyone I'd ever met. I'd found him sitting in one of the back booths with a cup of coffee and a pile of sheet music. The cat was on the opposite banquette, eating what looked suspiciously to me like scrambled eggs and salami.

Sam had moved his mug and the music out of the way, and I'd set the guitar case on the table. Elvis studied me for a moment and then went back to his breakfast.

"Who's your friend?" I asked, tipping my head toward the cat.

"That's Elvis," Sam said, flipping open the latches on the battered Tolex case with his long fingers. He was tall and lean, his shaggy hair a mix of blond and white.

"Really?" I said. "The King of Rock and Roll was reincarnated as a cat?"

Sam looked at me over the top of his dollar-store reading glasses. "Ha, ha. You're so funny."

I made a face at him. Elvis was watching me again. "Move over." I gestured with one hand. To my surprise the cat obligingly scooted around to the other side of the plate. "Thank you," I said, sliding onto the burgundy vinyl. He dipped his head, almost as though he were saying, "You're welcome," and went back to his scrambled eggs. They were definitely Sam's specialty. I could smell the salami.

"Is this the cat I've been hearing about?" I asked.

Sam was engrossed in examining the vintage Fender. "What? Oh yeah, it is."

Elvis's ears twitched, as though he knew we were talking about him.

"Why Elvis?"

Sam shrugged. "He doesn't seem to like the Stones, so naming him Mick was kinda out of the question." He waved a hand in the direction of the bar. "There's coffee."

That was Sam's way of telling me to stop talking so he could focus his full attention on the candy apple

red Stratocaster. I got up and went behind the bar for the coffee, careful to keep the mug well out of the way of the old guitar when I brought it back to the table. Elvis had finished eating and was washing his face.

"What do you think?" I asked after a couple of minutes of silence. Sam's head was bent over the neck of the guitar, examining the fret board.

"Gimme a second," he said.

I waited, and after another minute or so he straightened up, pulling a hand over the back of his neck. "So, tell me what you think," he said, setting his glasses on the table.

I put my coffee cup on the floor beside my feet before I answered. "Based on what the homeowner told me it's a 1966. It belonged to her husband. It's not mint, but it's in good shape. There's some buckle wear on the back, but overall it's been taken care of. I think it's the real thing and I think it could bring twelve to fifteen thousand."

Beside me Elvis gave a loud meow.

"The cat agrees," I said.

"That makes three of us, then," Sam said.

I grinned at him across the table. "Thanks."

When I got up to leave, Elvis jumped down and followed me. "I think you made a friend," Sam said. He walked me out to my truck, set the guitar carefully on the passenger's side, and then wrapped me in a bear hug. He smelled like coffee and Old Spice. "Come by Saturday night, if you're free," he said. "I think you'll like the band."

"Old stuff?" I asked, pulling my keys out of the pocket of my jeans.

"Hey, it's gotta be rock-and-roll music if you wanna dance with me," he said, raising his eyebrows and giving me a sly smile. He looked down at Elvis, who had been sitting by the truck, watching us. "C'mon, you. You're gonna get turned into roadkill if you stay here." He reached for the cat, who jumped up onto the front seat.

"Hey, get down from there," I said.

Elvis ignored me, made his way along the black vinyl seat and settled himself on the passenger's side, next to the guitar case.

"No, no, no, you can't come with me." I leaned into the truck to grab him, but he slipped off the seat, onto the floor mat. With the guitar there I couldn't reach him.

Behind me, I could hear Sam laughing.

I blew my hair out of my face, backed out of the truck and glared at Sam. "Your cat's in my truck. Do something!"

He folded his arms over his chest. "He's not my cat. I'm pretty sure he's your cat now."

"I don't want a cat."

"Tell him that," Sam said with a shrug.

I stuck my head back through the open driver's door. "I don't want a cat," I said.

Ensconced out of my reach in the little lean-to made by the guitar case, Elvis looked up from washing his face—again—and meowed once and went back to it.

"I have a dog," I warned. "A big, mean one with big, mean teeth." The cat's whiskers didn't so much as quiver.

Sam leaned over my shoulder. "No, she doesn't," he said.

I elbowed him. "You're not helping."

He laughed. "Look, the cat likes you." He rolled his eyes. "Lord knows why. Take him. Do you want him to just keep living on the street?"

"No," I mumbled. I glanced in the truck again. Elvis, with some kind of uncanny timing, chose that moment to tip his head to one side and look up at me with his big green eyes. With his scarred nose he looked . . . lonely.

"What am I going to do with a cat?" I said, bouncing the keys in my right hand.

Sam shrugged. "Feed him. Talk to him. Scratch under his chin. He likes that."

I glanced at the cat again. He still had that lonely, slightly pathetic look going.

"You two will make a great team," Sam said. "Like Lennon and McCartney or Jagger and Richards."

"SpongeBob and Patrick," I muttered.

"Exactly," Sam said.

I was pretty sure I was being conned, but, like it or not, I had a cat.

I looked over now toward the end wall of the store. My cat had apparently helped sell a mandolin. The young man was headed to the cash register with it. Elvis made his way over to me.

I leaned over to stroke the top of his head. "Nice

work," I whispered. I wasn't imagining the cat smile he gave me.

The woman who had been looking at the post office desk was headed for the door, but there was a certain smugness to Mac's expression that told me he'd made the sale. I walked over to him. "Go ahead, say 'I told you so,'" I said.

He folded his arms over his chest. "I can't. I'm fairly certain she's going to buy it. She just wishes it were black."

I laughed. "I guess black really is the new black," I said. "I'm about ready to leave. I have to pick up Charlotte, and Avery is going to get her grandmother. Do you need anything before I go?"

I was doing a workshop on color-washing furniture for a group of seniors over at Legacy Place. North Harbor was full of beautiful old buildings. It was part of the town's charm. The top floors of the old chocolate factory had been converted into seniors' apartments. There were a couple of community rooms on the main level, where the residents had various classes like French and yoga and got together to socialize. We were using one of them for the workshop since many of the class participants lived in the building. Eventually I wanted to renovate part of the old garage next to the Second Chance building for workshops; for now, when I did classes for the general public, I had to settle for renting space at the high school. Luckily the hourly rate was pretty good. This workshop was a freebie my gram had nudged me into doing.

Mac shook his head. "I've got everything covered." He narrowed his brown eyes at me. "Are you sure it's a good idea to make Avery go with you?"

"Actually she volunteered."

"Avery volunteered to help you teach a workshop for a bunch of senior citizens?" One eyebrow shot up. "Seriously?"

"Seriously. She's good with older people. They'll be feeding her cookies and exclaiming over her hair color, and before you know it she'll have wangled an invitation to go prowl around someone's attic." Avery had a thing for vintage jewelry, and thanks to her grandmother Liz's friends, was building a nice collection.

I pressed my hands into the small of my back and stretched. I was still kinked from crawling around that old house all morning. "You know, I used to hang around with some of those same women when I was Avery's age." I'd spent my summers in North Harbor with my grandmother as far back as I could remember. The rest of the time I'd lived first in upstate New York and then in New Hampshire. "Liz taught me how to wax my legs and put on false eyelashes."

"I could have gone the rest of my life not knowing that," Mac said dryly.

"And I know the secret to Charlotte's potpie," I teased.

"You're not going to say it's love, are you?"

I shook my head and grinned. "Nope. Actually it's bacon fat."

My father had been an only child and so was my mother, so I didn't have a gaggle of cousins to hang out

with in the summer. My grandmother's friends, Charlotte, Liz and Rose had become a kind of surrogate extended family, a trio of indulgent aunts. When I'd decided to open Second Chance, they'd been almost as pleased as my grandmother, and Charlotte and Rose had come to work for me part-time. Now with Gram out of town on her honeymoon, the three women fed me, gently nagged me about working too much and pointed out every single man between twenty-five and, well, death. When Gram had asked me to offer one of my workshops to her friends, how could I say no?

I glanced at my watch. "I don't expect to be more than a couple of hours," I said. "And I have my cell."

"Elvis and I can hold down the fort," Mac said. "Are you going to take another look at that SUV?"

I'd been thinking about replacing the aging truck we used to move furniture with an SUV, if I could get it for the right price. "I might," I said.

"Well, take your time," Mac said. "It's Monday afternoon. Nothing ever happens in this town on a Monday."

Of course he was wrong.

Sofie Kelly is a *New York Times* bestselling author and mixed-media artist who lives on the East Coast with her husband and daughter. She writes the *New York Times* bestselling Magical Cats Mysteries (*Hooked on a Feline, A Case of Cat and Mouse, A Night's Tail*) and, as Sofie Ryan, writes the *New York Times* bestselling Second Chance Cat Mysteries (*Totally Pawstruck, Undercover Kitty, Claw Enforcement*).